"An excellent presentation of dietary protocols! The material is anchored with practical examples so casual athletes (and parents of young athletes) will relate. And it's replete with guidelines for the coach or trainer. The scope is broad, the coverage in-depth and up-to-date—with virtually all stages of life and activity addressed. The Resource Guide in the Appendix alone is worth the price of the book."

Doris Brown Heritage
1984 Olympic Women's Team Track Coach
5 Time World Champion, Cross Country Running

"Sure to become a valuable resource for both professional and amateur dancers and athletes. [The authors] present a wealth of much needed information with the clarity and care they have always shown their patients."

Francia Russell
Artistic Director
Pacific Northwest Ballet

"A very useful tool for not only the elite athlete but all the way down the scale to the beginner. It is invaluable to the coach at all levels because it is concise, yet it answers all the questions concerning the often-experienced dilemma of a proper diet for each individual."

Ken Shannon
Track and Field Coach
University of Washington

Marilyn S. Peterson has been the consulting nutritionist for the Sports Medicine Clinic in Seattle for the past 24 years. She and her husband Keith founded the clinic, the oldest and largest privately owned sports medicine facility in the United States.

She received her bachelor of science degree in home economics from the University of Montana and her master of science degree in nutrition and physiology from the University of Washington. Early experience included teaching home economics at the junior high school level in Lincoln, Nebraska, and serving as a county extension agent in Missouri. She was also a food supervisor at the Neiman-Marcus restaurants in Texas.

Currently, Peterson is a consultant to the Seattle Mariners Baseball Club, Pacific Northwest Ballet, Bellevue Athletic Club, and numerous Seattle area high schools. She is also an Adjunct Professor at Seattle Pacific University, where she teaches graduate-level courses in nutrition, fitness, and weight control.

Peterson coauthored *The Athlete's Cookbook* and has written for *Young Athlete Magazine, The Physician and Sports Medicine, BAC-Vue News* and *Sportswatch.* She wrote the pamphlet *Nutrition, Health and Athletic Performance* for the American Heart Association.

Other activities have included serving as the nutritional consultant for the Women's 1984 Olympic Development Committee and as a volunteer in various community organizations. Peterson, her husband, and four children reside in Seattle, and all are enthusiastic about good food and fitness.

Keith Peterson is President and Director of the Sports Medicine Clinic in Seattle, Washington.

He received his bachelor of science degree from the University of Montana, and his DOM degree from Kirksville College of Osteopathic Medicine.

Peterson is currently a scout for the Cincinnati Reds baseball team. He is a board member of and frequent contributor to *The Physician and Sports Medicine.*

Eat to Compete
A Guide to Sports Nutrition

by
Marilyn S. Peterson, M.S., R.D.
and
Keith Peterson, D.O.

YEAR BOOK MEDICAL PUBLISHERS, INC.
CHICAGO • LONDON • BOCA RATON

1 2 3 4 5 6 7 8 9 0 KC 92 91 90 89 88

Library of Congress Cataloging-in-Publication Data

Peterson, Marilyn Shope, 1935–
  Eat to compete.

  Includes bibliographies and index.
  1. Athletes–Nutrition. I. Peterson, Keith.
II. Title. [DNLM: 1. Nutrition. 2. Sports Medicine.
QU 145 P485e]
TX361.A8P473 1988   613.2′024796   88–5532
ISBN 0-8151-6720-2

Sponsoring Editor: James D. Ryan, Jr.
Assistant Director, Manuscript Services: Frances M. Perveiler
Production Project Manager: Carol A. Reynolds
Proofroom Supervisor: Shirley A. Taylor

To the athletes in our lives

Preface

This book was written for those who want to know more about the relationship between nutrition and physical performance. The information is appropriate for both athletes and those who advise athletes.

Nutritional care for the athlete and the physically active person is generally provided by several different health professionals—the most prominant (and logical) being dietitians, nurses and physicians, and physical therapists. However, most nutrition education outside of the office and classroom is given by coaches, athletic trainers, sports physiologists and, to a great extent, by team members and parents.

In contrast to the many scholarly offerings that provide insight into the complexities of nutrition and performance, this book is brief and uncomplicated. Its subject is exciting and the information should be as helpful to the physician as to the parent of the Little League catcher. One chapter explains various methodologies of testing and analysis. Another discusses counseling techniques. Straightforward recommendations are given for all readers, regardless of their physical activity preference.

Even with a complete understanding of basic nutrition for performance, an athlete can find it difficult to adhere to a diet that is adequate for physiological needs. *Eat to Compete: A Guide to Sports Nutrition* addresses that problem.

An overview that is based on information on which most experts agree opens the book. This is followed by interpretation geared to the team setting. Finally, I offer an individual strategy to guide the advisor as well as the athlete who is preparing for performance. These final recommendations are based on current knowledge and my years of experience "working in the trenches" and in classroom and laboratory settings.

The chapter sequence follows the logical inquiry of the physician: gathering information, studying the results, sharing findings with, and giving recommendations to, the patient.

I hope the reader will find the book enjoyable and very, very useful.

Marilyn S. Peterson, M.S., R.D.

Acknowledgments

My role as author of *Eat to Compete* has been that of compiler of a huge amount of current data on nutrition and performance. There were countless hours spent documenting files, gathering and sorting, and digesting and discarding information that has been part of my internal philosophy and knowledge during the past 25 years. There was also the task of organizing this collection and then putting these facts on paper. For those who know me closely, they will remember that I spent as much time wandering around unguided and feeling very much alone, as I did quietly sheltered in my son's bedroom, typing away.

My co-author and I have always shared the belief that diet can play a role in success or failure in athletic achievement. And while he did not push the pen, he has been the driving force of this book. He introduced me, and others, to the many pressing concerns of sports medicine, especially for care and feeding of athletes. Without him, athletes would have been for me, but an occasional client. The legitimacy of this book can be regarded as partial acknowledgment of my indebtedness to him. I was advising athletes long before most coaches knew how to spell "dietitian" correctly. Looking back, I can only say thank you for the shove into and continual exposure to "the trenches," the reception of his esteem and enthusiasm, and for his gracious introduction to his friends and to membership into the American College of Sports Medicine. He's certainly made of fine stuff.

Many highly professional people took time from their busy

lives to give information and provide technical review of the beginning drafts. My thanks go out to Dr. Elaine Monsen, editor of the Journal of the American Dietetic Association, who returned my "manuscript" with encouraging remarks; to Kathleen Mahan, co-author of *Food, Nutrition & Diet Therapy*, who so willingly shared information and opened many doors in the publication world; and to Dr. Bonnie Worthington-Roberts who not only has been an inspiration, but is one of the finest athletes herself.

My special gratitude goes forth to Pat Fitch and Julie Seitz, both registered dietitians, who reviewed the text and added immensely to the reliability of the information. David Abrams and Jeff Droker, nutrition students who are now in the professional ranks, spent time in the library and at the computer, and were enthusiastic and supportive. I am indebted and in awe of my daughter Julie, who periodically reminded me that I was once again behind in my writing schedule, and who would casually redraw and retype my information with the greatest ease. I would be remiss if I did not mention my editor Jim Ryan, and Peter Raven, who presented me with the challenge of writing, and Christine White, who helped place all my thoughts in order. And a special note of thanks goes to Jon, Erik, and Chris, the athletes in my life, whose stories are sprinkled throughout the text.

The issue of food, nurture, and caring bring to mind an indebtedness of another time and order. I will always be grateful to my aunt, Erva Love Shope, for our love of food preparation; and to my cousin, Charlotte Davis Kasl, for her expert ear and generous commentary. I needed these great and good women to assure me that there are many special moments in our memories that are touched with life.

And to Peggy Machen and Susan Ingalina, who helped in the many ways they will never fully realize, a big thank you for cheerfully walking me through the writing of these pages.

Marilyn S. Peterson, M.S., R.D.

Contents

The Role of Nutrition in Sports

The subject of nutrition for the athlete is a fascinating one, partly because there is an athlete in all of us. Each of us has carried the winning touchdown or won the marathon, if only in our dreams. Because more and more of us are being introduced to physical activity today, we are enjoying the benefits of increased fitness and are interested in the factors involved in improving performance. Likewise, the athlete who trains every day for a specific event is becoming more aware of the advantages of proper nutrition.

HISTORICAL COMMENTARY

Athletes intent on winning will try anything to improve their performance, including consuming doses of extra vitamins and minerals or subjecting themselves to bizarre and impractical diet regimens. The situation is not unique to the present day. Diet choices for the pre-event meal date back so far that their origins are untraceable. We know, for instance, that early mankind believed that eating the flesh of selected animals could cause them to assume certain physical characteristics. Hence, the fleet footed may have chosen to dine on rabbit, whereas those involved in strength activities might have preferred lion steaks. As these athletes became legendary for their feats, their individualized diets became popular and were often proposed as part of training sequences. It was probably natural to connect a successful athletic accomplishment with a preceding event, namely, eating a particular food. Some of these beliefs remain today and are a mixture of superstition, mythology, and observation. Even though the scientific community has rejected most myths, there are still many athletes who ascribe to individual testimony and questionable advice in their pursuit of health, fitness, and performance.[1]

For example, our eyes and our logic tell us that athletes have more muscle than their same-age counterparts. Muscles are protein; therefore, athletes need more protein than other people. Right? Wrong. To maintain protein mass, the athlete needs only to replace the nitrogen lost each day or to eat about 1 gm of protein/kg of body weight. To increase muscle mass, the athlete needs to be in positive nitrogen balance or to eat a little more than 1 or 2 gm of protein/kg of body weight each day. But this is dependent on fast growth or intense muscular work. There is no way to add extra protein to muscle cells. All cells work by adapting to specific demands placed on them, so that if a muscle is worked and enough protein is available in the diet, the muscle will enlarge (hypertrophy). If the muscle is not worked and the protein and calories in the diet are not adequate, the muscle will become smaller (atrophy). Each athlete will respond physiologically on an individual basis.

Simple and straightforward? Definitely not! From a historical prospective, protein requirements have been a hot debate for many centuries, and future scientific research will continue to question the actual protein needs of the athlete.

Another myth is that the pre-event meal is the most important meal for the athlete. Certainly, it is acknowledged that what an athlete eats before competition does make a difference, both physically and psychologically. However, Christiansen and Hansen, Scandinavian physiologists, observed in the 1930s that the diet of swimmers directly before the competitive event did not seem to influence their performances.[2] This finding directly opposed the written instructions of Galen, the first sports medicine physician, to his gladiators[3] and Vince Lombardi's advice to his football team. They said, instead, that the diet in general and the total carbohydrates consumed in the 2 weeks previous to the event seemed to influence the endurance of the athlete. Their writings were the beginnings of the current emphasis on carbohydrate feedings and, at that time, were stimulating. Not only was the theory new but their justifications, based on observation, experimentation, and careful data collection, resulted in fresh revelations in the volatile fields of nutrition and athletics.

A BACKGROUND OF KNOWLEDGE FOR THE STUDY OF NUTRITION AND SPORTS

Every athlete seeks the winning combination of physical training, mental and emotional preparation, and diet that will ensure success in competition. Diet is especially important. Questions will continually arise as to the number of calories and fluids required, the influence of increased carbohydrates on endurance events, and what special nutrients will benefit performance.[4]

The volumes of scientifically valid data currently available are overwhelming in comparison with the relatively small amount of information available in historical medical writings. Yet, after study, one can still ask what diet will allow the dancer to execute a design on stage while retaining a slender image, or enhance the skill of the thrower, increase the anaerobic threshhold of the rower, or strengthen the solid brick wall of the defensive team. Each athlete has a unique job.

Diet must be individualized. However, a balanced regimen, using a wide variety of foods, will be appropriate to any phase or condition of an athlete's life—fast growth, injury, chronic or acute illness, pregnancy, lactation, aging, training, or participation.[5]

If diet has any relationship to performance, the study of diet cannot be limited to a single course of examination. Preparation for the field of sports nutrition must include basic nutrition, physiology, chemistry, psychology, food preparation, and an understanding of athletes. Continuation of study includes the ap-

plied sciences, statistics, and laboratory work. Finally, it is necessary to develop counseling and teaching skills with which to
address the needs of athletes.

NUTRITION IN THE LOCKER ROOM

There is no optimum setting for nutrition education for the
athlete. It depends on many factors. Many coaches view nutrition education as the province of the health education class or as
a response to a problem that has arisen because of the demands
of athletics. For example, weight loss is usually a compromising
situation for the growing athlete. He or she needs to be building
muscle tissue and adding height instead of losing weight. Appropriate information on protecting growth may have been given in
class, but limited time to reach standardized weight may promote
fasting and other harmful practices. The coach will need to in-
tervene if winning is the goal, because poorly nourished athletes
do not compete well.[6] The help of nutrition experts may also be
needed. In reality, athletes receive nutritional information in
small pieces in various settings throughout their careers, and it
can be effective as long as it is *correct, practical,* and *timely.*

Anyone can be a student of nutrition: the very young soccer
player experiencing dehydration for the first time, the elite female runner receiving weight gain forecasting during pregnancy, the dancer responding to counseling for food habit management, the professional ballplayer choosing a meal on the
road, or the mother receiving a phone message from the physician after her child's preseason physical examination. The setting depends on the reason for teaching, the location, the tools
available, the qualifications of the teacher, and the athlete.

Teaching opportunities are always present. Nutrition is often
integrated into the school curriculum, but informally lessons are
learned in the locker room. There is no set style or format for
teaching nutrition to an athlete. "I just grab them when I can,"
said one coach. Assessment of needs, the present knowledge base
of athlete and teacher, and the ability to learn and use information are considerations.

All athletes have the potential to learn how their bodies use food, and they will benefit from this knowledge for the rest of their lives. This is a learn by doing situation. Learning takes time, practice, and feedback.

The sequence of instruction is the same whether it is for diet modifications, a protocol for precompetition meals, or a class in health education. The teacher needs to:

1. Identify the learner's needs and the goal of instruction.
2. Assess knowledge of the learner.
3. Establish behavioral objectives.
4. Select an evaluation tool.
5. Choose format of instruction.
6. Organize information.
7. Teach.
8. Test and measure.

All teaching begins with identifying the needs of the learner and the goal of instruction. A critical factor is differentiating between the needs of the learner and the needs of the teacher. Many coaches (and dietitians) have left classrooms feeling satisfied with the chalk talk or lecture while the learners remained confused.

For instance, a young dietitian was asked to lecture to a track team about eating more carbohydrates during training. She emphasized the advantages of muscle glycogen storage, charted the conversion of glucose to glycogen, spoke of complex carbohydrate foods and absorption rates, and even mentioned that diet plays an important role in preparing the liver for the demands of distance running. What the team really needed to know, however, was specific food sources of carbohydrates, appropriate amounts to eat, and types of menus that would benefit runners who perform long-distance work. A practical discussion would have made it clear that proper nutrition can play an important role in distance running performance and that eating more foods from the grain and fruit and vegetable groups will increase the availability of carbohydrate for muscle energy!

The second step is assessing the knowledge of the learner.

Using graduate students in exercise physiology as study subjects is one matter; dealing with prepubertal dancers and the issue of weight gain is another. A pretest, such as that outlined in Appendix S, is a nonthreatening way to determine the athlete's knowledge base. Answers to questions that address the problem at hand give a counselor a good understanding of learner needs.

At this point, specific behavioral objectives can be established. They should be easy to achieve in a short period of time. Four components of an objective should be considered: performer, behavior, existing conditions, and outcome. For example, supplied with a list of grocery stores and fast-food restaurants near the ball park, players can pick food items or menus that are healthful. What's more, they will not go over their per diem. By establishing objectives, the coach has automatically fixed a point of evaluation. The players will either come back requesting more money or will start complaining about the food. Asking them to perform under limitations readily identifies whether the team needs more instruction or a new strategy needs to be developed to determine the task.

Once the objectives are established, an evaluation tool can be selected. Formal evaluations, such as tests, are usually not practical in the athletic area. Basic nutrition, nutrition for performance, and pre-event meals are topics that deal with food behaviors, past experiences, and time and money. The coach asked the players to perform a task, namely, choosing appropriate menus and foods from a local restaurant or grocery store. The point is that the players are performing behaviors they are expected to carry out during the season, and the question is whether they can achieve the task unassisted. Informal observations can be made by the coach or manager at shared meals.

Is this directive unrealistic? Several years ago, members of a major baseball team were having health problems (which may or may not have been related to their dietary habits). Traditionally, players slept late on game days, ate a large, high-fat breakfast, ate junk food at the ball park during warm-ups, and ate at fast-food restaurants after the game. It came as a surprise to the management that the players (many of whom made more money than the President of the United States) were getting less than 50% of the recommended dietary allowances (RDAs) and were overweight and overfat in comparison with other athletes. One objective was to improve the dietary habits of the players by providing a nutritious low-fat, pre-event meal on site. Because the meal was free as well as convenient, most of the players took advantage of it. It was later determined (by 24-hour dietary recall) that this meal alone provided more than 50% of the recommended nutrients for an adult male. Although it did not solve the team's health problems, it introduced improved nutrition via the pre-event meal and relaxed management a bit.

Once a format for teaching has been chosen, instruction can begin. A valuable and practical time to teach nutrition to athletes is during the team physical examination. The physical examination is actually quite an event. Usually several physicians, physical therapists, nurses, and other health specialists are present to screen team members for injuries, give general health recommendations and guidelines for the season, and administer the sports-specific tests that will yield useful data. It usually takes 4 to 6 hours to test a team, and there is a lot of free time between examinations. Handouts that outline general information are appropriate and can be read on site. Special problems, such as weight loss or gain, can be addressed immediately.

It is also a unique opportunity to gather information on nutritional habits, beliefs, food records, and caloric intake. Minilectures can be given on nutritional guidelines that are appropriate to a specific sport (e.g., caloric requirements for growth, metabolism, and training for an under–age 15 soccer team). Most athletes are interested in pre-event and postevent meals, fluid needs, and pros and cons about diet supplementation. A list of prepublished handouts and sources may be found in Appendix A. Some of these could be available in the waiting room. A tip sheet headed with the team's logo and listing dietary recommendations is an effective tool.

Young athletes learn best when the coach demonstrates good food choices and when there is parent involvement. Parent and coach seminars are an excellent way to teach nutrition. In addition, an introduction to nutrition for athletes can be taught in health science, home economics, or physical education classes. A course outline, list of teaching tools, and suggested testing methods are given in the Appendix.

AVOIDING THE MYTHS

Athletic performances have improved at astonishing rates over the past several decades. Competitive times have dropped, and standards of excellence have risen. Increased workloads, advanced medical care, and superior nutrition are some of the reasons athletes are better than ever. But is superior nutrition due to improved diet, or does it consist of consumption of foods, drugs, or extra nutrients that promise miraculous improvement? When athletes are surveyed, they frequently indicate that they think performance is improved by high-protein diets, that synthetic vitamins are inferior to natural vitamins, that salt tablets should be taken in hot weather, that amino acids stimulate the human growth hormone, and so forth. There is no area where fads and ignorance are more widely spread than in athletics. Here, faddism is flaunted.[8]

Many studies conclude with the recommendation that dietitians and nutritionists consider correcting the discrepancies between what is known and what is practiced. Yet, surprisingly, along with the coach and athletic trainer, the athlete's parents are still relied on for most nutrition education. The information they share with their children is often a continuation of the myths that were fostered in their playing days. It is difficult to break into this closed loop of learning. Those who know better seldom get into the locker room. And, as some athletes have noted, many health professionals are such poor representatives of fitness that it is not surprising that no one pays attention to what they say.

This situation is changing. More and more athletes are entering the health professions, and the medical practitioner may frequently be observed at the track! Times change and, since money is such an influencing factor in the sports world, athletes are demanding the best in everything, including sound nutritional advice.

Many events are won by fractions of seconds, so it is not surprising that athletes, coaches, and parents are susceptible to claims for improved performance. Virtually every food, at some time, has been promoted as an ergogenic aid, a substance reputed to enhance performance above the levels anticipated under normal conditions. The list is overwhelming and includes such items as wheat germ, honey, lecithin, all of the vitamins and minerals, bee pollen, and brewer's yeast. Many of the old standbys, such as protein powders, have reappeared as products in another form, namely, protein isolates.[9–11]

On the other hand, research has validated some of the dietary practices followed by athletes. For instance, it was fairly well known that some runners drank fluids containing caffeine before marathons. Studies later confirmed the ergogenic effects of caffeine[12] (for some individuals, not all). Surveys of weight lifters, body builders, and football players have disclosed the popular use of glandular products and amino acids purported to stimulate muscle growth. The hope has been, illogical though it be, that these substances will give the same effects as steroids[13, 14] but will prove less dangerous. It is true that amino acids are not detected in the urine, but that is because they are digested as protein and used for growth, development, and repair of tissue. However, excess protein is converted to fat, not muscle. Although the scientific data may support coffee drinkers and refute protein enthusiasts, only time will tell if the beliefs of athletes will change.

Supplemental vitamins and minerals are a big business in the United States. Nationwide, the retail sales of health food stores total billions of dollars, with vitamins and supplements accounting for nearly one third of total sales. Athletes are close behind the general population in consumption of vitamins and minerals. For the most part, those who use them have adequate diets, and those with less than adequate diets do not supplement. It is been observed that the vitamins most commonly supplemented, C and E, are often taken in megadose amounts. It is difficult to believe that any athlete can benefit from megadosing, yet if he or she is convinced that a certain food or vitamin will improve performance, there may, indeed, be a profound psychological advantage. Actually, many athletes do make poor nutrition choices, but if they meet their energy needs (which may require more than 4,000 kcal/day), their nutrient needs will be met by sheer volume of food. At the same time, the athlete with an intake of less than 1,200 kcal/day will be unable to meet the RDAs without supplementation. Malnutrition will be a factor if poor food choices are made.

Athletes perform incredible feats every day without knowledge of proper nutrition, and lack of advanced training or medical care. But long-term success results from a combination of talent, hard training, and plenty of preparation before competition. Obviously, the optimal situation is to capitalize on genetic talent and build on every advantage possible. Because one advantage is a proper diet, it is well to be realistic about the "guarantees" of ergogenic aids. If an athlete is relying on testimonies, miracles, and myths, it is better to question than to be fooled. If parents, coaches, and athletic trainers are the major influences in the nutrition decisions of athletes, they have the right and the responsibility to criticize health fraud and misrepresentation.

Before any purchase to optimize performance is made, evaluate the product, claim, or book by asking:[15, 16]

1. Who is selling it? Who wrote it?
2. What is his or her job, education, reputation and financial interest?
3. Is the information factual, specific, and clear or vague and highly emotional?
4. Is scientific data given to document the information, or is it based on a single case history?
5. Was it tested or evaluated?
6. Are references or quotations used and correctly identified?
7. Does it promise quick, dramatic, or miraculous cures and use testimonials to support claims?
8. Where was this manufactured or published?
9. When was it released?
10. Is it available in most pharmacies or public libraries? Is it supported by reputable health professionals?

Then, make an informed decision!

REFERENCES

1. Astrand PO, Rodahl K: *Textbook of Work Physiology,* ed 3. New York, McGraw-Hill Book Co, 1986.
2. Christiansen EH, Hansen O: Arbeitsfahigkeit and Ernahrung. *Scand Arch Physiol* 1939; 81:160.
3. Galen: *Encyclopedia Britannica* 1978; 7:849.
4. Smith M: Nutrition for physical fitness and athletic performance for adults: Technical support paper. *J Am Diet Assoc* 1987; 87:934.
5. Peterson MS: Nutrition, health and athletic performance. Washington State Heart Association, Seattle, June 1986.
6. Parr RB, Porter MS, Hodgson SD: Nutrition knowledge and practice of coaches, trainers and athletes. *Phys Sports Med* 1984; 12:127.
7. Peterson MS: Unpublished data, 1986.
8. Munnings FD: College athletes are losing to food quacks. *Phys Sports Med* 1986; 14:38.
9. Polk MR: The dietitian vs food faddism: An educational challenge. *J Am Diet Assoc* 1985; 85:1335.
10. Young HJ, Stitt RS: Nutrition quackery—upholding the right to criticize. *Food Technol* 1981; 12:42.
11. Stephenson M: *The Confusing World of Health Foods.* HEW Publication (FDA) 79-2108, US Government Printing Office, Washington, DC, 1979.
12. Powers SK, Dodd S: Caffeine and endurance performance. *Sports Med* 1985; 2:165.
13. Jarvis WT: Vitamin use and abuse. *Contemp Nutr* 1984; 9:1.
14. Todhunter E: Food habits, food faddism and nutrition. *World Rev Nutr Diet* 1973; 16:286.
15. Nutrition misinformation. *Dairy Counc Dig* 1981; 52:19.
16. Rogers CC: Of magic, miracles, and exercise myths. *Phys Sports Med* 1985; 13:156.

2

Digestion, Metabolism, and Energy Balance

DIGESTION: SUPPLYING THE CELLS WITH NUTRIENTS

In the training diet, the transition of the food on the plate to nutrients in a form capable of being absorbed and metabolized is known as digestion. The digestive tract is actually a long tube with an opening at either end that stretches and widens at intervals to receive food. It mixes food with the digestive juices and enzymes necessary to fraction the component parts (proteins, carbohydrates, and fats) before they can be absorbed. The movement of food along the length of this tube is accomplished by peristalsis, or contraction of the intestinal muscles. Other muscles churn and reduce the food to small particles, mixing them with digestive fluids. When all of the particles are small enough to enter the capillaries of the blood and lymphatic system, they are carried to the functioning cells of the body. Fragments of food that do not make this transition in size or form are gathered together in the large intestine and expelled.

In general, the digestive process is accomplished with great efficiency. About 95% of all food eaten is available to the body for energy and nutrient needs. However, in some cases, nutrients are poorly absorbed, as in disease states or during high levels of stress. For instance, in cases of traveler's diarrhea or in dehydration caused by high temperatures, the body's first need is for fluid, and any food eaten may be lost by vomiting. It is obvious in examining the demands placed on the athlete that the hazards of participation may interfere with the simple, involuntary act of digestion.

Normal Digestive Process

The complete digestive tract is shown in Figure 2–1. Chewing begins the digestive process. Food is cut into small particles by the teeth and mixed with saliva. Salivary amylase, an enzyme, begins the digestion of starches (e.g., rice or pasta), and the food begins its passage down the esophagus to the stomach.

Food is dumped into the stomach and, depending on the size and composition of the meal, stays there from 30 minutes to as long as 5 or 6 hours until it flows into the small intestine. Digestion of starch continues until the contents of the stomach become acidic, as hydrochloric acid and pepsin are pumped in. Hydrochloric acid activates the pepsin, and partial digestion of protein foods, such as fish or chicken, begins. Later, pancreatic and intestinal secretions will produce the enzymes necessary for complete digestion of protein within the small intestine (which is why hormones and enzymes cannot effectively be taken by mouth; they will be digested before reaching the absorptive phase).

Fat from protein foods or from pure forms of butter and oil are unaffected by the secretions. In high concentrations, fat will delay the emptying of the stomach. This is the reason that high-carbohydrate (and very low-fat) foods are recommended for pre-event meals.

Small amounts of food are then moved forcefully into the large intestine. Mixing of the food with secretions from the pancreas and liver occurs immediately in the small intestine. By this time, starch digestion is less than half completed, and chains of protein have been reduced to small chains of amino acids. When fatty foods are released from the stomach, bile is released from the gallbladder and enters the small intestine. Bile functions as

The Digestive System

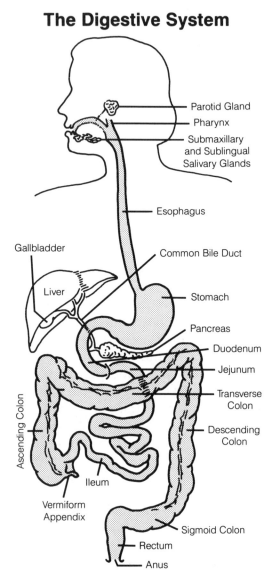

FIG 2–1.
Diagram of the digestive tract. (Redrawn from Jacob SW, Francone CA: *Structure and Function in Man,* ed 5. WB Saunders Co 1982.)

an emulsifier and, together with the contractions of the small intestine, reduces large fat globules into small fat droplets. Emulsification of fats enhances absorption into the blood. Pancreatic secretions include bicarbonates, which neutralize stomach acids; pancreatic amylase, which reduces the remaining starches to maltose; trypsin, which continues the breakdown of amino acids; and pancreatic lipase, which reduces triglycerides to monoglycerides and diglycerides. Final digestion occurs with the help of enzymes secreted by cells of the intestinal mucosa. At this point, carbohydrates are reduced to monosaccharides, proteins are reduced to individual amino acids, and fat is reduced to glycerol and fatty acids. For reduction to occur, each food element requires a specific hormone or enzyme and a specific pH.

The size of the surface area that absorbs nutrients is estimated to be one fourth of an acre (3,000 sq ft), or about the size of a basketball court. Most nutrients are completely absorbed by the time they reach the large intestine. These digestive products are taken directly into the blood through the capillaries in the intestinal villi. Fatty acids, cholesterol, and lipid substances, such as fat-soluble vitamins, are absorbed into the lymphatic capillaries. Water-soluble products of digestion, such as amino acids, monosaccharides, glycerol, and the water-soluble vitamins and minerals, are absorbed along with water into the blood. Some water and alcohol are absorbed directly from the stomach. All of these capillaries merge to form the portal vein, which leads directly to the liver. This gives the liver the first opportunity to extract nutrients from the blood. The liver cells process the three classes of energy nutrients: fats, carbohydrates, and proteins. Sugars are converted into glucose; storage glycogen and surplus sugars are converted into storage fat. Fatty acids and glycerol are reassembled into larger fat packages and coated with protein for transport. Amino acids are used in making proteins or converted to glucose or fat.

The new products are released into the bloodstream and circulated to all the other cells of the body. Surplus fat is deposited in fat cells, and glycogen, the reserve supply of the body's sugar, is stored in the liver or the muscle cells.

Two nutrients of current interest to athletes are iron and calcium. Iron uptake from the intestines is regulated by a mechanism that inhibits absorption. Proteins in the intestinal mucosal cells attach to absorbed iron and keep it in storage. When saturation occurs, no more iron can be absorbed. This mechanism can be overwhelmed by excessive intake of iron.

Calcium is absorbed through the upper end of the duodenum. Any situation that hastens food movement through the small intestine, such as stress or diarrhea, will interfere with calcium absorption. Oxalic acid and phytic acid from such foods as spinach and oatmeal combine with calcium and make it unavailable. The best insurance for adequate calcium absorption is a generous daily calcium intake.

Undigested food collects in the large intestine, where water is resorbed. Food enters the large intestine within 12 to 70 hours after eating and remains there as long as 18 hours before defecation.

Some of the influencing factors of digestion are controlled consciously, namely, food composition, variety, and volume, as well as chewing properly and swallowing small amounts at a time. Messages from millions of cells tell the brain when it is time for decision and action, such as hunger. The rest of the digestive process takes place automatically, part of a finely tuned system. When the intellect is actively involved, correct food choices (and an understanding and appreciation of the body) help influence energy metabolism.

METABOLISM: RELEASING THE ENERGY FROM NUTRIENTS

There are three energy nutrients (Table 2–1): carbohydrates, fats, and protein. *Carbohydrates* offer energy for all athletic participation; *fats* offer concentrated energy; and *proteins* can be an energy source when carbohydrate and fat are not available.

It is acknowledged that long-term nutrition will influence an athlete's performance, but the consequences of an athlete's diet immediately preceding and during competition continue to remain a controversial matter. The current questions involve levels of carbohydrate necessary for glycogen storage and what levels of carbohydrate can be tolerated during the event to protect ex-

TABLE 2–1.

Foods in Each of the Energy Categories

Carbohydrate	Protein	Fat
Fruits	Cereals/milk	Avocados
Beans	Cheese	Bacon
Bread	Eggs	Butter
Cookies	Fish	Mayonnaise
Cereals	Lean meat	Margarine
Legumes	Milk	Nuts
Potatoes	Poultry	Peanut butter
Syrups, sugars		Olives

isting storage. Although the percentage of fat in the diet is being deemphasized, protein levels continue to be investigated. The expectation for any pre-event or training regimen is for greatly improved performance.

The work of many physiologists indicates that increased carbohydrate in the diet, coordinated with a precise training schedule, definitely boosts an athlete's endurance for long-duration aerobic events. Improved performance is attributed to greater intracellular storage of glycogen, the storage form of carbohydrate.[2, 3] Participants in brief anaerobic events also recognize increased carbohydrate storage as an advantage.

Although controlled laboratory tests indicate that performance is enhanced by varying the amounts of glucose or carbohydrate in training, scientists are just beginning to collect information on large numbers of participants in field studies and competition (e.g., triathlon).[4] Controlled field studies are difficult to conduct. For instance, an athlete who attempts glycogen loading may find that the rigid demands of dietary management do not coincide with training schedules or that appropriate food choices are not available. Often athletes (e.g., weight lifters) may attempt improvement through unusual food choices and supplementation that do not satisfy their nutritional needs. In many cases, testimonies of increased endurance or strength do not give either valid scientific data on dietary intake or information suitable for large groups of athletes in various stages of growth. Then, when an individual attempts to duplicate a procedure, he or she meets with varying levels of success.

Measurement of glycogen storage or blood lactate or psychological profiles for field studies present other difficulties. Although multiple muscle biopsy or blood chemistry determinations[5] may be practical (and even exciting) feedback for physically mature subjects undergoing laboratory tests, they are inappropriate for immature subjects even if they are attempting peak physical performance. There is the matter of human subject consent, but also, there are just too many immeasurable outside influences.

Examples are erg scores in rowing versus actual performance in the shell and free throws during practice versus actual performance in the game. Who can measure the effects of weather, fan support, pressure from opponents, influence from the coach, or fatigue from travel? Therefore, indirect approaches that can relate the predictions to the performance must be used. The question will always be: how did they win?

The final step in implementing any dietary or training recommendation is the preparation of guidelines for the athlete. Foods must be identified as to composition, and menus must be prepared. Training schedules must be coordinated with other activities. And the problems of food availability, parent cooperation, and time and money must be addressed. With these taken care of, it usually becomes possible for an athlete to build maximal glycogen storage and achieve physical endurance without sacrificing nutrient adequacy.

The team or individual can benefit by knowing how energy is released from foods. Energy is generated by the metabolism of food, or the actual breakdown of the body's energy stores. Foods are converted in the body to glucose, fatty acids, and amino acids before they reach the cells. Within the cells these nutrients react with oxygen, finally forming carbon dioxide and water. This reaction consists of a long series of steps, with the rates controlled by various enzymes. The energy produced is used to form adenosine triphosphate (ATP), which provides energy instantly for muscle contraction, transport of material through cell walls, and syntheses of chemical compounds (Table 2–2).[6]

Also formed during the reaction is adenosine diphosphate (ADP) or adenosine monophosphate (AMP). They can be rephosphorylated to ATP by oxidative reactions. This process is

TABLE 2–2.

General Characteristics of the Energy Systems*

ATP-PC (Phosphagen) System	Lactic Acid System	Oxygen System
Anaerobic	Anaerobic	Aerobic
Very rapid	Rapid	Slow
Chemical fuel: PC	Food fuel: glycogen	Food fuels: glycogen, fats, and protein
Very limited ATP production	Limited ATP production	Unlimited ATP production
Muscular stores limited	By-product, lactic acid, causes muscular fatigue	No fatiguing by-products
Used with sprint or any high-power, short-duration activity	Used with activities of 1- to 3-min duration	Used with endurance or long-duration activities

*From Fox EL: *Sports Physiology*. Philadelphia, WB Saunders Co, 1984, p 22. Used by permission.

continuous. Adenosine triphosphate is the energy currency of the cell; it can be used and regenerated repeatedly. Creatine phosphate is another energy-rich compound and is considered the reservoir of high-energy phosphate because it is stored in the body in larger quantities. During exercise, ATP can be produced by three major metabolic pathways: the phosphogen system (ATP), anaerobic glycolysis (lactic acid), and aerobic metabolism (oxygen).[6]

Each muscle fiber has a quantity of ATP stored for immediate use, yet this supply is limited and will supply only enough energy for 3 to 5 seconds of "all out" work.

Anaerobic exercise or anaerobic glycolysis occurs without oxygen. The work is too intense for the respiratory and circulatory systems to supply the oxygen needed for muscular work. Anaerobic metabolism provides fuel for exercise that lasts less than 2 minutes. In anaerobic glycolysis, which would occur in high-intensity, near-maximal work, glycogen is used at a rate many times faster than during oxidative phosphorylation. Much of the lactic acid that accumulates as a by-product of anaerobic metabolism diffuses from the muscle and into the blood. This increase in blood lactate concentration inhibits lipolysis and enhances carbohydrate utilization, further increases lactic acid, and, eventually, contributes to fatigue.[1] The aerobic system is far more efficient than the anaerobic system with respect to ATP production. This metabolic state takes place within the mitochondria of the cell in the presence of oxygen and provides fuel for exercise that lasts longer than 5 minutes. By considering the vigor of the sport or activity and its duration, one can estimate which system is used for each activity (Table 2–3).

The body's energy needs increase during any bout of exercise. This increased need dictates changes in the pathways that supply oxygen and fuel to the muscles. Hormones, which act as chemical messengers in energy production, mobilize to influence the fuel supply to the muscles.

Exercise suppresses insulin secretion from the pancreas and stimulates secretion of glucagon from the duodenum, growth hormone from the anterior pituitary, and cortisol and catecholamines from the adrenal cortex (Fig 2–2). These hormones stimulate glycogenolysis and gluconeogenesis in the liver and lipolysis in fat cells, releasing glucose and free fatty acids into the blood, which carries them to the muscles. There, fatty acids are broken down through β-oxidation, which frees acetyl-CoA. The acetyl-CoA is further oxidized in the Krebs cycle. Meanwhile, glycogenolysis and glycolysis occur in the muscles, ultimately yielding lactate and acetyl-CoA. Lactate returns to the liver via the blood and is used in gluconeogenesis. In addition, exercise fosters catabolism of amino acids to some degree, fosters movement of alanine from muscles to the liver, and enhances hepatic glyconeogenesis.

Muscles contain thousands of long strands of fibers or filaments ranging from 1 to 45 mm and containing the contractile proteins actin and myosin. Muscles shorten and produce movement when the filaments slide across each other. This sliding is accomplished by tiny cross-bridges that extend from the thicker myosin to the thinner actin filaments. Movement produced in one location is added to that produced along the length of the fiber, and visible motion takes place. Because the muscles attach to bony lever systems, the shortening is multiplied to produce familiar movement patterns, like a pitcher throwing a ball.[7]

Muscle fibers contract at the command of the motor nerves (Fig 2–3). Each motor nerve branches many times. These nerves and fibers are called *motor units.*

TABLE 2–3.

Sports and Their Predominant Energy Systems*

Sports or Sport Activity	ATP-PC and LA†	LA-O_2‡	O_2§
	Emphasis According to Energy Systems		
Baseball	80	20	—
Basketball	85	15	—
Fencing	90	10	—
Field hockey	60	20	20
Football	90	10	—
Golf	95	5	—
Gymnastics			
Ice hockey			
Forwards, defense,	80	20	—
goalie	95	5	—
Lacrosse			
Goalie defense, attack men	80	20	—
midfielders, man-down	60	20	20
Rowing	20	30	50
Skiing			
Slalom, jumping, downhill,	80	20	—
cross-country,	—	5	95
pleasure skiing	34	33	33
Soccer			
Goalie, wings, strikers,	80	20	—
halfbacks or link men	60	20	20
Swimming and diving			
50-yd diving	98	2	—
100 yd	80	15	5
200 yd	30	65	5
400–500 yd	20	40	40
1,500–1,650 yd	10	20	70
Tennis	70	20	10
Track and field			
100–200 yd	98	2	—
Field events	90	10	—
440 yd	80	15	5
880 yd	30	65	5
1 mile	20	55	25
2 miles	20	40	40
3 miles	10	20	70
6 miles (cross country)	5	15	80
Marathon	—	5	95
Volleyball	90	10	—

*From Sports Nutrition: A Guide for the Professional Working With Active People, Sports and Cardiovascular Nutritionists. Chicago, American Dietetic Association, 1986. Used by permission.
†Anaerobic (phosphagen system).
‡Combination (lactic acid–oxygen).
§Aerobic (oxygen).

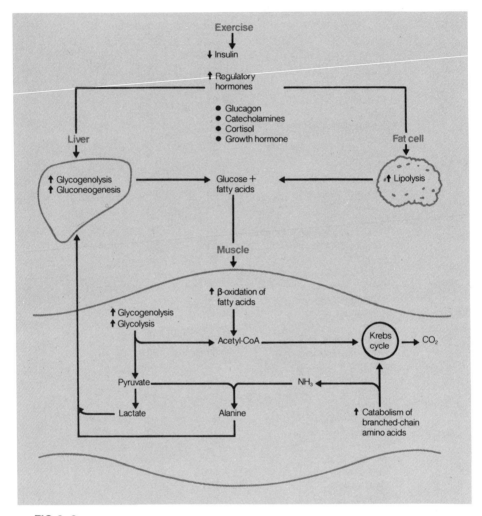

FIG 2–2.
Schematic diagram shows how hormones mobilized during exercise influence fuel supply
to the muscles and outlines the general metabolism of fuel within muscle tissue. Exercise
suppresses insulin secretion and stimulates secretion of glucagon, catecholamines, cortisol, and growth hormone. These hormones stimulate glycogenolysis and gluconeogenesis
in the liver and lipolysis in fat cells, releasing glucose and free fatty acids into the blood,
which carries them to the muscles. There, fatty acids are broken down through β-oxidation,
which frees acetylcoenzyme A *(acetyl-CoA).* The acetyl-CoA is further oxidized in the Krebs
cycle. Meanwhile, glycogenolysis and glycolysis occur in the muscle, ultimately yielding
lactate and acetyl-CoA. Lactate returns to the liver via the blood and is used in gluconeogenesis. In addition, exercise fosters catabolism of amino acids to some degree, and movement of alanine from muscles to the liver also enhances hepatic gluconeogenesis. (From
Phys Sports Med 1986; 14:111. Used by permission.)

The Muscle Structure

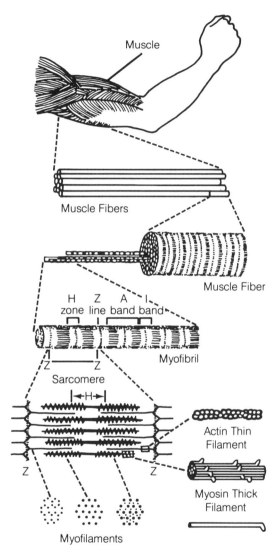

FIG 2–3.
Microscopic organization of skeletal muscle mass contains fibers, which, in turn, are composed of myofibrils, part of which are actin and myosin. (Redrawn from Vander AJ, Sherman JH, Luciano DS: *Human Physiology,* ed 2. New York, McGraw-Hill, Book Co, 1976.)

In recent years, investigators have shown that human skeletal muscles are composed of two distinct fiber types: slow twitch and fast twitch (Table 2–4 and Fig 2–4). Slow-twitch types are oxidative type I, or slow-oxidative, fibers that contract slowly and are slow to fatigue. They have a rich capillary supply and are well supplied with the chemistry required for long-duration endurance activities. They may also be classified as red fibers due to their high myoglobin content. Fast-twitch types are oxidative, glycolytic type IIA fibers that are fast contracting and quick to fatigue. They are larger, have fewer capillaries, and are best suited for short, intense effort. Another type of fast-twitch fiber is glycolytic type IIB, which are fast contracting, easily fatigued, and have a high anaerobic capacity. They may also be classified as white fibers.[8]

The ratio of fast-twitch/slow-twitch fibers in an individual depends on heredity. Athletes will usually gravitate to the sport where they experience success. World-class distance runners usually have more slow-twitch muscle fibers. Sprinters, long jumpers, and high jumpers have high percentages of fast-twitch fibers.[9]

Carbohydrates

Years of training will bring about a change in the size and oxidative capacity of the individual muscle fibers. The intensity

TABLE 2–4.

Characteristics of Muscle Fibers*

Characteristics	Slow-Twitch or Slow-Oxidative Type I	Fast-Twitch or Fast-Oxidative-Glycolytic Type IIA	Fast-Twitch or Fast-Glycolytic Type IIB
Average fiber percentage	50	35	15
Speed of contraction	Slow	Fast	Fast
Force of contraction	Low	High	High
Size	Smaller	Large	Large
Fatigability	Fatigue resistant	Less resistant	Easily fatigued
Aerobic capacity	High	Medium	Low
Capillary density	High	High	Low
Anaerobic capacity	Low	Medium	High

*From Sharkey BJ: *Physiology of Fitness*. Champaign, Ill, Human Kinetics Publishers, 1984. Used by permission.

Fast and Slow Twitch Muscle Fibers

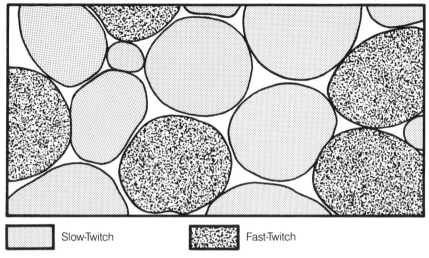

Slow-Twitch   Fast-Twitch

FIG 2–4.
Fast- and slow-twitch fibers intermingle in human muscle, the proportion of which probably remains constant throughout life. The predominant fiber type in specific muscles is an important factor determining success in particular sports or activities. (Redrawn from Sharkey BJ: *Physiology of Fitness,* ed 2. Champaign, Ill, Human Kinetics Publishers, 1984.)

and duration of the activity are determinants of which fibers are recruited during exercise. An athlete beginning at a slow warm-up, progressing to a run, and then into a sprint will recruit slow-oxidative, fast-oxidative, and then fast-glycolytic fibers to meet the varying demands of the workout. As the work load changes, so does the demand on the fuel supply. For example, with work loads up to 60% of maximal oxygen consumption on a normal mixed diet, about one half of the energy is derived from carbohydrate. As the work load is increased to 90% maximal oxygen consumption, the energy contribution of carbohydrate approaches 100%. During the first few minutes of any exercise, blood glucose is the major fuel source. To sustain the activity, the body utilizes glycogen found in the liver and muscle cells. Liver glycogen regulates blood glucose levels, whereas muscle glycogen stores are used directly by the muscle itself.

For example, a mature adult body may contain as much as 66 lb (30 kg) of muscle. If 60% of the muscle mass is involved in exercise, the potential caloric storage available for work can be estimated as follows:

> 30,000 gm of muscle (30 kg) × 1.75 gm glycogen
> per 100 gm of muscle × 4 kcal/gm glycogen
> × 0.60 (active muscle recruitment) =
> 1,260 kcal of potential energy

If all the stored glycogen could be used for exercise, there would be about 1,250 calories available, enough for a 12-mile run.

Increasing the amount of carbohydrate in the diet can affect initial glycogen stores. There is a straightforward correlation between these levels and time to exhaustion at a standard pace; however, glycogen use or depletion occurs at different rates in different fibers. Long-term, steady work probably depletes slow-twitch fibers at the beginning of the event. Fast-twitch fibers are recruited as the glycogen content of the slow-twitch fibers becomes depleted. Costill et al. reported that a loss of periodic acid–Schiff (PAS) staining (a test indicating the muscle glycogen level) is observed first in the slow-twitch fibers in all conditions of running.[10] Other fibers will be recruited for continued work; many of these may be fast twitch, and eventual use of most of the glycogen specific to that muscle group will occur. In all the studies reported from the laboratory or field examinations, the consensus is that the amount of glycogen stored in the muscle, previous to the work, is the major influencing factor in prolonged work at a standard rate of exertion.

When diet manipulations for the athlete are considered, it is important to realize that there are certain types of events in which increasing the ratio of carbohydrate to total calorie intake will improve performance. These include long-duration endurance sports such as swimming, running, soccer, and basketball.

Generalized recommendations to increase carbohydrate in athletes' diets have been acknowledged since the 1960s. Reported levels of an athlete's muscle glycogen may increase to 5 gm/100 gm of wet muscle tissue, with a corresponding increase in the subject's performance in controlled exercise procedures. Since there is substantial evidence that subjects on high-carbohydrate diets can maintain work loads longer than those on mixed- or low-carbohydrate diets, evidence alone merits consideration for recommending more carbohydrates.

Some disagreement occurs when examining sparing of glycogen by ingestion of glucose-rich fluids during performance.[11] In general, small amounts of low-carbohydrate solutions, drunk frequently during competition, will usually enhance bicycling performance. Higher levels of either glucose or polymers have caused nausea and a feeling of fullness. Again, it seems better to try out a possible performance enhancer during training than to wait until competition. Commercial products may, indeed, prolong the high-quality performance of an athlete. About 240 to 500 calories in the form of glucose polymers (80–125 gm/L) seem to be well tolerated by most distance athletes. Since some events, such as the triathlon and marathon, require at least 2,600 calories or more, an added form of energy during competition provides a logical alternative to burning fat (or muscle protein).[12, 13]

Training also enhances the muscles' glycogen storage ability. Gollnick et al. examined men selected to represent different age groups, states of physical fitness, and types of training programs.[14] The investigators examined the enzyme activity and fiber composition in skeletal muscle of trained and untrained men and made comparisons within each training segment. Slow-twitch fibers predominated in the muscles of the endurance athletes, although a wide range of fiber composition existed in all groups. Oxidative capacity of both fiber types was greater in the endurance groups, and muscle glycogen storage was highest in the trained subjects. It is interesting to note that the training required to elicit a change in metabolic response in the subjects involved 5 months of pedaling 1 hour/day, 4 days/week, at a load intensity representing 75% of maximum aerobic power. Maximum volume of oxygen uptake (maximum VO_2) increased an average of 13% over the 5-month period. These results suggest that trained athletes with large muscle mass composed predominantly of slow-twitch fibers who compete in long-endurance events may benefit most from increased carbohydrate intake.

Piehl et al. indicated in an early work that well-trained subjects have higher glycogen levels in their muscles than untrained individuals[15] and that training can induce a local increase in glycogen level or an increased ability for glycogen storage in muscles. Exercise caused a parallel glycogen decrease in trained and untrained muscle, but the untrained muscle had lower initial glycogen levels. Therefore, at the end of identical depletion routines, the trained muscle still contained one third of the initial glycogen. A matter to consider, then, is that training induces a local increase in muscle glycogen levels independent of diet. In their study, Piehl et al. emphasized that a subject must allow at least 3 days for muscles to regain preexercise glycogen levels.

Glycogen repletion presents a problem to the athlete who is attempting high-glycogen levels during training and competition. The usage of glycogen during training often exceeds the ability to replace it. It is necessary to decrease training and concentrate on a diet high in carbohydrates. Complex carbohydrates—fruits, vegetables, whole grains, cereals, legumes—are necessary for resynthesizing glycogen. Simple sugars or refined carbohydrates may cause cramps, nausea, gas, and bloating. Ingestion of concentrated glucose solutions, such as colas or fruit juices, up to 45 minutes before competition results in decreased performance because of a tendency of the pancreas to secrete insulin. This higher insulin level prevents the body from using fat, and, therefore, glycogen must be used exclusively.

When the ability of individual carbohydrates to raise blood sugar levels following consumption was studied, it was found that dried legumes produced the smallest rise in blood glucose level and potatoes and carrots produced a blood glucose elevation similar to or greater than that produced by refined sugar. Breads, cereals, grains, and fruits produced a lower elevation than sugar. Fructose has been shown to produce a lower insulin response than does sucrose for most individuals.[16]

Figure 2–5 suggests that a gradual decline in muscle glycogen in combination with a low-carbohydrate diet (40% of calories) may be directly related to the chronic fatigue experienced by athletes immediately before competition and after successive days of heavy training. A high-carbohydrate diet (70% of calories) can replace muscle glycogen during training. If enough carbohydrate is eaten, even muscles severely emptied of glycogen can be adequately refilled within 24 hours.[17]

Piehl also examined the time needed for glycogen repletion

Muscle Glycogen Levels

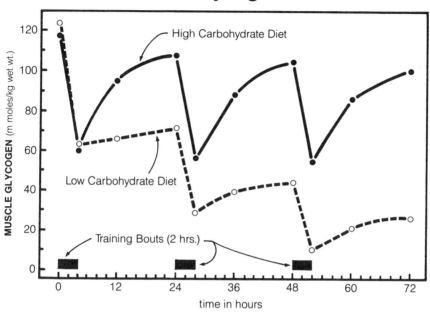

FIG 2–5.

A graded decline in muscle glycogen may be related to the chronic fatigue often experienced by athletes during repetitive strenuous training. The effect is reduced speed, precision, and endurance. A high-carbohydrate diet encourages glycogen resynthesis, returning the muscle stores to near normal levels for each succeeding day of training. (Redrawn from Costill DL, Miller JM: Nutrition for endurance sport: Carbohydrate balance. *Int J Sports Med* 1980; 1:2.)

in individual human muscle fibers after exercise-induced glycogen depletion[19] and evaluated the correlation between glycogen repletion and the amount and time of carbohydrate intake. Her subjects consumed a diet in which carbohydrate contributed 60% of total calories. Caloric intake was 4,000 kcal/24 hours, or approximately 57 kcal/kg of body weight/24 hours, during the 46 hours after depletion. The most pronounced recovery of glycogen was during the first 10 hours of the experiment. It appeared that, on this initial schedule, the entire carbohydrate intake was converted to muscle glycogen.

It is recognized that depletion occurs on a regular basis during any training protocol. To take advantage of the resynthesis of glycogen stores, a carbohydrate-rich diet should be available to the athlete as soon as possible after depletion, regardless of the level of depletion. It is also suggested that the diet continue for at least 3 days and that training be greatly decreased immediately after depletion for maximum resynthesis. This is especially important in preparation for competition.

Key points to remember are:

1. Athletes with well-developed muscles will be able to store more glycogen.

2. Well-trained muscles have the ability to store more glycogen.

3. Large, trained muscles plus a diet rich in carbohydrates will produce an even greater storage of glycogen.

4. Hard physical training depletes the stores of glycogen in the muscles. If repletion does not occur quickly, chronic fatigue will result.

5. Repletion is successful when athletes follow a diet that is more than 60% carbohydrate. Meals should not be skipped; they should always be eaten within 10 hours of exhaustive exercise.

6. When planning the high-carbohydrate training diet, one should remember that cereals, breads, pasta, legumes, muffins, pancakes, rolls, and all other grain products are excellent sources of carbohydrate. Fruits, juices and vegetables are good sources, and milk, yogurt, ice milk, milkshakes, and ice cream also have carbohydrate. All high-protein foods, such as meats, have very little carbohydrate. Desserts and regular soft drinks are high in carbohydrate but low in all other nutrients.

7. During preparation for competition, it will be necessary to decrease training levels up to 3 days prior to the event to protect glycogen stores in the muscles. Carbohydrate should contribute at least 70% of the calories consumed.

8. Sugary drinks, large quantities of honey, or candy bars are not recommended immediately before competition, although drinking low concentrations of glucose or glucose

polymer solutions during the event may spare glycogen stores.

9. Recovery of fatigue will be greatly enhanced by post-event feedings of carbohydrate within 10 hours.

Fats

Intense exercise requires glycogen as fuel; moderate exercise can be maintained by fat. Training increases the capacity of skeletal muscle to utilize fat. A highly trained long-distance runner, working at a level of 70% of maximum V_{O_2}, will be using fat about 75% of the run. Any regimen that will spare muscle glycogen and force fat to be used will result in increased endurance.

Fat is a concentrated source of energy, providing about 9 kcal of energy/gm. Fats in the diet are digested, producing fatty acids and glycerol. After absorption they are converted to triglycerides, the storage form of fat found in adipose tissue. When needed by muscles, fat from adipose tissue is released and transported by the blood to the muscles, where it is oxidized.[19]

During light to moderate aerobic exercise, stored fat supplies 50% to 60% of needed energy. Trained athletes can use the abundant supply of fat in their bodies as fuel and spare glycogen. Another way to increase free fatty acid concentration in the blood is to consume caffeinated drinks containing 250 to 350 mg (or about 8 oz of coffee or cola). It takes 20 or 30 minutes from the time an athlete starts to exercise until enough fat is available to be used as fuel.

Along with carbohydrate loading to prolong exercise duration, fat loading has also been suggested for events in the ultrasports. Dietary fat is increased for several days before the event. There is an increased utilization of plasma-free fatty acid and a decreased utilization of muscle glycogen. However, it has been observed that performance from athletes on this diet is significantly impaired and, therefore, fat loading is not recommended. It is currently recommended that all individuals restrict total fat calories to less than 30%. The Pritikin diet and the American Heart Association advise lowering fat even further.[21] Whether or not this is possible for the general population, the athletic segment might do well to follow any dietary suggestions aimed at reducing the risk of heart disease, cancer, and obesity.

Protein

The major function of protein in the diet is to furnish the materials for new growth, to maintain and repair tissue, and to build such body proteins as hemoglobin, enzymes, hormones, and antibodies. Protein is required for the formation of materials that transport fat, to maintain the proper amount of fluid in the blood and tissues, and to provide energy if there is a shortage of the other energy nutrients (e.g., during severe dieting, starvation, or when glycogen stores are depleted).

When protein is used as a fuel source, it is used at considerable expense to the body because protein is then drawn away from its structural and regulatory roles. When amino acid components are degraded for energy, the amine group is incorporated by the liver into urea and sent to the kidney for excretion. Excess volumes of water are lost in this process, and the body can become dehydrated quickly. This is the rationale for many quick weight loss diets. The remaining carbon, hydrogen, and oxygen can be used as glucose and fat to build carbohydrate. If necessary, protein can help maintain a steady blood glucose level.[20]

Because protein is such a valuable nutrient for the body, it is understandable why it is so revered in the world of athletics. However, the athlete handles protein no differently than the nonathlete, and, consequently, the standard protein recommendations are much the same for both (Table 2–5). To determine the RDA for protein, determine ideal weight, convert pounds to kilograms by dividing by 2.2, and multiply by the correct gram per kilogram value.

Protein requirements may be higher during periods of intense training or in heavy lifting, but there is no supporting evidence for the need of more than the RDA. If there is an increased need, it can easily be met by a well-balanced diet, with 15% to 20% of calories provided by protein.

For athletes on a vegetarian diet, the problem of meeting daily protein needs takes on another dimension. Knowledge of

TABLE 2–5.

Recommended Dietary
Allowances for Protein*

Age (yr)	RDA† (gm/kg)
0–0.5	2.2
0.5–1	2.0
1–3	1.8
4–10	1.1
11–14	1.0
15–18	0.9
19 and older	0.8

*From Food and Nutrition Board, National Academy of Sciences: *National Research Council Recommended Dietary Allowances,* rev. Washington, DC, National Academy of Sciences, 1980.
†The recommended dietary allowance (RDA) increases by 30 gm/day during pregnancy and by 20 gm/day during lactation.

complementary protein is needed to provide the combination of amino acids equivalent to that of complete protein. Complementary protein combinations for the vegetarian include:

1. Legumes with grains (peanut butter sandwich, beans and tortillas, pea soup and cornbread)
2. Grains with milk (oatmeal and milk, rice pudding, macaroni and cheese)
3. Seeds with vegetables (sunflower seeds and broccoli, nut butters on raw vegetables, sesame seeds with green leafy vegetables)

Guidelines for the lacto-ovo vegetarian are:

1. Decrease empty calories.
2. Replace meat with eggs, legumes, nuts, seeds, and meat analogs.

3. Use low-fat milk products.
4. Select whole-grain or other nutritious grain foods.
5. Include a variety of fruits and vegetables in the diet.

The vegetarian athlete will need to eat more calories to meet protein needs because many food choices provide only about one half as much protein as a serving of meat. Quite often, the bulk of a vegetarian diet is so large, there is not enough time to eat or even room in the stomach to include all needed nutrients. Additional attention must be given to vitamins D and B_{12} when the diet excludes dairy products.

ENERGY BALANCE

At some point the question will arise as to the best way to determine ideal body weight and how to calculate the energy needed to either maintain or change it. The cost of individual energy is determined by basal metabolic requirements, muscular activity, and assimilation of food. These values are never absolute; they are only estimates. This is difficult to accept when we want to be exact about calculating the calories needed for sport or growth needs. The reality is that athletes do not sit in quiet collection chambers or participate while wearing Douglas bags (which collect the amount of expelled air). Their basal metabolism changes during the day, if not moment by moment. For these reasons, charts and tables are compelling reading and valuable in presenting information to the athlete (see Appendix B). All diet orders are based on scientific observation, which continues when the athlete accepts information and tries suggestions (Table 2–6).

Basal metabolism is expressed as the quantity of energy used by the body at rest. Most energy supports the metabolic work of the body's cells: heartbeat, breathing, temperature maintenance, nerve transmission, and hormonal messenger systems. All of these needs must be met before there is any energy left over for

TABLE 2–6.

Median Energy Consumption and Corresponding Daily Food Requirements of Groups
of Elite Male Athletes*

Selected Sports Category 1	Expenditure of Energy/kg of Body Weight/Day (kcal) 2	Average Body Weight (kg) 3	Normative Daily Net Needs Based on Computed Energy Requirements (Column 2 × Column 3) (kcal) 4	Optimal Daily Gross Requirements With 10% Added for SDA Effect (kcal) 5
Group A				
Cross-country skiing	82.14	67.5	5.550	6.105
Crew racing	69.21	80.0	5.550	6.105
Canoe racing	72.72	75.0	5.450	5.995
Swimming	69.87	76.0	5.300	5.830
Bicycle racing	80.39	68.0	5.450	5.995
Marathon racing	79.07	68.0	5.400	5.940
Average values (men)			5.450	5.995

Rounded-off norm: 6.000 kcal

Also belonging to sports of group A are skiing, Norwegian combination, middle-distance racing, walking, ice racing, modern pentahlon, equine sports, military, and touring (alpine climbing).

Group B				
Soccer	72.28	74.0	5.350	5.885
Handball	68.06	75.0	5.100	5.610
Basketball	67.93	75.0	5.100	5.610
Field hockey	69.18	75.0	5.200	5.720
Ice hockey	71.87	68.0	4.900	5.390
Average values (men)			5.130	5.643

Rounded-off norm: 5.600 kcal

Also belonging to group B are rugby, water polo, volleyball, tennis, polo, and bicycle polo.

Group C				
Canoe slalom	67.16	68.0	4.550	5.005
Shooting	62.71	72.5	4.550	5.005
Table tennis	59.96	74.0	4.450	4.895
Bowling	62.69	75.0	4.700	5.170
Sailing	63.77	74.0	4.700	5.170
Average values (men)			4.590	5.049

Rounded-off norm: 5.000 kcal

Also belonging to group C are circuit cycle racing (1,000–4,000 m, fencing, ice sailing, and gliding.

Group D				
Sprinting	61.77	69.0	4.250	4.675
Running: short to middle distances	65.62	65.0	4.250	4.675
Pole vault	57.83	73.0	4.200	4.620
Diving	69.24	61.0	4.200	4.620

TABLE 2–6.   (cont.)

Selected Sports Category 1	Expenditure of Energy/kg of Body Weight/Day (kcal) 2	Average Body Weight (kg) 3	Normative Daily Net Needs Based on Computed Energy Requirements (Column 2 × Column 3) (kcal) 4	Optimal Daily Gross Requirements With 10% Added for SDA Effect (kcal) 5
Boxing (middle and welter weight to 63.5 kg)	67.25	63.0	4.250	4.675
Average values (men)			4.230	4.653

Rounded-off norm: 4.600 kcal

Also belonging to group D are hurdle races, broad and high jump, hop-skip-and-jump, ballet swimming, figure skating, figure roller skating, and skiing, ski jump, bobsled, and tobogganing.

Group E1				
Judo (lightweight)	72.92	62.5	4.550	5.005
Weight lifting (lightweight)	69.15	67.5	4.650	5.115
Javelin	56.95	76.0	4.350	4.785
Gymnastics with apparatus	67.14	65.0	4.350	4.785
Steeplechase	63.96	68.0	4.350	4.785
Ski: Alpine competition	71.29	67.5	4.800	5.280
Average values (men)			4.508	4.959

Rounded-off norm: 5.000 kcal

Also belonging to group E1 are wrestling, automobile rallies, motor racing, gymnastics, acrobatics, parachute jumping, equine sports shows, decathlon, and bicycle gymnastics.

Group E2				
Hammerthrow	62.46	102.0	6.350	6.985
Shot put and discus	62.47	102.0	6.350	6.985

Rounded-off norm: 7.000 kcal

*From *Sports Nutrition: A Guide for the Professional Working With Active People, Sports and Cardiovascular Nutritionists.* Chicago, American Dietetic Association, 1986, p 42. p 42. Used by permission.

growth, repair, digestion, or athletic activity, which is why dietitians maintain that the body's first need is for energy.

A substantial amount of energy is required to keep the body functioning and it is influenced by a number of factors: (1) age and sex, (2) physical states, (3) pregnancy, and (4) climate.

Age and Sex.—In general, the younger a person, the higher the basal metabolic rate, probably because of increased activity of cell division. It is most pronounced during growth spurts but also because children and adolescents have a greater ratio of surface area to weight. The greater the body surface area, the faster the metabolism. Males usually have a higher metabolic rate than females due to a greater percentage of lean tissue.

Physical States.—Disease, starvation, chronic undernutrition, or low-calorie diets decrease the metabolic rate because of the loss of lean tissues and the shutdown of functions the body cannot support. The latter may underlie the reason why some dieters have problems losing weight when severely limiting calories. Stress can increase epinephrine levels, increase the energy demands of every cell, and temporarily raise the metabolic rate. These would account for the weight loss that some people experience during high stress, although it is not unusual for weight gain to occur, because binge eating may temporarily relieve stress. The activity of the thyroid gland has a direct influence on the metabolic rate. The less thyroxin secreted, the lower the energy requirement. In cases of starvation diets as experienced in anorexia, fractions of the thyroid hormone may be suppressed. Again, it is a protective mechanism for the body.

Pregnancy.—At any age, pregnancy raises the metabolic rate. Increased cell activity and increased cardiac output and respiratory rate are responsible.

Climate.—Metabolic rates increase in colder weather. This is a factor to consider when very young athletes compete in winter sports or when the playing season extends into cold weather.[20]

PHYSICAL ACTIVITY

Physical activity does not make a large contribution to energy requirements, as explained in Appendix B. In general, people today tend to overemphasize their activity. During the early part of this century, the U.S. Department of Agriculture described a sedentary woman as a farm wife who walked only 2 miles daily. But unlike basal metabolism, which changes infrequently, physical exercise can be increased, and energy demands may range from as little as an extra 2 calories/minute for leisurely canoeing to more than 14 calories/minute for cross-country racing. The number of calories needed for an activity depends entirely on the involvement of the muscles and the demands of respiration and heartbeat. The greater the amount of muscular work, the heavier the weight being moved; the longer the time the activity takes, the more calories are necessary.

The kilocalorie is used to approximate the number of calories used by the body during a particular exercise. The range of energy for an individual may vary from as little as 50 calories/activity to more than 800. This range acknowledges the immense differences in metabolism among people in skill and efficiency levels and, perhaps, in health status.

Each person needs to work out his or her own energy balance, knowing that there is a wide range to consider. There is an easy way to do this—weigh-ins! But then comes the hard part. If an individual is overweight, he or she must take in fewer calories than are burned, which means selecting foods that contain fewer calories and increasing activity.

Energy output can be expressed either as kilocalories per minute, milliliters per minute per kilogram of body weight (MET), or a training heart rate. The oxygen intake is used in research; the heart rate is used as the indicator of exercise intensity.

OTHER FACTORS THAT DETERMINE FUEL UTILIZATION

Along with difficulties in determining individual caloric needs to maintain body weight, many other factors influence fuel utilization, caloric needs, and expenditures.

Alcohol

Alcohol not only replaces necessary nutrients with empty calories but also adversely affects the physiologic mechanisms and pathways that are involved in metabolizing energy. Unlike protein, fat, and carbohydrate, all of which pass from the stomach into the small intestine before moving into the bloodstream, alcohol is absorbed quickly and directly from the stomach. Alcohol, or ethanol, is such a small molecule that it is not necessary to break it down to smaller components before it enters the circulatory system. That portion of alcohol not absorbed directly from the stomach goes through the small intestine.

The body recognizes alcohol as a drug and tries to eliminate it quickly. A small amount leaves via urine, perspiration, and expired air. It is easy to detect with a breath analyzer or by simply taking a good whiff of a person who has been drinking. The rest of the alcohol is either metabolized by the liver or processed in the stomach and small intestine. Disordered liver metabolism occurs because alcohol converts to acetaldehyde and hydrogen instead of a more usable fuel such as glucose. However, it is possible for some maintenance energy to be derived from the calories in consumed alcohol. For example, 20 oz of 86-proof liquor provides 1,500 kcal, or about one half to two thirds of the daily caloric requirement, but it provides no protein, vitamins, or minerals.

Alcohol causes inflammation of the stomach, pancreas, and intestine and begins interfering with the normal processes of digestion and absorption, resulting in malabsorption of nutrients, and secondary malnutrition. Absorption of thiamin, vitamin B_{12}, folic acid, and ascorbic acid is depressed in the presence of alcohol. Alcohol decreases the activity of the enzymes lactase, sucrase, maltase, and alkaline phosphatase. Lactose intolerance may explain milk aversion in heavy drinkers. Negligible lactase activity has been found in both black and white alcoholics. Silent, genetically determined lactose intolerance may become noticeable after alcohol ingestion.

Because the liver can work on only a few grams of alcohol per hour, alcohol starts to accumulate in the blood stream and affect other organs, notably the brain (which has a high priority on glucose or any available fuel). There it acts as a narcotic, actually putting nerve cells to sleep. This effect begins in the areas of the brain that control behavior, eliminating inhibitions that usually regulate words and actions.

As the blood alcohol level rises, other brain centers become depressed. Vision blurs, speech becomes slurred, and walking or driving becomes difficult. Finally, the entire conscious brain dozes off; the individual passes out and will not remember any actions taken. It is even possible to disturb the brain's unconscious centers, those that control breathing and heart rate.

Of all the complications of alcohol consumption, the most deleterious to the athlete are hyperlipidemia, high blood lactic acid levels, and low blood glucose levels. Moderate drinking can increase the body's requirement for B complex vitamins (which are needed to metabolize alcohol) and magnesium. Carbohydrate metabolism is also altered, the conversion rate of glycogen to glucose is slowed, and protein stores will be mobilized for energy.[20] It is estimated that 1 out of every 10 Americans who drink is an alcoholic, so it would be absurd to give the standard advice for moderation. Instead, it may be more appropriate to classify the situations in athletes when and when it is not appropriate to drink.

There is evidence of a relationship between alcohol intake and the state of a person's blood vessels. There is conjecture that moderate drinking may even reduce the incidence of coronary disease. The mechanism by which alcohol alters coronary artery disease is still unknown. Alcohol has multiple effects that may contribute to the protection that occurs. Perhaps a glass of wine with dinner lowers the stress of everyday life. Sheehan has remarked, "I find that drinking a couple of beers is a good way to end my day. They restore my inner climate to normal."[21] Many ballplayers agree—just so they do not believe that beer also restores hydration, because it does not! For the most part, there is agreement that alcohol in any amount has a deleterious effect on athletic performance. The position statement of the American College of Sports Medicine makes five major points[22]:

1. The acute ingestion of alcohol can have a deleterious effect on many psychomotor skills, such as reaction time, hand-eye coordination, accuracy, balance, and complex coordination. Performance will be affected most seriously in sports involving rapid reactions to changing stimuli.

2. Acute alcohol consumption substantially influences metabolic or physiological functions crucial to physical performance, such as energy metabolism, maximal oxygen consumption, heart rate, stroke volume, cardiac output, muscle blood flow, arteriovenous oxygen difference, or respiratory dynamics. It may impair body temperature regulation during prolonged exercise in a cold environment.

3. Acute alcohol ingestion will not improve and may decrease strength, power, local muscular endurance, speed, and cardiovascular endurance. Thus, alcohol ingestion will not improve muscular work capacity and may decrease performance levels.

4. Alcohol is the most abused drug in the United States, and prolonged excessive consumption can lead to cellular changes in the liver, heart, brain, and muscle.

5. All of those associated with athletes and athletic events should make serious and continuing efforts to educate athletes on the adverse physiological effects of alcohol and advise against its use in conjunction with athletic contests.

Keep in mind that there are varying reactions to alcohol ingestion not only among individuals but also within an individual, depending on the circumstances.

Athletes can still perform the morning after ingesting alcohol, but muscle glycogen levels at rest will be significantly lower following alcohol consumption compared with nonconsumption. Although alcohol does not impair lipolysis during exercise, it may decrease glucose output, decrease the potential contribution from liver gluconeogenesis, elicit a greater decline in blood glucose levels (leading to hypoglycemia), and decrease the leg muscle uptake of glucose during the latter stages of a long run.

Situations where alcohol ingestion is definitely not appropriate are pregnancy, lactation, childhood, premenstrual syndrome (PMS), hypertension, diabetes, weight loss, and driving.

Pregnancy.—Alcohol reaches the unborn baby's blood at the same concentration as the mother's within 15 minutes. At a very high level of chronic intake, it causes a number of defects known as *fetal alcohol syndrome*. Moderate drinking may be linked to miscarriages, stillbirths, and low birth weight.

Lactation.—Alcohol can inhibit the letdown reflex that leads to milk secretion. Although the level of alcohol in breast milk is lower than the level in the mother's own blood, an infant can become intoxicated after its mother has had a few drinks.

Childhood.—The smaller the body, the greater is alcohol's effect. A 160-lb man would have to have four or five drinks over the course of 1 or 2 hours to reach a blood alcohol level of legal intoxication, but it would take less than four drinks for a 120-lb woman to reach the same blood alcohol level. It would take only two and one half drinks to intoxicate a 90-lb child, and at that level, the alcohol may be lethal. In addition, why encourage a habit that may lead to problems later in life?

Premenstrual Syndrome.—Alcohol metabolism tends to be slowest right before the menstrual period, making a woman more likely to be affected by a drink then. Along with increasing fiber and drinking more water, avoiding alcohol makes sense for women who have problems with PMS.

Hypertension.—Not only does alcohol appear to be involved in the development of hypertension, but it may also aggravate an existing condition. People with high blood pressure should limit their drinks to no more than two per day.

Diabetes.—Alcohol interferes with blood glucose metabolism; can raise blood triglycerides; and may interact with oral medication, such as chlorpropamide (Diabinese), which can result in flushing, nausea, a quickened heartbeat, or impaired speech.

Weight Loss.—Drinking is not compatible with dieting. A major problem restricting calories is to get the necessary nutrients. Alcohol is a limited source of energy and has virtually no nutrients.

Driving.—Those responsible for the safe delivery of athletes to and from the playing field should not drink. They need their psychomotor skills just as much as the quarterback does. After alcohol enters the bloodstream, there is no way to speed up its metabolism. It will not do any good to walk around the block, because muscles do not use alcohol for fuel. Coffee or cold showers will not help either.[23]

Aspirin

Aspirin is an anti-inflammatory that is used often in athletics. It can lessen joint stiffness and increase mobility. Taken several hours before exercise, it masks slight pain that would otherwise be aggravated by movement. Usually the advice is to exercise to pain and not through it. Pain should be the signal to stop exercising, to rest and start icing. After the pain subsides, its cause should be determined.

Blood Doping

In the real world of athletics, blood doping is seldom used. However, when muscles are required to work over an extended period of time, the amount of oxygen carried to muscle by blood is possibly a limiting factor. Removing blood from the athlete, storing the red blood cells, and then reinfusing them into the same donor increases hemoglobin concentration and augments oxygen-carrying capacity. Several studies have found that aerobic performance was enhanced by this method.[24]

In practical terms, blood banking facilities are needed, and infections can be acquired by the recipient. The fact that blood doping represents an attempt to artificially boost performance makes this practice illegal and unethical. Hopefully, other ways to boost hemoglobin, such as increasing iron intake, will interest future researchers and athletes.

Caffeine

Caffeine is a central nervous system stimulant found in coffee, tea, cola drinks, chocolate, and many over-the-counter products that are sold to combat drowsiness or diminish feelings of fatigue and is among the most common substances ingested by exercisers.[25] Some research suggests that doses of caffeine (as little as that found in 8 oz of coffee) will bolster the body's ability to withstand long endurance events by increasing the muscles' capacity to burn fat as fuel, thus sparing glycogen. Some athletes report beneficial effects, but many find no benefit at all. The dose frequently cited as effective is 2 to 3 mg of caffeine/kg of body weight.

Frequently reported side effects are consistent restlessness, tremor, and irritability at high doses. Such side effects could be disastrous for those high-skill sports that require precision of movement and calm, such as archery, riflery, and gymnastics. Other side effects include diuresis. Attempts to increase caffeine to spare glycogen should be tried out in training or long before key performances.

Caffeine is on the International Olympic Committee's list of banned drugs. The threshold is 15 μg/ml of urine, an amount that allows an average level of caffeine from moderate coffee and soft drink use.

Carbohydrate Loading

Glycogen, the body's store of carbohydrate, is the preferred fuel for long-distance work. Although body fat makes significant energy contributions during long events, initial glycogen stores determine performance. When these stores are depleted, the athlete must either stop or slow down.

Depletion on a continual basis is a problem during competition that lasts more than 3 hours or during heavy training schedules when use of glycogen exceeds the body's ability to replace it. During training, more than one half of all calories in the diet should come from carbohydrate. Then, at least 3 days prior to the event, carbohydrate intake should be boosted to 70% to 80% of calories. It is also necessary for the athlete to rest or taper off during this time.[26]

Drugs, Steroids, and Stimulants

The successes of record-breaking athletes invariably raises the issue of performance-enhancing drugs. Because all of the substances in question are readily available all of the time, most athletes can do exactly what they want to do most of the time. Suppliers include teammates, coaches, physicians, trainers, pharmacists, and sports fans.

The big concern is not that drug use is banned from international competition but that many drugs can cause damage to overall health and longevity. Athletes are tested routinely at high-level contests, but use or dependence usually begins when an athlete is just beginning to appreciate the fact that there is a special place in the winner's circle for him or her.

Very young developing athletes are now experiencing the trend to expand and extend serious training programs. These young people are under tremendous performance pressure and are especially vulnerable to claims for any product that can boost strength, endurance, and reaction, increase the body's muscle-building capacities, blunt stage fright, or hasten weight loss. What these athletes are often too young to understand is that no drug is without risk, as shown in Table 2–7. Those taking steroids still need increased calories and protein for growth effects. Amphetamine users will need more calories. Marihuana users seldom eat well, and depressant users need a lower caloric intake.

Fasting

Metabolic changes occur within 24 hours of fasting. It is a severe and rapid way to lose weight and is often used by wrestlers, crew members, dancers, or any athlete faced with the ultimatum of making weight in a short time. There is usually enough time to reach standardized weight, but because dieting is not fun, caloric restriction is put off until the very last minute. Often fasting is used along with spitting, intense exercise, or other methods of dehydration. Fasting may also be intentional, as a dietary treatment for diarrhea, to provide rest to the gastrointestinal tract, or during holy days. Intentional fasting may occur on road trips when food is not available; the team may dislike the pre-event meal; or there may be simply not enough time to eat and play ball. The latter cases are usually the result of poor planning, but they can be nightmares. Every team

TABLE 2–7.

Drugs Commonly Used in Sports

Drug	Rational	Possible Side Effects
Anabolic steroids	Increases strength and muscle mass	Acne, baldness, increased facial hair, deepening voice, closure of epiphyses, decreased sperm production, decreased testosterone, decreased high-density lipoprotein, increased liver tumors, increased aggressiveness
Growth hormone	Increased height	Possible acromegaly, cardiac disorders, bone disorders
Amphetamines	Decreased fatigue, appetite suppression, increased endurance	Anorexia, restlessness, tremor, confusion, hypertension
Cocaine	Increased endurance	Psychological dependency, damage to nasal mucosa
Marihuana	Increased well-being	Increased metabolic rate, airway obstruction, bronchitis, sinusitis, asthma, tachycardia, decreased oxygen carrying, decreased sweating, decreased psychomotor function, decreased coordination, decreased memory, decreased attention span, confusion
Depressants	Decreased tremors, sleep inducers	Habit forming

*Amphetamine users will need more calories.

trainer has a few stories to tell about them and what happened to performance.

Even at rest, cells require energy. Fuel must be delivered on a 24-hour basis. After a meal, glucose and fat supply immediate energy. After a few hours glucose is used up, and storage glycogen maintains the glucose supply. When glycogen is gone, cells must depend on fatty acids. Fatty acids work for a while, but the brain and the central nervous system require glucose. Body protein will begin to break down to supply amino acids, a fairly wasteful reaction that also produces amine groups. This process is described by Whitney[19]:

> To make matters worse, body fat is hopelessly inefficient as a glucose source; only the tiny glycerol backbone in each giant triglyceride molecule can be converted to glucose and it takes two glycerols to make a single glucose unit. Fatty acids cannot be con-

verted to glucose. Using glycerols from fat this way obligates the body to dispose of the large quantities of fatty acids released at the same time. For energy from fatty acids to be released, carbohydrates must enter the energy cycle simultaneously. During fasting, after glycogen stores are exhausted, there is no available glucose in the body for this function. Therefore, the fatty acid fragments are converted into ketone bodies. As the fast continues, the body adapts by condensing the fragments derived from fatty acids into ketones. An adaptation takes place in the brain as well. Some of the nerve cells become able to use the ketones as fuel. Ketone production rises until it is meeting about half of the brain's energy needs. Still, many areas of the brain rely exclusively on glucose and body protein continues to be sacrificed to produce it. A hazard of ketoses is that ketones may be produced in greater quantities than can be used or excreted in the urine, so they accumulate in the blood. Because they are organic acids, their accumulation leads to acidosis. Simultaneously, the body drastically reduces its energy output in order to conserve both its fat and lean tissue. As the lean organ tissue shrinks in mass, it performs less metabolic work, reducing energy needs. Because of slower metabolism, the loss of fat falls to a bare minimum. Thus, although weight loss during fasting may be quite dramatic, fat loss may be less than when a low calorie diet is eaten.

During training, the athlete may need from 500 to 5,000 extra kcal/day above basal metabolic demands. Fasting to meet weight expectations is just not a good idea. The metabolic rate drops, and fatigue sets in quickly. Some body builders, for example, fast prior to competition in the hope that the definition of their muscles will be greater. It is part of their magic eating formula, part of the mystique of the muscle bound. These athletes are not attempting real work, which requires calories and carbohydrates.

Fatigue and Stress

Muscle fatigue is accelerated by vigorous exercise that overwhelms the aerobic system. At that point, little oxygen reaches the muscle cells, lactic acid accumulates, and exhaustion occurs. It may be intentional, as when an athlete attempts to boost the anaerobic threshold. The ability to judge a running pace that will allow sufficient oxygen to reach the muscles will prevent fatigue. Relaxing or taking the tension off specific muscle groups, as in alternating hard and easy workouts, will allow lactic acid to be disposed of by the liver. Preventing fatigue caused by overtraining is a matter of anticipating other stresses and monitoring them to minimize the risk of a breakdown.

Fatigue is a common, and often nonspecific, symptom of underlying physical or emotional disorder. Its presence is a source of concern for the physician, coach, and athlete. Relief usually comes with a reduction or alteration in training pace or complete rest.

In fatigue, the body experiences a conservation withdrawal, a lowering of metabolic and physical activity, in an attempt to conserve energy. This stage usually continues until energy stores of glycogen are repleted or the threat of energy depletion passes. Factors capable of evoking fatigue include the aftermath of a physical or emotional crisis, which leads to loss of competitive desire, decreased enthusiasm for training, poor nutrition, diminished sleep, or disease. The physiological responses to fatigue are similar to those observed during sleep, diminished sympathetic nervous system activity, decrease in muscle tone and activity, and slower heart rate, cardiac output, and respiration. Gastrointestinal blood flow, secretions, and peristalsis decline, as well as adrenocorticotropin hormone and growth hormone secretion. The net result is an overall slowing of biochemical activity, with a switch to anaerobic metabolism. Fatigue is seldom the sole symptom or single complaint of the athlete; it is probably a multitude of physiological alterations.

Various measurements are used to diagnose overtraining. They are rarely done on a timely basis and may be related only to the normal physiological responses to heavy training. The first step in the evaluation of fatigue is separating the organic from the psychological. The defining complaints of being "tired out, can't go on with training" or "unable to maintain training schedule" may be accompanied by other symptoms.[27] For example, fever, cough, or weight loss may indicate a biological disease. Insomnia may be caused by exercise-induced allergies. In the fatigued athlete, careful attention needs to be given to blood parameters (anemia), endocrine balance (thyroid, diabetes), renal conditions (renal insufficiency or chronic infection), and other symptoms as necessary. The athlete's medication, drug, and alcohol history must be examined.

A complete diet history may reveal a lack of thiamin, which could cause nausea, severe exhaustion, and loss of appetite; iron deficiency, which would involve oxygen-carrying capacity and motivation to persist in tasks; vitamin B_{12} deficiency; dehydration; or lack of enough calories to cover energy expenditure. Physical and environmental stresses, such as exercising in heat, cold, noise, or confusion, are capable of producing extreme fatigue. For example, body heat is lost about two to four times as fast in cool water as in air of the same temperature. Even with moderate exercise in cold water, the metabolic heat generated is often insufficient to counter the large thermal drain. Repeated days of hard training cause a gradual reduction in muscle glycogen. Unless the athlete consumes large quantities of carbohydrates during training, muscle and liver glycogen reserves will be depleted, leaving the muscle fibers incapable of generating energy.

Unresolved emotional conflicts, anger, anxiety, depression, grief, and lack of sleep may raise the body's caloric needs. High levels of stress, diminished self-worth, helplessness, hopelessness, suicidal tendencies, or a recent loss (or anniversary of a loss) are usually accompanied by a drastic change in diet. Fast foods or foods with a lower nutrient density are often eaten rather than the quality diet that might alleviate some of the underlying disorders.

Therefore, if the athlete does not feel well, the diet should be checked. A rule of thumb is that at least 17 nutritious foods should be consumed every day, and total calories should equal the requirements for basal metabolism, growth, and exercise. The athlete should rest or engage in some form of low-intensity exercise, such as walking. Remember, too, that at the end of the season or the quarter term, there is nothing wrong with a few days of relaxing.

Nicotine

When people start exercising, they usually change lifestyles.[28, 29] A few athletes still smoke, but this is rare, because smoking is associated with a decrease in maximum Vo_2. Nicotine is considered a toxic drug. It constricts the terminal bronchioles of the lungs, causes swelling of the epithelial lining, and decreases fluid secretion in the bronchial tree. Nicotine paralyzes the cilia on the surfaces of the respiratory epithelial cells, which normally remove excess fluids and foreign particles.

Tobacco can be smoked, chewed, or placed between the lip and gum. Nicotine in smoke passes across the alveolar membrane into circulation, where it acts as a mild stimulant to the central nervous system. It increases attention span but also relaxes skeletal muscles. A former smoker may gain weight abruptly with the decrease in basal metabolic rate. Nicotine is a vasoconstrictor and will elevate blood pressure. The contact of tobacco with the oral mucosa will damage gums (baseball players frequently have lesions on the inside of their mouths) and is associated with cancer of the mouth. Even the most moderate exerciser will feel the respiratory strain during exercise if he or she continues to smoke.

REFERENCES

1. Guyton AC: *Human Physiology and Mechanisms of Disease*, ed 4. Philadelphia, WB Saunders Co, 1987.
2. Bergstrom J, Hermansen L, Hultman E, et al: Diet, muscle glycogen and physical performance. *Acta Physiol Scand* 1967; 71:140.
3. Hermansen L, Hultman E, Saltin B: Muscle glycogen during prolonged severe exercise. *Acta Physiol Scand* 1967; 71:129.
4. Costill DL, Gollnick PD, Jansson ED, et al: Glycogen depletion patterns in muscle fibers during distance running. *Acta Physiol Scand* 1973; 89:374.
5. Hagerman F: Personal communication, 1987.
6. Fox EL: *Sports Physiology*. Philadelphia, CBS College Publishing, 1984.
7. McArdle WD, Katch FI, Katch VL: *Exercise Physiology*. Philadelphia, Lea & Febiger, 1986.
8. Sharkey BJ: *Physiology of Fitness*. Champaign, Ill, Human Kinetics Publishers, 1984.
9. Saltin B, Blomquist G, Mitchell JH, et al: Fiber types and metabolis potentials of skeletal muscles in sedentary men and endur-

ance in runners, *The Marathon*. New York, New York Academy of Sciences, 1977.

10. Costill DL, Jansson E, Gollnick PD, et al: Glycogen utilization in leg muscles of men during level and uphill running. *Acta Physiol Scand* 1974; 91:475.

11. Maughan RJ: Metabolic and circulatory responses to the ingestion of glucose polymer and glucose/electrolyte solutions during exercise in man. *Eur J Appl Physiol* 1987; 56:356.

12. Langenfeld MD: Glucose polymer ingestion during ultraendurance bicycling. *Res Q* 1983; 54:411.

13. Ivy JL, Miller W, Dover V, et al: Endurance improved by ingestion of a glucose polymer supplement. *Med Sci Sports* 1983; 15:466.

14. Gollnick PD, Piehl K, Saubert CW, et al: Diet, exercise and glycogen changes in human muscle fibers. *J Appl Physiol* 1972; 33:421.

15. Piehl K, Adolfsson S, Nazar K: Glycogen storage and glycogen synthetase activity in trained and untrained muscles of man. *Acta Physiol Scand* 1974; 90:779.

16. Krause M, Mahan LK: *Food, Nutrition and Diet Therapy*. Philadelphia, WB Saunders Co, 1984.

17. Costill DL, Miller JM: Nutrition for endurance sport: Carbohydrate and fluid balance. *Int J Sports Med* 1980; 1:2.

18. Piehl K: Time course for refilling glycogen stores in human muscle fibers following induced glycogen depletion. *ACTA Physiol Scand* 1974; 90:297–302.

19. Hamilton EM, Whitney EN: *Nutrition*, ed 2. St Paul, Minn, West Publishing Co, 1982.

20. Pritikin N: *The Pritikin Promise*. New York, Simon & Schuster, 1983.

21. Sheehan G: Moderate drinking OK. *Phys Sports Med* 1985; 13:42.

22. American College of Sports Medicine: *The Use of Alcohol in Sports*. Indianapolis, Indiana, American College of Sports Medicine, 1980.

23. To drink or not to drink? *Tufts Newslett* 3:86.

24. Gledhill N: Blood doping and related issues: a brief review. *Med Sci Sports Exerc* 1982; 14:183.

25. Slavin JL: Caffeine and sports performance. *Phys Sports Med* 1985; 13:191.

26. Hargreaves M, Costill DL, Coggan A, et al: Effect of carbohydrate feedings on muscle glycogen utilization and exercise performance. *Med Sci Sports Exerc* 1984; 16:219.

27. Anonymous: Overtraining: Physiological and psychological effects of training overload. American College of Sports Medicine, Symposium, Las Vegas, Nevada, May 1987.
28. Sheehan G: Running and smoking don't mix. *Phys Sports Med* 1986; 14:69.
29. Renaud AM, Cormier Y: Acute effects of marihuana smoking on maximal exercise performance. *Med Sci Sports Exerc* 1986; 18:685.

3

Conditions Affecting Performance

THE CHILD ATHLETE

More and more children and adolescents are becoming involved in athletic training and competition. Female gymnasts and ballet dancers begin lessons at 3 to 4 years of age and become serious performers by the time they are 8 or 9. There have been baseball and basketball leagues for the 6-year-old for a long time, and now there are soccer leagues as well.[1]

Although athletics is usually viewed as good, healthy fun and as motivation and discipline for improved nutrition, there are concerns regarding young athletes. These concerns go beyond the most obvious—that some coaches are not well trained to work with the immature, that injuries occurring at this time can be devastating, and that equipment often does not fit properly. Psychological traumas as well as nutritional dilemmas also need to be dealt with.[2]

It is socially acceptable to be a child athlete. More than 20 million children and adolescents participate at some level in organized athletic activities. The questions raised today, however, are much different than those of a generation ago. Now, often the parent asks: "Can my daughter play on the boys' football team? Will dieting to lose weight harm my 9-year-old? Will my babysitter agree to drive the carpool? What type of breakfast should I feed my little athlete? Will snacks be beneficial? Will fluids be available at the playing field?"

Children should be given the opportunity to train and compete in a variety of sports, but it is best to accept the fact that children are not miniature adults and start with a preparticipation evaluation.

A physical examination is not legally required by most school organizations until a child becomes a member of a team. Some states currently require only one physical examination per athlete per high school career (an injury requires permission before a student can return to further team participation). Reasons given for this apparent laxity are to reduce family expense and to avoid possible exclusion of low-income students from sports. Wrestlers, however, must be certified annually for maximum allowable weight reduction. The biggest objection to the present practice is that many athletes do not receive any sort of annual physical examination. Healthy adolescents rarely have reason to be examined for illness and are likely to forego preseason examinations if they are not required. Another consideration is that youth is a time of rapid physical growth and vast psychological changes that can have implications for sports participation.

It is always unfortunate to discover a problem in midseason that might have been detected earlier. Findings frequently include a multitude of musculoskeletal disorders. Medical problems have also included hypertension, diabetes, amenorrhea, ulcers, infections, and so forth. But immunizations, allergies, and emergency information should be reviewed often. If any child is playing for more than just fun, an examination that includes a major health evaluation, developmental profiling, and injury screening is recommended. A nutritional assessment should be built into it as well. Such questions as the following need to be addressed[3]:

1. Will the child need to change weight to improve performance or to make the team?
2. How often does he or she practice and for how long?

3. Does the player eat anything before practice?
4. Is he or she drinking anything during practice?
5. How much weight does the child lose during practice?
6. Is he or she taking any medications or supplements (what and why)?

One assumes that these are common sense questions to ask any athlete, but consider what reality is for a 6-year-old.

The American Academy of Pediatrics, the American College of Sports Medicine, and the American Osteopathic Academy of Sports Medicine[4] offer guidelines on conducting health evaluations and suggest criteria to use when counseling athletes and their parents on participation in specific sports. Recommendations are for general age-appropriate evaluations that are divided into sections that will provide data for either selection or elimination of an individual from a sport. Other aspects of examinations should include growth analysis, sexual and physical maturation, cardiopulmonary examination, biochemical evaluation, flexibility and strength estimates, body composition, and nutritional advice.

Body composition is difficult to measure because children are not chemically mature. Adult-identified nomograms or formulas are not appropriate. Heights and weights within acceptable ranges or the triceps skinfold thickness assessment from the National Center for Health Statistics (which gives mean and standard deviations) are more suitable (Tables 3–1 and 3–2).

Weight monitoring and caloric intake stabilization are recommended for children who need to change weight. Individual needs and circumstances must be addressed, and identifiable cases of pathogenic food behavior should be referred to a specialist.

Caloric Support.—Young children need about 36 to 40 calories/lb/day (see Appendix C). Because children use more energy at all levels of activity than adults, it is very important to monitor weight during the athletic season. A young athlete is likely to compete in more than one sport at the same time (e.g., soccer at

TABLE 3–1.

Triceps Skinfold Thickness: Youth, 1–17 Years, United States, 1971–1974*

Triceps Skinfold (mm) — Males

Race and Age (yr)	No. in Sample	Estimated Population in Thousands	Mean	Standard Deviation	Percentile								
					5th	10th	15th	25th	50th	75th	85th	90th	95th
White													
1	211	1,402	10.7	3.0	7.0	7.0	7.5	8.0	10.0	12.0	14.0	15.0	16.5
2	217	1,461	9.9	2.6	6.0	6.5	7.0	8.0	10.0	12.0	12.5	13.0	14.7
3	226	1,536	9.9	2.6	6.5	7.0	7.0	8.0	10.0	11.0	12.5	13.5	14.5
4	229	1,547	9.6	2.4	6.0	7.0	7.0	8.0	10.0	11.0	12.0	12.5	14.0
5	207	1,319	9.8	3.2	6.0	6.5	7.0	7.5	9.0	11.0	12.5	13.5	15.0
6	126	1,343	8.9	3.1	5.5	5.6	6.0	7.0	9.0	10.0	12.0	12.5	14.0
7	125	1,718	9.1	3.5	5.0	5.5	6.0	7.0	8.0	10.5	12.0	13.5	17.0
8	116	1,644	9.1	3.3	5.0	5.5	6.0	7.0	8.5	10.5	12.0	13.0	16.0
9	117	1,636	11.1	4.8	5.5	6.5	6.5	7.5	10.0	14.0	17.0	17.0	19.0
10	148	1,909	11.1	4.2	5.5	6.0	7.0	8.0	10.0	14.0	15.5	17.0	19.5
11	132	1,823	12.5	6.5	6.0	6.0	7.0	8.0	10.0	15.0	19.0	20.5	24.5
12	152	1,970	12.4	6.1	6.0	6.0	7.0	8.5	11.0	14.0	18.0	21.0	27.0
13	129	1,697	11.7	6.7	5.0	6.0	6.0	7.0	10.0	14.0	19.0	22.0	25.5
14	134	1,730	10.9	6.4	4.0	5.0	6.0	7.0	9.0	13.0	18.0	20.0	24.0
15	124	1,728	10.2	6.1	4.0	5.0	6.0	6.0	8.0	12.0	15.0	19.0	24.0
16	128	1,752	10.1	5.2	4.0	5.0	5.0	6.5	9.0	12.5	15.0	17.0	22.0
17	139	1,831	9.3	5.4	4.5	5.0	5.5	6.0	7.5	11.0	13.0	15.0	19.0
Black													
1	72	280	9.4	3.4	4.5	6.0	7.0	8.0	8.0	11.0	12.0	13.0	15.0
2	77	267	10.1	3.2	4.5	6.0	6.5	8.0	10.0	12.0	14.0	15.0	15.0
3	72	212	9.1	2.6	6.0	6.5	6.5	7.0	9.0	10.5	12.0	12.0	13.0
4	74	260	8.0	2.6	5.0	5.0	5.0	6.5	7.0	9.0	10.0	10.5	15.0
5	64	226	7.7	3.4	4.5	5.0	5.0	5.0	7.0	9.0	10.0	12.0	15.5

Females (continued)

Age	n	N	Mean	SD									
6	52	321	7.1	1.8	4.0	4.0	5.0	6.0	7.0	8.0	9.0	9.0	9.0
7	38	253	7.5	3.2	4.0	4.0	4.0	5.0	6.5	9.0	11.5	13.0	15.0
8	33	203	7.8	3.4	4.0	5.0	5.0	6.0	6.5	10.0	11.0	11.0	12.5
9	52	383	8.2	3.9	3.5	4.0	4.5	6.0	7.0	8.0	12.0	13.0	18.0
10	33	251	9.1	5.3	5.0	5.0	6.0	6.0	7.5	8.5	13.0	15.0	20.0
11	43	313	8.0	5.0	4.0	4.0	5.0	6.0	6.0	10.7	11.0	12.0	15.0
12	47	316	9.4	7.0	4.0	4.0	4.5	6.0	7.5	8.5	11.0	15.0	24.0
13	45	281	8.2	4.4	4.0	5.0	5.0	5.0	7.0	7.0	11.0	19.0	19.0
14	39	282	6.6	2.6	3.5	3.5	3.5	5.0	6.5	9.0	8.0	9.0	12.0
15	43	310	8.9	6.1	4.0	4.5	5.0	5.0	6.5	7.5	10.0	21.0	21.0
16	41	267	7.2	4.8	4.0	4.0	4.0	5.0	6.0	10.5	8.0	11.0	15.0
17	35	235	8.7	5.8	3.5	3.5	5.0	5.0	7.0		12.0	12.0	23.2

White

Age	n	N	Mean	SD									
1	189	1,328	10.2	2.8	6.0	7.0	7.0	8.0	10.0	12.0	13.0	13.5	15.5
2	203	1,434	10.6	2.6	7.0	7.5	8.0	9.0	10.0	12.0	13.5	14.0	15.0
3	211	1,438	11.1	2.6	7.0	8.0	8.5	9.0	11.0	13.0	13.5	14.0	15.0
4	204	1,339	10.8	2.6	7.5	8.0	8.0	9.0	10.5	12.0	13.0	14.5	16.0
5	224	1,416	10.7	3.7	6.0	7.0	8.0	8.5	10.0	12.0	13.0	15.0	17.5
6	125	1,445	10.6	3.3	6.5	7.0	7.5	8.0	10.5	12.0	13.0	14.0	16.0
7	122	1,507	10.9	4.2	4.0	6.0	7.0	8.0	11.0	15.0	15.0	15.5	17.5
8	117	1,507	12.4	4.7	7.0	8.0	8.0	9.0	11.5	16.0	16.5	18.0	22.0
9	129	1,751	13.6	4.6	7.5	8.0	9.0	10.0	13.0	15.5	18.0	20.0	22.0
10	148	1,855	13.4	4.8	7.5	8.0	8.5	10.0	12.5	17.5	19.0	20.0	23.0
11	122	1,569	14.9	6.1	8.0	8.5	9.0	10.0	13.0	18.5	20.5	24.5	28.5
12	128	1,506	15.2	5.6	8.0	9.0	10.0	11.0	14.0	20.0	20.0	23.0	26.0
13	153	1,886	16.2	6.8	7.0	8.0	10.0	11.5	15.0	21.0	24.0	25.0	28.5
14	132	1,731	17.8	7.3	9.0	9.5	10.5	13.0	16.7	21.0	24.0	28.5	33.0
15	125	1,752	17.7	6.7	9.0	10.5	11.0	13.0	17.0	21.0	24.0	25.0	28.5
16	141	1,933	18.2	6.6	10.0	10.5	12.5	14.0	17.0	24.0	24.0	26.0	32.1
17	117	1,549	19.8	8.0	10.0	12.0	12.5	13.5	19.0		26.5	29.5	35.0

Continued.

TABLE 3-1. (cont.)

Triceps Skinfold Thickness: Youth, 1–17 Years, United States, 1971–1974*

Race and Age (yr)	No. in Sample	Estimated Population in Thousands	Mean	Standard Deviation	Percentile								
					5th	10th	15th	25th	50th	75th	85th	90th	95th
Black													
1	73	257	10.0	3.0	5.5	5.5	7.0	8.0	10.0	12.0	13.0	14.0	15.0
2	66	261	10.0	2.3	7.0	8.0	8.0	8.0	10.0	11.0	12.0	14.0	15.5
3	78	245	9.7	2.9	6.0	7.0	7.0	8.0	10.0	11.0	12.0	13.0	14.0
4	73	246	8.8	2.7	5.0	6.0	7.0	7.0	8.0	10.5	12.0	13.0	14.0
5	88	265	9.4	3.9	5.0	5.0	6.5	7.0	8.0	10.0	12.0	13.5	17.0
6	50	336	9.0	3.1	5.5	6.0	6.0	8.0	8.0	10.0	11.5	12.0	13.0
7	46	241	10.1	4.0	5.0	6.0	7.0	7.5	9.0	11.0	17.5	18.0	18.0
8	35	293	11.5	5.1	5.0	6.5	7.0	8.0	10.0	13.5	18.0	18.0	23.0
9	41	247	10.2	5.1	5.5	6.0	6.0	6.5	8.0	12.0	18.0	18.0	20.0
10	48	303	11.7	5.6	6.5	6.5	7.0	7.5	10.0	16.0	18.0	19.0	24.0
11	42	315	12.7	6.4	4.0	5.0	6.5	7.5	10.0	18.0	22.0	23.0	23.0
12	47	284	13.6	7.6	5.5	6.0	6.0	7.5	12.0	17.0	22.0	25.0	30.0
13	44	287	16.1	7.0	7.0	8.5	10.0	11.0	14.0	18.0	24.0	24.0	33.5
14	50	265	15.9	6.7	8.0	8.0	9.0	10.5	14.0	20.5	24.0	24.5	24.5
15	46	411	14.0	7.6	6.5	6.5	8.0	10.0	12.5	16.0	16.5	20.0	32.8
16	33	203	18.9	8.0	8.0	8.0	10.0	12.0	19.0	24.0	24.5	33.0	33.1
17	39	239	16.9	6.6	7.5	9.0	11.0	12.0	14.5	20.0	24.0	28.0	31.0

*From the National Center for Health Statistics, Department of Health and Human Services: *Health and Nutrition Examination Survey I, 1971–1974.* Washington, DC, US Government Printing Office, 1974.

TABLE 3–2.
Triceps Skinfold Thickness: Adults, United States, 1971–1974*

Race and Age (yr)	No. in Sample	Estimated Population in Thousands	Mean	Standard Deviation	Percentile									
					5th	10th	15th	25th	50th	75th	85th	90th	95th
Triceps Skinfold (mm)														
Males														
White	4,344	54,694	12.2	5.8	5.0	6.0	6.5	8.0	11.0	15.0	18.0	20.0	23.0
18–19	203	3,206	11.3	5.9	5.0	5.5	6.0	7.0	9.0	15.0	18.0	20.0	23.0
20–24	423	7,094	11.5	6.0	4.0	5.0	6.0	7.0	10.0	15.0	18.0	21.0	23.0
25–34	672	11,594	12.7	6.2	5.0	6.0	6.5	8.0	12.0	16.0	18.5	21.0	24.0
35–44	569	9,516	12.6	5.4	5.0	6.0	7.0	9.0	12.0	15.5	17.5	20.0	23.0
45–54	628	10,039	12.6	5.9	5.5	6.5	7.0	8.5	11.0	15.0	18.0	20.0	26.0
55–64	505	8,275	11.7	5.0	5.0	6.0	7.0	8.0	11.0	14.0	16.5	18.0	21.0
65–74	1,344	4,970	12.0	5.4	5.0	6.0	7.0	8.0	11.0	15.0	17.0	19.0	22.0
Black	847	5,753	10.6	7.0	3.5	4.0	4.5	6.0	8.5	13.0	16.0	20.0	23.0
18–19	52	404	8.9	6.7	2.0	4.0	5.0	5.1	7.0	8.0	12.0	21.0	24.0
20–24	80	866	10.0	7.9	3.0	4.0	4.0	6.0	8.0	11.0	13.0	18.0	24.0
25–34	119	1,232	11.8	8.4	4.0	4.0	4.0	5.0	10.0	15.0	20.0	22.0	23.0
35–44	87	1,005	11.3	6.5	4.0	4.5	5.0	7.0	10.0	14.0	17.0	18.4	22.0
45–54	130	1,057	10.0	5.1	4.0	4.0	5.0	6.0	10.0	12.5	14.0	16.0	20.0
55–64	85	703	10.7	7.2	3.0	4.0	4.5	5.0	8.0	14.0	20.0	22.0	26.0
65–74	294	486	9.7	5.4	4.0	4.5	5.0	6.0	9.0	12.0	14.0	15.0	19.5

Continued.

TABLE 3-2. (cont.)

Triceps Skinfold Thickness: Adults, United States, 1971–1974*

Race and Age (yr)	No. in Sample	Estimated Population in Thousands	Mean	Standard Deviation	Percentile								
					5th	10th	15th	25th	50th	75th	85th	90th	95th
Females													
White													
	6,757	59,923	22.9	8.1	11.0	13.0	14.5	17.0	22.0	28.0	31.0	34.0	37.0
18–19	208	3,159	18.9	6.6	9.5	12.0	13.0	14.5	18.0	22.5	24.0	26.5	33.5
20–24	956	7,972	19.8	7.7	10.0	11.0	12.0	14.0	19.0	24.0	27.9	30.5	34.0
25–34	1,539	12,161	21.8	8.0	11.0	12.5	14.0	16.0	20.5	26.0	30.0	33.0	36.5
35–44	1,302	10,111	23.7	8.3	12.0	14.0	15.9	18.0	22.5	29.0	32.0	35.1	38.5
45–54	705	10,879	25.3	8.1	13.0	15.0	17.0	20.0	25.0	30.0	33.5	35.5	39.5
55–64	551	9,037	24.6	7.9	11.5	14.5	16.0	19.0	24.0	30.0	33.0	34.1	38.0
65–74	1,496	6,603	23.3	7.3	12.0	14.0	16.0	18.0	23.0	28.0	31.0	33.0	35.5
Black													
	1,557	7,302	23.7	10.3	9.0	11.0	12.0	15.5	23.0	30.5	34.0	36.6	41.0
18–19	70	504	16.2	7.3	8.0	9.0	9.0	11.5	14.0	20.0	25.0	29.0	32.0
20–24	259	1,073	19.3	8.7	9.0	10.0	11.5	12.5	17.0	24.5	28.6	32.0	36.0
25–34	335	1,646	22.5	9.6	8.5	10.0	12.0	14.0	22.0	30.0	32.6	34.1	40.0
35–44	334	1,318	25.8	9.2	11.5	13.0	16.0	20.0	25.5	32.0	35.0	36.5	41.0
45–54	126	1,237	26.8	9.8	12.0	14.0	17.0	20.0	26.0	34.0	37.1	40.0	42.2
55–64	115	871	28.2	12.9	10.0	11.0	13.0	19.0	28.0	34.0	40.0	45.0	51.5
65–74	318	652	23.8	9.0	7.5	11.5	15.0	17.5	24.0	30.0	32.2	35.5	40.0

*From the National Center for Health Statistics, Department of Health and Human Services: *Health and Nutrition Examination Survey I, 1971–1974.* Washington, DC, US Government Printing Office, 1974.

school and tennis on weekends) and often will participate each season, all year long, until self-selection occurs.

The important questions facing parents with children who are athletes is (1) *how much* to feed them (ideal body weight × 36–40 cal/day + 1.5 − 2 × the specific activity factor; see Appendix B), (2) *when* to feed them (breakfast, school or sack lunch, snack every 1.5 hours, dinner, and bedtime snack), and (3) *how* to fit feedings around hectic practice schedules.

A commonly used estimate of energy expenditure for children (reference child weighs 100 lb) is the following:

1. *Low-energy output:* Baseball, cycling (up to 9 miles/hour), bowling, light calisthenics, moderate football, gymnastics, horseback riding (sitting to trot), table tennis, tennis doubles, and walking; uses less than 4 kcal/minute, or 240 kcal/hour.

2. *Moderate-energy output:* Basketball, cycling (10–13 miles/hour), touch football, hiking with pack (3 miles/hour), ice hockey, horseback riding (posting and gallop), mountain climbing, roller skating, running more than 12 minutes/mile, and ice skating (9 miles/hour); uses 4 to 7 kcal/minute, or 330 kcal/hour.

3. *High-energy output:* Cycling (more than 14 miles/hour), vigorous calisthenics (e.g., in some aerobic dance), judo, karate, and running activities (less than 6 miles/hour); uses more than 7 kcal/minute, or 420 kcal/hour.[5]

One busy family with three boys (ages 10, 11, and 13 years) on three different soccer teams and one daughter (age 7 years) in dance made the following arrangements. The mother was responsible for breakfast and dinner. All of the children made double lunches the evening before school, were taught to make pasta with various sauces, and kept snack stashes in their lockers at school. The day's nutrition included a substantial breakfast; frequent trips to lockers for snacks, one lunch eaten at the regular time, and usually a half lunch eaten before practice or dance. One boy was able to come home before practice. The remainder of the lunches was eaten on the way home, and dinner was ready just barely in time to ward off starvation. Another sandwich or a milkshake accompanied homework.

Although this diet seems to contain a great deal of food, the importance of good nutrition became very apparent when one boy missed his carpool one day, took the bus home, and arrived hot, thirsty, and dizzy. After that, chocolate flavored Ensure Plus, along with canned juice or Diet 7Up was kept in the children's gear bags, healthful snacks that also solved the food safety question. Concern about the pre-event meal was solved by one of the youngsters. He became the pasta chef of the neighborhood.

Fluid Needs.—The bodies of young children and adolescents are inefficient in thermoregulation.[6, 7] Their skin surface areas are much greater in comparison with body weight than those of adults. They also produce less perspiration than adults and take longer to acclimatize. Most heat injury problems that occur in children are the result of the oversight of the adults in charge of an activity. Special supervision is necessary at the beginning of and during the season; fluids at the field or gym are a must; and frequent breaks between practice bouts are advisable. Children should be fully hydrated before each physical session and allowed to drink every 15 minutes of practice.

Several members of a youth football team were hospital bound after this scenario. The summer had been extremely warm, and the boys had experienced more air conditioning than usual. Everyone wore new, full gear during early practice sessions. The water faucet was close to the gym but not to the playing field, and no attempt was made by the coach to restrain the excitement, intensity, and duration of exercise.

Iron and Calcium.—Small children have special iron needs.[8] Young athletes need to be screened for anemia in each preseason examination. The iron necessary to allow efficient oxygen transport can be supplied by iron-fortified cereals and grains, heme-iron foods such as red meats and oysters, and in supplement form (10 mg/day). Milk and water intake have been decreasing due to the popularity of diet sodas. Ice cream, cheeses, yogurts, and puddings are favorite calcium-rich foods of youngsters, and they should be encouraged to eat four servings/day.

Carbohydrate.—Often, by the end of the week, a young athlete will complain of being too tired to play. Increasing high-carbohydrate foods may solve this fatigue. Smaller, growing muscles cannot store glycogen as efficiently as the larger, stronger muscles of older athletes. Carbohydrate foods take a lot of time to chew and are often abandoned in favor of juice, pop, or milk. Therefore, ensuring that breakfast includes cereals, breads, and fruits and that lunch contains pasta, vegetables, or a hearty chili or soup will help satisfy carbohydrate need. Potatoes or rice, fruit salad, and an oatmeal cookie or two will add more carbohydrate at dinner time.

Weight Monitoring.—There is growing opinion that exact weight should not be an issue in athletics until after fast growth has ceased. Until there is more information, common sense (often not available in large quantities in younger athletes) needs to be the rule. A gradual weight gain or loss of 1 to 2 lb/week or month, combined with a supervised aerobic exercise program, is effective for the desired change. An athlete should never be informed that he or she needs to make a weight change without adequate follow-up. Young people do not have the necessary judgment to monitor weight changes; incidental anorexia or bulimia may result.

Muscle Mass.—Attempts to increase muscle mass are usually successful if athletes are scheduled into a well-supervised program of weight training combined with an increased intake of 500 to 1,000 kcal/day over basal plus growth plus activity calories, which may be as much as 5,000 to 7,500 kcal/day! For safety, it must first be determined if the youth has arrived at a level of maturation at which larger and stronger muscles can respond to increased work. Guidelines for adolescent weight training include the use of only well-maintained equipment, adequate instruction and supervision, and a program that includes an overall aerobic fitness regimen. Sessions should be preceded by easy warm-ups and stretching and followed by a cool-down period using the full range of joint motion. Maximum lifts are prohibited. Training is recommended two to three times/week for 20- to 30-minute periods (see Appendix D).

Conclusion

The message that should be understood well by the physician, the coach, and the trainer is to give nutrition and proper eating the appropriate priority in the training program. The goals of competition by children and adolescents should be fun, enjoyment, and healthy self-images. "Winning is everything" pressure has no place at this age.

THE YOUNG ADULT

For the well-nourished young adult, exercise sessions do not require additional nutrients except when he or she is exercising in hot weather (more fluids) or is in long-duration training (more calories and carbohydrate).

As work and family become more important, actual time spent in athletic activities decreases for most adults. In these circumstances, healthful eating patterns with attention to special needs will suffice. With habitual training or in those work levels that induce a training effect (i.e., high mileage and intense exercise modes), B complex vitamins; minerals (iron, zinc, magnesium, and calcium); electrolytes; and specific ratios of carbohydrate, protein, and fat need to be addressed (see Chapter 5).

During a recent observation, a group of single, employed, female athletes training for distance or triathlon events had difficulty managing caloric intake and quality of diet.[9] All of the women trained 6 days/week, with an average range of increased expenditure of 500 to 1,000 kcal/day. Initial screening revealed that all received less than 40% of their calories from carbohydrate and that their iron and calcium intakes were low. Each athlete responded well to counseling and later reported consuming more food portions from the carbohydrate and mineral sources listed on a food frequency questionnaire.

It is fairly common for athletes to concentrate so hard on training that they forget about food. For example, caloric intakes appear to be low for women running 10 or more miles/day, although they are usually above the recommended dietary allowances (RDAs) for sedentary women.

THE WHEELCHAIR ATHLETE

Training for athletic competition requires vigorous exercise. Generally recognized benefits are maintenance of weight, decreased risk of cardiovascular disease, and lower levels of tension and stress. Other advantages are the lowering of body fat due to increased caloric demands and possible improvement in glucose tolerance. Increased muscle activity improves calcium metabolism. These benefits are also available to handicapped athletes and provide a decrease in some of the problems peculiar to wheelchair dependence, such as pressure sores, as well.

The level of previous injury or the individual's disorder influences the participation of these athletes, which, in turn, influences their cardiovascular respiratory responses to changes. Other considerations are possible decreased vital capacity, lower stroke volume, and reduced maximal heart rate. Venous return is lessened because of loss of muscle and muscle tone in the legs. However, maximum oxygen utilization does improve with arm exercises alone.

Wheelchair athletes are just as likely as runners to become dehydrated. Interference with normal temperature mechanisms is usual in an individual with a spinal cord injury in which autonomic or cardiac output mechanisms are compromised. Venous return also tends to be hampered. Because their ability to shiver is limited, wheelchair marathoners may also be extremely vulnerable to lower temperatures.[10]

AMENORRHEA

The mechanism of amenorrhea is unclear but seems to involve primarily the hypothalamus. With heavy physical exercise, particularly in an athlete whose body weight is low, the hypothalmic rhythm may be altered. The ovaries may be understimulated, leading to reduced secretion of estrogen; then oligomenorrhea or amenorrhea results. These disturbances cannot be automatically attributed to exercise, since athletes are as likely as nonathletes to develop conditions in which amenorrhea is a symptom: stress, tumors, weight loss, or thyroid disorders. All other causes must be ruled out before an athlete's amenorrhea can be blamed on her exercise pattern alone.[11, 12] If the patient with secondary menstrual alterations and exercise-related hormonal abnormalities does not want to reduce her exercise or increase her body weight, estrogen and progesterone replacement is required.[13, 14] These substances protect the skeletal mass and the endometrium. She needs to understand that bone structure integrity depends on an adequate estrogen level.

Primary amenorrhea is very common among elite adolescent athletes. When congenital abnormalities, genetic problems, or eating disorders are ruled out, exercise is the most likely cause of delayed menarche. There are concerns that young girls with prolonged hypoestrogenism may jeopardize their bone development. In any case, a 15-year-old world-class runner is not likely to stop training so that her periods can start. However, if a young woman reaches age 18 without experiencing menarche, or if the duration of secondary amenorrhea is longer than 6 months, determination of estrogen status is very important.

PREGNANCY

The normal courses of pregnancy and lactation need not hinder the female athlete, but the duration and intensity of activity will decrease because pregnancy affects work output. Other physiological changes also occur, such as a lower maximum volume of oxygen (maximum VO_2), increased heart rate, and certain inconveniences during activity, such as frequent urination, balance, and flexibility alterations.[15] Furthermore, any consideration of the pregnant athlete's response to exercise must also take into account its influence on the fetus.

Though there are inconsistencies in the guidelines for maternal athletic activities, there is a general rule: nothing new and nothing excessive. Activities with a risk of trauma (skin diving, bicycle racing, mountain climbing, hang gliding, etc.) should be avoided; exercise performed in the supine position should be very limited after the first 4 or 5 months of pregnancy. Women who are not in top athletic condition should limit their activities to walking and exercises that strengthen the back and abdomen. Workouts should be restricted to 30 minutes. Although these recommendations are conservative, most women athletes report physical limitations while exercising during pregnancy, which tend to keep their caloric usage close to that advised for all pregnant women.

Pregnancy and lactation exert the greatest effects on nutrient needs. As shown in the RDA chart, increased nutritional needs go straight across the board. Obvious increased needs are for protein, iron, calcium, and folic acid. The added daily energy costs of pregnancy are about 300 kcal after the first trimester.

Counselors need to consider the patient's current pregnant weight when estimating energy expenditure for a particular kind of exercise (Table 3–3). As pregnancy progresses, more calories are required to perform the same activities. During nutritional counseling of a pregnant teenaged athlete, emphasis must be placed on the dietary energy intake because of its overall influence on the nutritional status of both mother and child (protein utilization and tissue synthesis). The teenager should consume an additional 300 kcal/day for the last 30 weeks of pregnancy if her weight is appropriate for height at the time of conception. Energy needs are slightly less if she is above average weight for height at this time.[16, 17]

An appropriate weight gain for either exercising or nonexercising pregnant women is approximately 24 to 30 lb. In general, exercising women gain less than nonexercising women, and their newborns' weight is less. Daily energy needs of an exercising woman can be estimated as 2,000 kcal/day (reference woman), plus 300 kcal (cost of pregnancy), plus cost of exercise, or close to 2,800 to 3,000 kcal/day. Heat is generated with exercise and is cumulative; the more exercise, the more heat produced. Elevated maternal temperatures and dehydration are the consequences of exercising, especially in warm climates. A single-

TABLE 3–3.

American College of Obstetricians and Gynecologists Guidelines for Exercise During Pregnancy and Postpartum*

Pregnancy and Postpartum	Pregnancy Only
1. Regular exercise (at least three times weekly) is preferable to intermittent activity. Competitive activities should be discouraged. 2. Vigorous exercise should not be performed in hot, humid weather or during a period of febrile illness. 3. Ballistic movements (jerky, bouncy motions) should be avoided. Exercise should be done on a wooden floor or a tightly carpeted surface to reduce shock and provide a sure footing. 4. Deep flexion or extension of joints should be avoided because of connective tissue laxity. Activities that require jumping, jarring motions, or rapid changes in direction should be avoided because of the instability of the joints. 5. Vigorous exercise should be preceded by a 5-minute period of muscle warm-up. This can be accomplished by slow walking or stationary cycling with low resistance. 6. Vigorous exercise should be followed by a period of gradually declining activity that includes gentle stationary stretching. Because connective tissue laxity increases the risk of joint injury, stretches should not be taken to the point of maximum resistance. 7. Heart rate should be measured at times of peak activity. Target heart rates and limits established in consultation with the physician should not be exceeded. 8. Care should be taken to rise from the floor gradually to avoid orthostatic hypotension. Some form of activity involving the legs should be continued for a brief period of time. 9. Liquids should be taken liberally before and after exercise to prevent dehydration. If necessary, activity should be interrupted to replenish fluids. 10. Women who have led sedentary life-styles should begin with physical activity of very low intensity and advance activity levels very gradually. 11. Activity should be stopped and the physician consulted if any unusual symptoms appear.	1. Maternal heart rate should not exceed 140 beats/minute. 2. Strenuous activities should not exceed 15 minutes in duration. 3. No exercise should be performed in the supine position after the fourth month of gestation has been completed. 4. Exercises that employ the Valsalva's maneuver should be avoided. 5. Calorie intake should be adequate to meet not only the extra energy needs of pregnancy but also of the exercise performed. 6. Maternal core temperature should not exceed 100.4°F.

*From American College of Obstetricians and Gynecologists: *Exercise During Pregnancy and the Postnatal Period* (ACOG Home Exercise Programs). Washington, DC, 1985, p 4. Used by permission.

use, paper thermometer is convenient to monitor changes in body temperature. Pregnant exercising women need to be continuously aware of the importance of hydration while exercising.

LACTATION

Caloric needs of lactation can be estimated by adding the energy needs of lactation (500 kcal/day) to the energy needs of basal metabolism and exercise. The minimal intake for full lactation support is in the range of 2,000 to 2,200 kcal/day. There is usually an overwhelming desire to lose weight and get back into shape quickly after childbirth. In addition, some of the benefits reported by exercising pregnant women include better control of weight and less postpartum depression. Lactation presents the major nutritional assault to the body.[18] Not only does the mother need extra calories and protein to produce milk, but the diet needs to be one that supplies more of every nutrient except vitamin D.

About 900 kcal of energy are required for the production of 1 quart (32 oz) of milk. During pregnancy, most women store approximately 5 to 8 lb of body fat, which can be mobilized to supply a portion of this energy. The remainder must be supplied daily from the diet. If lactation continues beyond the initial 3 months, or if maternal weight falls below ideal weight for height, extra energy must be supplied for nursing to be effective. This is not the time to be on a weight loss diet!

General recommendations for the exercising nursing mother include:

1. Cover energy needs for lactation, exercise, and ideal body weight. A calorically reduced diet is not recommended unless weight is more than 10% of ideal body weight for height. (Extra nutritional requirements [see Appendix C] can be covered by adding an extra cup (8 oz) of milk, another serving from the bread and cereal group, one extra meat serving, and one more fruit serving than is recommended for pregnancy.) The level of water- and fat-soluble

vitamins in human milk generally reflects maternal intake. Avoid alcohol; limit caffeine intake to less than two cups (16 oz) of coffee/day.

2. Drink at least 2 quarts (64 oz) of fluids daily. Increased intake does not affect human milk volume (as does inadequate caloric intake), but fluid and temperature regulation are still major concerns for any exercising female.

3. Continue taking a prenatal vitamin supplement for several weeks after delivery. Maternal iron supplementation may be required to replenish stores lost during pregnancy and parturition. This does not change the iron concentration of breast milk. (Be aware that some "mom" athletes have been described as "chronically undernourished.")

4. Nurse or express milk before exercising. Activity often encourages the letdown response. Change bra after exercising and allow nipples to dry before replacing the flaps of a nursing bra.

Very few superwomen athletes can live up to their reputation after the baby arrives. The first few weeks are relatively easy compared with the mother's return to full-time employment. Then she must juggle job, baby, husband, household, and her own personal needs. Too often she becomes exhausted, nervous, and overscheduled. Exercise should take place at the same time each day. Having the babysitter come early and stay until after cool-down exercises, shower, and dinner preparation would be one way to accomplish that.

Wise heads say, "Save your strength for yourself and for enjoying your baby. You have lots of time to regain your former endurance and conditioning status. Your child will be your responsibility for many years, and there will always be another big race next year."

THE OLDER ATHLETE

There is really no definition of an older athlete. George Sheehan said, "We're not doing this because we're older, we're doing this because it's fun!" However, even Peter Pan had to grow up, and as we age, we change. Muscle mass decreases along with physical working capacity; gut absorption decreases, and there is a high incidence of poor food choices, which may or may not be related to decreased taste sensitivity. Dehydration, weight loss, osteoporosis, general vigor, and flatulence are common notations on the physician's chart. Regardless of all of these, there are still lots of older folks running around out there. Ivor Welch, age 86, finished a marathon in 5 hours, 40 minutes; Ed Benham, age 76, finished in 3 hours, 34 minutes. Clinical evidence points out that there is not only an increased sense of well-being when activity levels remain high but such physical factors as glucose tolerance and muscles respond well to work.

Considerations in diet planning include:

1. Yearly physical examinations to screen for such major disorders as heart disease, stroke, and cancer.

2. A general range of appropriate body weights for activity levels.

3. Definite guidelines for training. Most older athletes are able to increase their aerobic capabilities but, without proper supervision, have problems in increasing muscle strength and flexibility.

4. Monitoring of caloric content and quality of the diet. (Increased activity allows for extra calories and, hopefully, a better quality diet.) Decreased caloric intake is usually recommended for older persons in adjustment to age-related decreases in physical activity and basal metabolic rate. However, increased calcium intake (1,200–1,500 mg) is always recommended for older women to counter decline in bone mass.

5. Drug-nutrient interactions. These may alter nutritional requirements. For example, diuretics used to treat hypertension may induce potassium depletion. Hypocholesterolemic drugs decrease absorption of fat-soluble vitamins, vitamin B_{12}, and iron. Antimicrobial drugs can decrease absorption of folic acid and vitamin B_{12}. Drugs can also alter nutritional status by impairing appetite or by modifying nutrient metabolism (see Appendix E).

6. Hypothermia. As people age, their temperature regulation is affected by various factors. They are at risk for hypothermia due to defective heat conservation, decreased heat production, and malnutrition and are more susceptible to various diseases that disrupt neuroendocrine function.

7. Normal consequences of aging. Loss of friends and relatives, lower income, decrease of self-esteem, longer time to recover from injuries and surgery, frequent urination and constipation, and lower back problems go hand in hand with aging. On a more positive note, grandmothers are now training for 6-mile (10-km) runs and marathons and, several years ago, a senior came to me for "the latest info on carbohydrate feedings for marathon training." He didn't even mention that he was blind.

As life expectancy continues to rise, and the percentage of elderly in the population grows, there will be an increased need for improving exercise modes and facilities—and for another category in the RDAs! Goals for health care givers should be for optimal physiological function of their patients and postponement of age-related disease. Exercise makes goals more attainable.[19–21]

ENVIRONMENTAL FACTORS

Several years ago, Seattle Pacific University's soccer team, the Falcons, began to prepare for its fourth attempt to be number 1 in NCAA Division 2 soccer league. They had been defeated the year before by Alabama A. & M. University.

The previous year's loss had been a particular grievance to the coach (Cliff McCrath) and the entire team because the game had gone into overtime. The final score was 2 to 1. The game was played in 90° F weather, with a relative humidity of 85%. The day had been hot, and the playing surface was warm to the touch. There was no wind. The team was wearing new lightweight cotton-polyester, long-sleeved uniforms. Fluids were available at the field, but in the excitement of the match, few players drank anything until they became thirsty or developed headaches. The team became more heat exhausted as the December day wore on.

Back in Seattle, the team analyzed the situation by "replaying" all the predisposing factors to prepare for next year's contest. First they identified all team members who had been most affected by the high temperature and humidity. They turned out to be the youngest members; one player who had traveler's diarrhea; those who always complained about heat (wherever they played); those who had trained less or had poorer performances during the season; and those who were dehydrated going into the final game.

Because the site was predetermined, there was nothing that could be done about the location of the next game. It would again be played in the South. The Falcons' season had been played up and down the West Coast in relatively cool, familiar territory all year.

The Falcons decided on the following strategy:

1. The uniforms were replaced by short-sleeved mesh shirts, with socks down and shirts out.

2. Team members began training in the heat, exercising on bicycle ergometers at 50% of maximum V_{O_2} for at least 15 minutes at 90° F in the school sauna and monitoring heart rate and body temperature.

3. Before the big game, Coach McCrath announced at a sports writers' luncheon that if the Falcon team won, he would crawl on his hands and knees all the way from the school to the Space Needle (2.7 miles).

4. The entire team began drinking more water the week before the game and drank fluids on the airplane. The trainer brought juices, fruits, and vegetables to workouts, and extra fluids were consumed before and during the game.

5. Any players who complained of early symptoms of heat problems (headaches, excessive sweating, nausea, or dizziness) were substituted and were treated immediately.

On December 2, 1978, the Falcons again played Alabama A. & M. University. The temperature was 92° F, the humidity was 89%, and the Seattle team won in triple overtime, 1 to 0. And the coach had sore knees, shoulders, and wrists for quite some time.[22, 23]

There have been a myriad of studies examining our adaptation to heat and cold and altitude. There are a few conflicting observations, but the data have produced helpful information. Everyone from hikers on a mountain picnic to elite athletes can prepare for outdoor activities by imagining the worst case situation.

No one plans to become disabled or lost or to place oneself where he or she is unable to cope with sudden changes. This can include instances where a runner has to call for a ride home after a fast run in Hawaiian heat, when hikers fall into mountain streams, or where cyclers see strange objects in the road during bike training at Pike's Peak. The example can also be extended to people driving through winter storms, equipped to stay warm only as long as their car runs. In other words, sports drinks are of no use to the runner if they are left in the refrigerator, and extra clothing left at home is of no value when hypothermia occurs.

High Altitude

Three major factors affect our response to altitude: (1) elevation, (2) speed of ascent, and (3) length of stay. Other critical variables include age, sex, general health, previous experience at high altitudes, and diet and level of hydration.[24]

Recreational skiers, mountain climbers, tourists, or athletes often drive or fly from low to moderately high elevations within a few hours. About one out of three will experience mild to moderate symptoms of nausea, headache, weakness, sleep disturbance, and lethargy. A few become so dehydrated they need medical care. Individuals may also suffer decreased memory, poor performance, and lack of good judgment at higher altitudes.

Careful consideration should be given to each day's food supply. Anyone who exercises at higher elevations needs about 500 to 1,000 extra calories/day (more or less, depending on length of exertion). A recreational skier may need 500 extra calories/day to support exercise needs; a cross-country skier may need more than an extra 1,500 kcal/day. Fluid intake is especially important. Every effort should be made to stay well hydrated. (Restricting alcohol and caffeine will have some benefits but may not be compatible with a skier's idea of vacation pleasures.)

Going higher and working harder may cause *hypoxia*. One of the symptoms of oxygen deficiency is anorexia, along with weight loss and malnutrition. Climbers have lost as much as 25% of their total body weight over a short period of time. Even though ample food is usually available on major expeditions, climbers often fail to eat properly. Fat and carbohydrate absorption are then impaired, and the body burns muscle protein to keep up with glucose demand.

Considerations when planning meals for mountain climbers include:

1. Climbers need 5,000 to 6,000 kcal/day, about 55% from carbohydrates, 30% from fats, and 15% from proteins (the same amount needed by endurance athletes).[25]
2. Foods that are easy to prepare and that provide variety should be planned. High-calorie snack foods should be included. Cooking time doubles for each 5,000-ft increase in elevation; a meal that takes 10 minutes to cook at sea level will take about 40 minutes at 10,000 ft. Everything should be prepackaged and stored by meal, which will keep decision making down to a minimum when everyone is tired and hungry. There should be one stove for each three people and 4 oz of fuel/person/day for cooking. Climbers should eat often; digestion takes longer at high altitudes.
3. Fluid needs should be estimated ahead of time and a daily intake goal set (it may be as high as 5 L/day, or double the consumption at sea level).
4. There are no specific vitamin helpers for climbers, but iron supplementation may be of assistance. The combination of loss of appetite plus inadequate dietary iron intake may precipitate an iron deficiency (affecting oxygen transport and utilization by iron-containing enzymes).

It is helpful to keep a diet history or record of foods preferred (and amounts eaten) to simplify planning for the next trip. Macaroni and cheese is a standby, but all kinds of commercially prepared freeze-dried foods, dried fruits, instant soup mixes, Stove Top dressings, dried potatoes, precooked rice, plain noodles, instant cereals, granola, cereal bars, cookies, bagels, pita bread, pasta dinners, snack crackers, and flavored gelatins can be considered. Check the grocers' shelves for other treats (e.g., individual trail mixes). Remember, too, that if your ski trip is in the Rocky Mountains, you will be hiking to the chair lift at about 6,000 to 10,000 ft.[26–28]

Temperature Control

One of the most powerful regulators of body temperature is behavioral control. When the body's temperature becomes too high or too low, signals from the preoptic area of the brain give the psychic sensation of being overheated or chilled. Then one takes off a shirt or reaches for a coat.

Cold Environments

In extremely cold environments, we adapt by putting on more clothing and spending less time outdoors. But if exposure is unavoidable (or acceptable because of the athletic arena), how does one maintain body temperature? The body has the capability to maintain its temperature by increasing heat production or decreasing heat dissipation. Shivering increases heat production. Heat loss takes place primarily through the skin and depends on the sweating mechanism, vascular activity, and the amount of insulation provided by subcutaneous fat. Individuals can improve their ability to withstand cold by effective vasoconstriction and improved insulation to minimize heat loss, but they can also impair it by drinking alcoholic beverages, causing vasodilatation and a greater loss of heat.[29]

Energy.—Energy expenditure in cold climates is higher than that in temperate ones. Cross-country skiing uses an average of 18/kcal/minute, whereas running at a comparable pace on a track probably uses only 10 to 11 kcal/minute. Even tasks that involve only sitting or standing (usually classified as low expenditure) require higher energy when performed in the cold.

Body Composition.—Whereas climbers on major expeditions often lose body weight and percentage of body fat as well as muscle, persons restricted to camp in cold regions (e.g., Antarctica) usually gain weight and increase their skinfold thickness, which is probably due to restricted activity and increased food intake. Since the complications of frostbite, hypothermia, and other cold injuries (tissue damage or respiratory tract irritations) may demand hospitalization, prevention is extremely important.[30]

Cold Weather Clothing.—The mesh and layering of cloth fibers work to trap air. The thicker the zone of trapped air next to the skin, the greater the insulation. Caps and hats conserve heat; at least 30% to 50% of body heat is lost through the head. Wet clothing loses most of its insulating properties and facilitates heat transfer from the body because water conducts heat faster than air. One of the problems of working strenuously in cold weather is that heat dissipates quickly through clothing. The ideal winter clothing system may be a Gore-Tex outer garment—parka and pants—over several light layers of wool, synthetics, or both.

Warm Environments

The various ways in which heat is lost from the body include radiation, conduction, evaporation, and convection. As long as body temperature is greater than that of the surrounding air, heat is lost by radiation and conduction. When the temperature of the air is greater than that of the skin, the body gains heat from its surroundings. Under these conditions, the body can cool off by evaporation.

When the body becomes heated, large quantities of perspiration are secreted onto the surface of the skin by the sweat glands to provide rapid evaporative cooling. In cold weather, the rate of sweat production is slow; in very warm weather, the rate ranges from 0.7 to 2 L/hour. Although runners attempt hydration before and during an event, it is not unusual for them to lose as much as 5% to 10% of their total body water in a long-distance event such as a marathon.

A factor that limits an athlete's performance is the degree of hydration.[31] Dehydrated persons are unable to tolerate exercise and heat stress and are forced to slow their pace. Heart rate and body temperature begin to rise, plasma volume is lost, and blood flow to the skin and muscles is reduced. These are the circumstances in which athletes collapse, with the usual signs of heat exhaustion. Problems with heat occur more often during hot days with high humidity, when there is little wind, and when there is a radiation effect from playing surfaces. The first hot day of spring usually catches athletes and their trainers off guard.

Heat-susceptible individuals are usually overweight and unfit, dehydrated, unacclimatized to heat, very young, or very old (perhaps those who are taller) or have had a recent illness. Persons with a history of heatstroke or hyperthermia should proceed with caution.

Human perspiration has been described as a *filtrate of plasma* because it contains many of the ions present in the water portion of the blood, such as sodium, potassium, magnesium, calcium, and iron. It is a very hypotonic or dilute version of body fluids. During heavy sweating, the body loses more water than minerals, and the first line of defense is to drink water often during exercise of any kind. Drinking will minimize dehydration, lessen the rise in internal body temperature, and reduce the stress placed on the circulatory system (as little as 4 oz of water may lower core temperature by 1° F).

Many factors affect the rate that water or other fluids are accepted by the stomach, pass into the intestine, and enter the blood:

1. Emptying of the stomach occurs at different rates among individuals. It is usually comfortable to drink 4 to 6

oz at 10- to 15-minute intervals during activity. This amount will empty easily into the intestine.

2. Cool drinks leave the stomach more rapidly than warm fluids. Liquids in the range of 38° F to 40° F are appropriate and will not cause stomach cramps.

3. Concentration of the liquid, or *osmolality,* is a consideration in emptying. More concentrated fluids will leave the stomach slowly (sports drinks or juices should be diluted by one half or more before they are considered as fluid replacements). Because carbohydrate sources are also important in long-distance work, glucose polymer drinks, which provide energy at low osmolality, should be considered.

Warm Weather Clothing.—Cottons and linens absorb moisture, whereas sweatsuit material and rubber or plastic produce a high relative humidity next to the skin, retarding cooling. Warm weather clothing should be loose fitting to permit circulation between skin and air. Dark colors absorb light and add to heat gain, whereas light colors reflect heat rays. An example of an athlete at great heat compromise because of clothing is the football player. Wrappings, taping, padding, and helmet seal off at least 50% of the body surface from evaporative cooling. This is compounded by equipment that may weigh more than 5 lb and whose surface may retain heat. The physical bulk of these athletes, with their relatively small surface area/mass ratios and higher percentages of body fat, also contributes to thermoregulation problems.

Conclusion

Heat illnesses are common in many competitive and recreational sports. One should remember that body weight fluctuations will indicate the amount of fluid to replace and should try to predict which situations are likely to promote dehydration—heavy suits and protective padding, high temperature and high humidity, air travel, heavy and long-term training, and lengthy competition. Then fluids should be consumed before dehydration occurs.[31–34]

ERGOGENIC AIDS

An ergogenic aid is a substance or food reputed to enhance performance above the levels anticipated under normal conditions. It is not surprising that along with the public and its enthusiasm for pursuing health and fitness, athletes would be susceptible to claims for special effects. The list of substances touted as ergogenic aids is a long one—everything from glandular products to megadoses of vitamins. Actually, it would be difficult to name those foods that have not been promoted at some time as ergogenic aids.

When we are convinced that certain foods, dietary regimens, or supplements will improve performance, those substances have a profound psychological effect on us. Many people tried zinc a few years ago. Now interest is centered around isolated amino acids. Regardless of the current trend or fad, one should question the need for ergogenic aids. What is their dollar cost? Are there risks and benefits associated with their use? Do they really work? Will their use replace a sound nutrition program that may actually benefit performance?

Costs

Several years ago, an entrepreneurial group began promoting nutritional supplements. The company stated that it was on a mission, "born out of necessity: a dedicated response to the growing dangers to our health from toxic pollution, stressful lifestyles and nutrient deficiencies from mass food processing." In its quantum leap into nutritional care, the operation pulled in revenues in excess of $27 million in 6 months.[35] The customer was sold pills, fiber bars, and a health drink for an average monthly cost of $135. Not only were the customers offered "better health," but they could earn money by becoming salespersons. Soon the sales force zoomed to 100,000 people who were selling products that did not acknowledge the existence of the RDAs; that contained amounts of vitamin A and β-carotene that could, over time, cause toxic symptoms; and that promoted a formula that did not contain iron.

Perhaps most objectionable was the marketing scheme itself. The company distributed copies of a videotape that was designed to convince consumers and health professionals of the need for its products. The narrator discussed the research and rationale for the products and presented medical and scientific experts who served as advisers. The company paid the advisers up to $20,000 in annual consulting fees, whether they consulted or not. Athletic endorsers were superstars such as Chris Evert-Lloyd, Joe Montana, and Steven Garvey. A number of the endorsers have since objected to the way their names were used.

Risks and Benefits

Statistics show that there is a new wave of steroid abusers. Why, when the American College of Sports Medicine, the American Medical Association, and the American Osteopathic Association (and most former users), have gone on record against it, is steroid use increasing? The numbers point to the women's and teenager's markets.[37]

Steroids may help to develop muscle; that is their questionable benefit. Risks, however, far outweigh any advantage. First, these drugs are illegal for use in national and international competition. The United States Olympic Committee has stated that any substance that gives an athlete unfair advantage over those who do not use it is illegal, and doses can be determined by either urine or blood tests. In addition, the side effects of steroids can be dangerous and irreversible. In women, there are risks of being afflicted with an enlarged clitoris, acne, increased facial hair, and reduction of breast tissue. Men can experience a decrease in testicle size and sperm production, premature baldness, and growth of breast tissue. Both sexes may become prone to an increase in aggressiveness, liver disorders, cardiovascular problems, drug addiction, depression, and effects on stature.[38] Finally, it will cost well over $1,000 yearly for the steroid user to maintain muscle mass once it is gained.

Education and testimonials from former users are prime ways to address steroid use. According to the National Federation of State High School Associations, some high schools include information in their curriculums on the dangers of steroids. A few states have passed laws requiring gyms to display posters detailing the medical and legal dangers of using steroids. There is also a growing interest in reclassifying anabolic-androgenic steroids under federal law as controlled substances.

On August 28, 1986, Tina Plakinger, a former Ms. America who had used steroids since her early twenties, entered the Ms. Olympia contest, the Super Bowl of women's professional body building competitions. "I was standing in the women's room, sticking a 2-inch needle into my rear end," she said. "I looked in the mirror and I saw myself covered with zits, and bloated, and I thought, 'This isn't what I want to do. No wonder I'm not happy.' So I withdrew from the contest. And I haven't touched steroids since."

Do Ergogenic Aids Work?

The information in Table 3–4 was prepared by Bonnie Worthington-Roberts, Ph.D. (professor and director of Nutritional Sciences and chief nutritionist in the clinical training unit at the University of Washington's Child Development and Mental Retardation Center). The contents will undoubtedly change over time, but one thing will remain constant: the expectation placed in substances above and beyond normal food intake. The seemingly eternal hope is that supplementation will cure nutrient deficiency symptoms and also alleviate similar symptoms, no matter what their cause.

As for claims of improved athletic ability, you have only to wander through the health food store or drugstore aisles or check the back pages of the muscle magazines to encounter promises of increased prowess. Consult the guide on vitamins and minerals (Tables 3–5 and 3–6), compare the probable toxic doses (Tables 3–7 and 3–8), and come to your own conclusions.[42, 43]

TABLE 3–4.

Analysis of Popular Health Foods

Product	Composition	Product Claims	Proved Assets	Side Effects	Comments
Alfalfa	Dried, ground, and sold in powder or tablet form; rich in protein, calcium, and trace minerals, carotene, vitamins E and K, all water-soluble vitamins, and vitamin D if sun cured.	Promoted for nutritional value; also marketed by health food enthusiasts for treatment of diabetes.	Alfalfa saponins reduce intestinal absorption of cholesterol and prevent the expected rise in cholesterol-fed rats and monkeys.	May reactivate symptoms in patients with quiescent systemic lupus.	
Aloe vera	Derived from the leaves of the aloe vera, a cactus-like plant of the lily family; most forms are not meant to be taken internally; aloe vera juice is a fair source of vitamin C and provides moderate amounts of potassium, calcium, manganese, and iron.	Claims for cures of pain, insomnia, baldness, burns, ulcers, tuberculosis, and a host of other maladies; also used in cosmetics, pain-reducing ointments, fungicides, and even used as food additive; reputation gained through personal testimonials.	Scientifically, no reported value of oral consumption has appeared in the literature; antibacterial and anti-inflammatory properties have not been proved in human studies; no scientific evidence to support effectiveness as a treatment for cancer, diabetes, or any other serious disease.	Dried latex (fluid from the leaves), an approved internal medication, is a severe cathartic; no serious toxic reactions reported from ingesting the raw plant or commercial preparation; caution is needed because quality control of product may be questionable.	Despite batteries of tests focused on discovering a basis for the reported efficacy of aloe vera, the limited data explain why FDA has not approved it for any ailment except minor first aid.

Continued.

83

TABLE 3–4. (cont.)

Product	Composition	Product Claims	Proved Assets	Side Effects	Comments
p-Aminobenzoic acid (PABA)	Folic acid component essential for producing folic acid in bacteria; often classified as a B vitamin, has no nutritional significance in man and cannot be substituted for folic acid.	Aid suntanning; prevent sunburn and cure gray hair, infertility, and impotence; somewhat effective in darkening hair, but 6 to 24 gm/day are required.	The only accepted medical use for PABA today is as a sunscreen in suntan lotions.	Intakes more than 10 gm/day of PABA may cause nausea, vomiting, acidosis, blood disorders, and sensitivity reactions; potentially can inhibit action of sulfa drugs used to treat bacterial infections.	
Bee pollen	A mixture of bee saliva, plant nectar, and pollen; sold as loose powder, compressed into tablets of 400 to 500 mg with or without other nutritional supplements, or as capsules; the protein varies from 10% to 36% with an average of 20%; the essential amino acid content is reasonably high; simple sugars make up 10% to 15% of the content; contains small	A vast body of literature extolls pollen's curative powers in diseases ranging from colitis, premature aging, and renal diseases to skin blemishes and obesity.	Scientific evidence for healthful properties of bee pollen is almost nil; reports of health benefits are entirely anecdotal.	Recently three patients were reported to experience systemic reactions after eating bee pollen; another patient was reportedly treated after anaphylactic reaction following ingestion for allergic rhinitis; since bee pollen contains nucleic acids, high intakes are not recommended for those predisposed to gout or with signs of renal disease.	

	quantities of fats and significant amounts of minerals.				
Blackstrap molasses	By-product of cane or beet sugar manufacture; the third and final extract; strong flavor and more of the minerals than light or medium molasses; fair, but variable and unreliable iron source; low levels of vitamins.	Popular press claims curative properties for cancer and other disorders; scientific literature does not support these claims.	A laxative; sometimes a good source of iron and calcium.	None reported.	Some find the licorice taste too strong when taken alone.
Bran	Outer coarse coat of grain; wheat, rice, and corn bran are most common; rich in fiber (especially cellulose and hemicellulose); has a significant portion of vitamin and mineral content of grain.	Abundance of literature extolls virtues of dietary fiber; relieves constipation.	A high-fiber diet is the treatment of choice in simple uncomplicated diverticular disease; use of coarse wheat bran usually lends to gradual reduction of diverticular disease symptoms; oat bran may have hypocholesterolemic properties; wheat bran may or may not depress the lithogenicity of bile in those with cholelithiasis.	Gut blockage after eating large amounts of nondigestible matter could occur; continual production of gas may increase risk for sigmoid volvulus; the phytic acid in bran may bind minerals, thereby reducing the amount of mineral available for absorption from the gut.	Response to the laxative effects of bran varies among individuals; some develop considerable gas and diarrhea when first adding it to the diet; bran should be introduced gradually to adapt to its effects less distressingly.

Continued.

TABLE 3-4. (cont.)

Product	Composition	Product Claims	Proved Assets	Side Effects	Comments
Brewer's yeast	Nonfermentative, nonextracted yeast (*Saccharomyces*); a by-product of brewing beer and ale; generally sold in dry forms since fresh form spoils easily; "debittered" is better choice.	Promoted as natural potent source of protein, vitamins, minerals, and nucleic acids; claims for usefulness in diabetes related to GIF-chromium content.	Rich supplemental source of B vitamins; good source of fair-quality protein, contains a minimum of 35% crude protein; rich in chromium and selenium, minerals limited in diets of some Americans.	Rich in nucleic acids, so those prone to gout should use cautiously; systemic *Saccharomyce* yeast infections have resulted from daily oral intake; use only dead yeast.	
Cranberry juice	Self-explanatory	Scientific and lay publications describe the suspected value of cranberry juice in reducing risk and severity of urinary tract infections.	Despite their relatively high acidity, cranberry products in palatable quantities are not reliable for sustained, consistent lowering of urinary pH.	None reported.	
Desiccated liver	An excellent source of chromium, selenium, copper, iron, vitamin B_{12}, and some other nutrients normally stored in this organ; rich in fat and cholesterol unless defatted.	Marketed as a good iron and vitamin B_{12} supplement.	Two teaspoons of liver powder/day provide plenty of extra minerals and vitamin B_{12}.	High–nucleic acid content makes it undesirable for those with gout; may promote positive results in tests for occult blood in stools.	

86

Continued.

| Eicosapentaenoic acid (EPA) | Analog of arachidonic acid found in fish, some other marine oils, and perhaps seaweed; available as capsules. | Made recent news as possible preventers of some cardiovascular problems. | Investigators have reported possible cardiovascular protective properties of marine fatty acids; University of Oregon group found that a 10-day diet of salmon, which contains ω-3 fatty acids, lowers plasma cholesterol levels by up to 17% in presumably healthy volunteers and by 20% or more in hyperlipidemic patients; triglyceride levels fall by as much as 40% in healthy volunteers and as much as 67% in hyperlipidemics; currently believed that EPA inhibits platelet aggregation probably by inhibiting the platelets' manufacture of | Appropriate dosage level not clearly defined; possible adverse effects from long-term consumption of EPA-rich regimen are unknown. |

TABLE 3–4. (cont.)

Product	Composition	Product Claims	Proved Assets	Side Effects	Comments
Fructose	Monosaccharide occurring naturally in a variety of foods; before 1975 fructose was not widely commercially available; expensive, but still used in increasing amounts in foods and in sugar bowls.	The greater availability of fructose has focused attention on use as a special dietary component or as treatment modality in a variety of diseases (obesity, diabetes, reactive hypoglycemia, dental caries, and alcohol intoxication).	May have useful role in the dietary management of diabetes mellitus, since substitution of fructose for other simple carbohydrates leads to reduced postprandial glucose levels; however, most data have been obtained from short-term studies; thus, there is insufficient information to determine if fructose or any other carbohydrate benefits long-term dietary management of diabetes; fructose incorporated into diabetic diet should	Large doses (70–100 gm) may cause abdominal pain and diarrhea; serum uric acid levels may also increase; in experimental animals, fructose may convert to fatty acids at a greater rate than sucrose.	Limited data from patients with reactive hypoglycemia suggest that symptoms may be averted with controlled use of fructose as a glucose or sucrose substitute; no convincing evidence that fructose aids weight reduction, but its sweetness may encourage smaller servings; fructose is somewhat less cariogenic than sucrose; fructose does not elevate plasma triglyceride levels even when consumed in large amounts (up to 120

thromboxane A_2, an aggregating agent, and the synthesis of prostaglandins.

			not exceed the average amount of sucrose used in the diet (75 gm/day).		gm/day); although fructose given orally or intravenously is generally reported to accelerate ethanol oxidation, this does not necessarily correlate with rate of improvement or in intensity of physical symptoms of alcohol abuse.
Garlic	Cloves derived from an underground bulb, a well-known seasoning, available in tablet with and without parsley, which supposedly neutralizes its odor; also available as odorless capsules, syrup, tincture, and essential oil.	Recommended for topical and internal use for various ailments, including athlete's foot, hay fever, arthritis, sleep disorders, sinus problems, and lung ailments; also claimed to retard aging and prevent cancer and heart disease; garlic oil has been said to inhibit platelet aggregation when taken in large amounts, but four normal subjects on a 10-day course of	Has mild hypoglycemic properties and works moderately well as a diuretic and vasodilator; may be useful in preventing atherosclerosis, stroke, and high blood pressure; in animals, garlic prevents plaque formation and may prevent a rise in plasma cholesterol after a high-fat feeding; an ether extract of garlic juice (taken with a	Nothing is known about optimal intakes; since many of the components in garlic have not been identified, it is not possible to make clear statements regarding toxic effects when garlic is consumed in large amounts; large doses of garlic produce flatulence, damage the stomach, and also produce a garlicky breath and body odor.	Although more scientific data are available about garlic than about many other "nutritional aids," evidence is not strong enough to promote this plant derivative as medicinal. The possible value of garlic as an anticancer agent has been suggested by several investigators for 30 yr; one report described the

Continued.

89

TABLE 3–4. (cont.)

Product	Composition	Product Claims	Proved Assets	Side Effects	Comments
		proprietary garlic capsules (six/day) showed no change in platelet aggregation.	fatty diet) can decrease plasma cholesterol and triglyceride concentration and increase fibrinolytic activity and blood coagulation time, increase high-density lipoprotein (HDL) and decrease low-density lipoprotein (LDL) fractions; when garlic was administered after introduction of virulent cells, tumors were either delayed in appearing or prevented from development as long as administration of garlic continued.		antitumor effect of garlic in mice; administration of garlic along with tumor cells resulted in a substantial delay of death from 16 days to 6 mo. Similarly, total inhibition of mammary tumor development was demonstrated in mice given complete garlic, but loss of the antitumor effect was noted when the compound allicin was destroyed. In most reported experiments, garlic was used in large enough amounts to consider it a drug, not a food.
Gerovital H3	Consists of a 2% procaine hydrochloride (Novocain; a local	Promoted as an effective antiaging nutritional factor beneficial for almost	Although many uncontrolled studies describe great benefits from its	Topical or systemic applications of Gerovital have resulted in	One report concluded that Gerovital H3 is of no value in retarding aging or

	anesthetic) solution with small amounts of benzoic acid (a preservative), potassium metabisulfide (an antioxidant), and diethylaminoethanol; some claims for Gerovital are attributed to PBA, but the amount is insignificant compared with that normally found in the diet.	any disease associated with premature aging, arthritis, atherosclerosis, angina pectoris, and other heart disease, deafness, neuritis, Parkinson's disease, depression, senile psychoses, and impotence; stimulates hair growth and repigments gray hair.	use, controlled, double-blind studies fail to show any improvement in the physical and mental status of elderly patients; in one study, Gerovital had an antidepressant effect, but this could not be confirmed and may be attributable to a unique subject population.	sensitivity reactions to procaine.	for the treatment of prevention of any disorder in the elderly.
Ginseng	Root of the ginseng plant sold in capsules, extract, instant powder, paste, tea (sometimes made with leaves), and whole root; growing popularity is attributed to pharmacological stimulants; contains peptides, steroids, and many unidentified	General tonic for digestive troubles, impotence, and overall lack of vitality.	Reports of effectiveness are largely anecdotal; the amounts consumed (1 teaspoon, or 5 gm) are too small to contribute nutrients. Recently, however, extracts from ginseng root powder were shown to lower cholesterol in birds, an effect attributed to	Two to 3 gm needed to elicit behavioral stimulation; recently, the ginseng abuse syndrome has been described. At doses as low as 3 gm, hypertension and neurological symptoms (insomnia, nervousness, feelings of depersonalization,	Most ginseng sold in the United States is derived from a North American plant related to the original *Panax ginseng* plant; though little work has been done, evidence indicates that extracts from the original plant may not have the same pharmacological

Continued.

TABLE 3-4. (cont.)

Product	Composition	Product Claims	Proved Assets	Side Effects	Comments
	substances that appear responsible for stimulant effect.		saponins (ginsenosides).	confusion, and depression) have been reported; skin eruptions, edema, and diarrhea are seen; abrupt withdrawal may lead to hypotensive crises.	effects as those from related plants.
				Reported to produce a physiological estrogen-like effect on the vaginal mucosa, and mastalgia with diffuse mammary nodularity in postmenopausal women, and experimentally, stimulation of corticotropin secretion and altered RNA hepatic metabolism.	
Honey	Glucose and fructose dissolved in 4% to 20% water with minor amounts of organic acids and traces of vitamins	Acquired special reputation as nutritional food or medicine; supplies a concentrated source of calories,	No less cariogenic than sucrose but is sweeter and therefore may be consumed in smaller amounts;	Recently, associated with infant botulism; *Clostridium botulinum* spores are ubiquitous and found in honey fed	

	and minerals; derived from flowering plant nectar the honey bee collects; bee supplies invertase enzyme to convert sucrose to glucose and fructose; color, flavor, and proportion of sugars vary with source of nectar.	but there are only traces of other nutrients; used alone or with vinegar as home remedy for variety of common problems, but supportive data only anecdotal.	no evidence supports claims that honey supplies quick energy.	to stricken infants; infants susceptible only in the first year, most physicians and nutritionists recommend that babies less than 1 year old not get honey.	
Lactobacillus acidophilus and acidophilus milk	Bottled suspensions of *L. acidophilus* and powder and tablets made from dried, viable bacteria. Acidophilus milk is pasteurized, usually low fat or skim, cultured with *L. acidophilus*; sweet acidophilus milk is now produced by adding frozen or freeze-dried *L. acidophilus* culture to milk and refrigerating to prevent fermentation.	Intestinal infection; lactose intolerance	Used to regenerate intestinal floral after antibiotic treatment or other conditions upsetting the gut's microfloral balance; *L. acidophilus* may liberate natural antibiotics and hydrogen peroxide to inhibit a number of pathogenic and nonpathogenic bacteria; lactobacilli inhibit the proliferation of tumor cells in animals and reduce growth of existent tumors.	None reported.	Acidophilus milk contains as much lactose as regular milk and has not been proved useful for lactose-intolerant people.

Continued.

93

TABLE 3–4. (cont.)

Product	Composition	Product Claims	Proved Assets	Side Effects	Comments
Lecithin	Phospholipid found in all living things; mixture of diglycerides of the fatty acids stearic, palmitic, and oleic combined with choline ester of phosphoric acid. The body synthesizes lecithin, but it is also ingested in a variety of foods; predominant commercial source of lecithin is soybeans; is an FDA-approved food additive to stabilize and emulsify margarine, dressings, chocolate, frozen desserts, and baked goods.	Supplemental lecithin proposed to prevent or cure arthritis, gallstones, heart disease, nervous disorders, and skin problems; most of these claims not supported by scientific investigations.	Attention has been given to role of lecithin in reducing risk of heart disease and gallstones; although several authors have reported lowered serum triglyceride and cholesterol levels and raised bile lecithin levels after oral administration of lecithin, others have not confirmed these reports; supplemental lecithin or choline may increase levels of acetylcholine in specific brain parts and thereby explain improvement seen in patients with tardive dyskinesia and Alzheimer's disease; studies of value of lecithin supplements in managing of other	Because high intake of lecithin or choline produces acute gastrointestinal distress, sweating, salivation, and anorexia, people probably will not have lasting health problems from taking of either compound; but depression or supersensitivity of dopamine receptors and disturbance of the cholinergic-dopaminergic-serotonergic balance may result from prolonged, repeated doses of large amounts of lecithin.	No evidence at this time that lecithin has any nutritional significance.

Life extension supplements	In the book called *Life Extension* by Durk Pearson and Sandy Shaw (Warner Books, 1982), use of large doses of butylated hydroxyanisole (BHA) and butylated hydroxytoluene (BHT) is advocated to retard aging; small amounts of these antioxidants commonly used by the food industry as stabilizing additives in vegetable oils and with other edible fat products.	Two grams of BHT or BHA daily are recommended to combat genital herpes, prevent cancer, and retard aging.	neurological disorders were only mildly successful. No reported effectiveness.	Research completed in 1957 showed that BHA or BHT in daily doses of 1 gm had deleterious effects on rabbits; the animals became weak and died after 2 weeks; BHT level calculated for humans taking 2-gm doses is only 10 times less than level lethal to rabbits.	
Lysine	An amino acid essential to humans; intake in the United States is about 6 to 7 gm/day.	Promoters claim lysine treats cold sores or fever blisters caused by herpes simplex type 1.	Interest began when research showed high concentrations of lysine, or high lysine/arginine ratio in tissue culture media, inhibited growth of herpesvirus; in a study of 10 patients, 390 mg of	Effects of long-term intake of lysine are unknown; large doses of single amino acids potentially can interfere with the absorption of other amino acids.	Since some patients may benefit from lysine treatment, further study is necessary; however, lysine is not a cure but a prophylactic, and therefore, patients would require daily intake.

Continued.

95

TABLE 3–4. (cont.)

Product	Composition	Product Claims	Proved Assets	Side Effects	Comments
			lysine/day caused rapid resolution of lesions; a large uncontrolled study using 312 to 1,000 mg/day got similar results; however, two double-blind, placebo-controlled studies using 1,000 mg of lysine/day showed no effect on the rate of healing of lesions or on their appearance; though one study found that patients fed lysine had fewer recurrences, the great interindividual and intraindividual variation in the frequency and course of recurrent herpes makes evaluating clinical studies difficult, especially since lesions usually		

Nucleic acids	RNA and DNA.	Received much attention as antiaging factors and promoted as a cure for degenerative diseases (atherosclerosis, diabetes, and senility) claimed to prevent gray hair and produce healthier shine.	disappear spontaneously within 10 days. None of the clinical studies of nucleic acids therapy were free from potential bias or placebo effects; a double-blind study with 10 patients found no effect of 20 gm/day of RNA on dementia; obviously, exogenous RNA cannot rejuvenate old cells and tissue.	Can increase serum uric acid levels.	When eaten, nucleic acids are broken down in the gastrointestinal tract and *not* absorbed intact; the body makes them, therefore, not essential nutrients.
Pancreatic enzymes	Self-explanatory.	Promoted to aid digestion and relieve indigestion.	Malabsorption usually does not occur until pancreatic enzyme secretion is reduced more than 90%; when true digestive problems exist from intestinal or pancreatic disease, enzyme therapy may be useful.	None reported.	Very susceptible to inactivation by acid environment of stomach; though coated for protection in the stomach, unlikely to benefit the normal person whose digestive tract is more than able to meet digestive demands.

Continued.

TABLE 3-4. (cont.)

Product	Composition	Product Claims	Proved Assets	Side Effects	Comments
Papaya/papain	Enzyme from the green fruit and leaves of papaya; is proteolytic and has been used to tenderize meats, clear beverages, prevent adhesions during wound healing, and aid digestion; sold in tablet and powder form.	Most frequently sold as digestive aids.	For individuals who truly need help with digestion and absorption, papaya tablet or powder may be useful; most Americans do not need it.	Therapy of gastric phytobezoars (concretions of food and fiber) with Adolph's Meat Tenderizer associated with hypernatremia and confusion in at least one case; allergic response to inhaled papain also reported.	
Protein supplements	Liquids, powders, and tablets; either contain all the essential amino acids to make a "high-quality" protein or contain only specific amino acids.	Improve physical performance, help in weight loss, or build skeletal muscles.	No evidence that athletes or physically active people require more protein than American adolescents or that extra protein improves physical performance.	Excess protein intake can lead to ketosis, dehydration, a tendency for gout, and an increase in urinary excretion of calcium.	Most Americans consume far more protein than they can use; excess protein can be converted to fat.
Royal jelly	Milky white substance produced by worker bees to nourish the queen bee; sold in capsule form as a nutritional	Promoters of royal jelly imply it will do as much for humans as it does for queen bees: increase size,	A rich source of certain B vitamins (like pantothenic acid) but not shown to have any recognizable	None reported.	Queen bees differ from worker bees: they are twice as big, live up to 8 yr (40 times longer than worker bees),

Name	Description	Claims/Uses	Evaluation	
	supplement but also is an ingredient in some expensive cosmetics.	longevity, and fertility.	preventive, therapeutic, or rejuvenating effects.	and lay 2,000 eggs/day (female worker bees are infertile). Although the egg of the queen starts out like all the others, the royal jelly fed to this bee accounts for the difference occurring during growth.
Seaweed (kelp)	Any plant that grows in the sea is seaweed or, botanically, algae; the best of the harvest is reserved to produce kelp tablets and seaweed powder for humans, and the bulk of the crop is marketed for livestock feed. Norwegian Seaweed Institute reports the composition of seaweed as: Protein 5.7% Fat 2.6% Fiber 7.0% Nitrogen-free extract 58.6% Ash 15.4%	Alleviating constipation, gastric catarrh, mucous colitis, and other disorders; claims have not been substantiated through properly conducted, controlled studies. Spirulina (*Spirulina maxima*) has been promoted heavily during the past few years; sold as a "natural diet pill," a remedy for various ailments, such as hypoglycemia and hay fever, but evidence to prove these claims is lacking.	Satisfactory source of iodine; vitamin B_{12} content of spirulina has been over emphasized; recent analyses of representative spirulina products show that 80% of the vitamin B_{12} activity described in spirulina products resides in analogs of vitamin B_{12}, which have no biological activity.	Dried seaweed has more than eight times as much iodine as iodized salt; large amounts eaten for a prolonged period may be harmful; fortunately, however, almost every brand of kelp tablet contains an amount of iodine equal to the U.S. RDA (150 gm/day) in each tablet. The possibility that some of the vitamin B_{12} analogs in spirulina could be harmful to humans is under investigation. Contrary to claims sometimes made, seaweeds are low in protein, and the protein is of very poor quality; a number of minerals are found in seaweed along with carotene, vitamin D, vitamin K, and most of the water-soluble vitamins. Although spirulina may be a satisfactory source of nutrition to the consumer, few people could afford to eat enough of it to significantly affect their nutritional status; *Continued.*

100

TABLE 3–4. (cont.)

Product	Composition	Product Claims	Proved Assets	Side Effects	Comments
	Moisture 10.7% / 100.0%			Spirulina is rich in nucleic acids, so consumption could lead to urinary stone formation or gout in susceptible people.	typical West Coast spirulina buyers pay $10 to $23 for the same amount of protein available in 75¢ worth of peanuts.
Superoxide dismutase (SOD)	Enzyme found in most cells of the body; catalyzes the breakdown of superoxide-free radicals—oxygen and hydrogen peroxide; protects cells from toxic effects of oxygen since these superoxide radicals damage DNA and age and destroy cells; deactivation of these superoxide radicals is called dismutation; hence, the name superoxide dismutase.	Some promoters claim SOD tablets prevent cancer and aging and lessen the effects of air pollution; the tablets contain a partially purified enzyme from cattle liver and other enzymes with antioxidant activity, including catalase and glutathione peroxidase.	As with any protein eaten, a person probably would digest it, and it would not enter the circulation intact; reports conflict about giving SOD parenterally. Injected into animals, it may have modified the toxicity of agents generating O_2; in most cases it would not penetrate the cell membranes; more promising evidence is accumulating that when parenterally given, the drug form of copper-zinc	None reported.	The FDA has approved SOD for animal use; human use is for research only. Several European nations permit its use for rheumatoid arthritis, osteoarthritis, urological disorders, and the side effects of radiation treatment; however, in the United States, some health food stores and mail order businesses sell SOD as a compound to reverse aging and degeneration.

					SOD, orgotein, is effective in treating arthritis without producing severe side effects; more research is still needed to determine clinical efficacy.
Tryptophan	Essential amino acid for humans; metabolized to the B vitamin, niacin; a precursor for a neurotransmitter serotonin; average daily intake about 1 to 2 gm; brain tryptophan levels dependent on food intake; the amount of tryptophan in the brain can control serotonin synthesis.	Advertised as nature's "sleeping pill" and natural sedative; also said to be an antidepressant and hypnotic.	A number of studies have reported the effects of 5 to 15 gm of tryptophan on sleep in normal subjects; despite variability in results, the major observations are a short time to fall asleep and a slight change in sleep patterns; the response to tryptophan may be related to circadian rhythm; effects on sleep were noted only if tryptophan was given at night, not in the morning.	Long-term safety when given in megadoses is uncertain; megadoses can produce nausea; in experimental animals, tryptophan and its metabolites promote tumors, and some of its metabolites may be hepatic and bladder carcinogens.	The antidepressant effects of tryptophan remain controversial, despite its use as adjunct therapy in Great Britain; present evidence indicates tryptophan does not benefit the treatment of depression.

TABLE 3–5.

The Important Minerals in the Body, Their Recommended Daily Intake, Dietary Sources, Major Bodily Functions, and the Effects of Deficiencies and Excesses*

Mineral	Amount in Adult Body (gm)	RDA for Healthy Adult Male and Female (mg)†	Dietary Sources	Major Body Functions	Deficiency	Excess
Calcium	1,500	800 800	Milk, cheese, dark-green vegetables, dried legumes	Bone and tooth formation, blood clotting, nerve transmission	Stunted growth, rickets, osteoporosis, convulsions	Not reported in humans
Phosphorus	860	800 800	Milk, cheese, meat, poultry, grains	Bone and tooth formation, acid-base balance	Weakness, demineralization of bone, loss of calcium	Erosion of jaw (fossy jaw)
Sulfur	300	(Provided by sulfur amino acids)	Sulfur amino acids (methionine and cystine) in dietary proteins	Constituent of active tissue compounds, cartilage and tendon	Related to intake and deficiency of sulfur amino acids	Excess sulfur amino acid intake leads to poor growth
Potassium	180	1,875–5,625	Meats, milk, many fruits	Acid-base balance, body water balance, nerve function	Muscular weakness, paralysis	Muscular weakness, death

Element		Amount	Food source	Function	Deficiency symptoms	Toxicity symptoms
Chlorine	74	1,700–5,100	Common salt	Formation of gastric juice, acid-base balance	Muscle cramps, mental apathy, reduced appetite	Vomiting
Sodium	64	1,100–3,300	Common salt	Acid-base balance, body water balance, nerve function	Muscle cramps, mental apathy, reduced appetite	High blood pressure
Magnesium	25	350 300	Whole grains, green leafy vegetables	Activates enzymes, involved in protein synthesis	Growth failure, behavioral disturbances, weakness, spasms	Diarrhea
Iron	4.5	10 18	Eggs, lean meats, legumes, whole grains, green leafy vegetables	Constituent of hemoglobin and enzymes involved in energy metabolism	Iron-deficiency anemia (weakness, reduced resistance to infection)	Siderosis, cirrhosis of liver
Fluorine	2.6	1.5–4.0	Drinking water, tea, seafood	May be important in maintenance of bone structure	Higher frequency of tooth decay	Mottling of teeth, increased bone density, neurologic disturbances
Zinc	2	15 15	Widely distributed in foods	Constituent of enzymes involved in digestion	Growth failure, small sex glands	Fever, nausea, vomiting, diarrhea

Continued.

103

TABLE 3–5. (cont.)

Mineral	Amount in Adult Body (gm)	RDA for Healthy Adult Male and Female (mg)†	Dietary Sources	Major Body Functions	Deficiency	Excess
Copper	0.1	2 2	Meats, drinking water	Constituent of enzymes associated with iron metabolism	Anemia, bone changes (rare in humans)	Rare metabolic condition (Wilson's disease)
Silicon Vanadium Tin Nickel	0.024 0.018 0.017 0.010	Not established	Widely distributed in foods	Function unknown (essential for animals)	Not reported in humans	Industrial exposures: Silicon—silicosis Vanadium—lung irritation Tin—vomiting Nickel—acute pneumonitis
Selenium	0.013	0.05–0.02	Seafood, meat, grains	Functions in close association with vitamin E	Anemia (rare)	Gastrointestinal disorders, lung irritation
Manganese	0.012	Not established (diet provides 6–8/day)	Widely distributed in foods	Constituent of enzymes involved in fat synthesis	In animals: poor growth, disturbances of nervous system, reproductive abnormalities	Poisoning in manganese mines: generalized disease of nervous system

Element	Amount in body	Recommended intake[†]	Food sources	Function	Deficiency	Excess/toxicity
Iodine	0.011	0.15	Marine fish and shellfish, dairy products, many vegetables	Constituent of thyroid hormones	Goiter (enlarged thyroid)	Very high intakes depress thyroid activity
Molybdenum	0.009	Not established (diet provides 0.4/day)	Legumes, cereals, organ meats	Constituent of some enzymes	Not reported in humans	Inhibition of enzymes
Chromium	0.006	0.05–0.2	Fats, vegetable oils, meats	Involved in glucose and energy metabolism	Impaired ability to metabolize glucose	Occupational exposures: skin and kidney damage
Cobalt	0.0015	(Required as vitamin B_{12})	Organ and muscle meats, milk	Constituent of vitamin B_{12}	Not reported in humans	Industrial exposure: dermatitis and diseases of red blood cells
Water	40,000 (60% of body weight)	1.5 L/day	Solid foods, liquids, drinking water	Transport of nutrients, temperature regulation, participates in metabolic reactions	Thirst, dehydration	Headaches, nausea, edema, high blood pressure

*Adapted from Scrimshaw NS, Young VR: The requirements of human nutrition. *Sci Am* 1976; 235:50–73; and *Recommended Dietary Allowances*, revised. Washington, DC, Food and Nutrition Board, National Academy of Sciences–National Research Council, 1980. From the National Dairy Council. Used by permission.
†First values are for males.

TABLE 3–6.
Water- and Fat-soluble Vitamins, Their Recommended Daily Intake, Dietary Sources, Major Bodily Functions, and Effects of Deficiencies and Excesses*

Vitamin	RDA for Healthy Adult Male and Female (mg)†	Dietary Sources	Major Body Functions‡	Deficiency	Excess
Water-soluble					
Vitamin B₁ (thiamine)	1.4–1.5 1.0–1.1	Pork, organ meats, whole grains, legumes	Coenzyme (thiamine pyrophosphate) in reactions involving the removal of carbon dioxide	Beriberi (peripheral nerve changes, edema, heart failure)	None reported
Vitamin B₂ (riboflavin)	1.6–1.7 1.2–1.3	Widely distributed in foods	Constituent of two flavin nucleotide coenzymes involved in energy metabolism (FAD and FMN)	Reddened lips, cracks at corner of mouth (cheilosis), lesions of eye	None reported
Niacin	18–19 13–14	Liver, lean meats, grains, legumes (can be formed from tryptophan)	Constituent of two coenzymes involved in oxidation-reduction reactions (NAD and NADP)	Pellagra (skin and gastrointestinal lesions, nervous, mental disorders)	Flushing, burning and tingling around neck, face, and hands
Vitamin B₆ (pyridoxine)	2.2 2.0	Meats, vegetables, whole-grain cereals	Coenzyme (pyridoxal phosphate) involved in amino acid metabolism	Irritability, convulsions, muscular twitching, dermatitis near eyes, kidney stones	None reported

106

Vitamin	Amounts		Food sources	Functions	Deficiency symptoms	Toxicity
Pantothenic acid	4–7	4–7	Widely distributed in foods	Constituent of coenzyme A, which plays a central role in energy metabolism	Fatigue, sleep disturbances, impaired coordination, nausea (rare in humans)	None reported
Folacin	0.4	0.4	Legumes, green vegetables, whole-wheat products	Coenzyme (reduced form) involved in transfer of single-carbon units in nucleic acid and amino acid metabolism	Anemia, gastrointestinal disturbances, diarrhea, red tongue	None reported
Vitamin B_{12}	0.003	0.003	Muscle meats, eggs, dairy products, (not present in plant foods)	Coenzyme involved in transfer of single-carbon units in nucleic acid metabolism	Pernicious anemia, neurologic disorders	None reported
Biotin	0.10–0.20	0.10–0.20	Legumes, vegetables, meats	Coenzyme required for fat synthesis, amino acid metabolism, and glycogen (animal starch) formation	Fatigue, depression, nausea, dermatitis, muscular pains	None reported
Vitamin C (ascorbic acid)	60	60	Citrus fruits, tomatoes, green peppers, salad greens	Maintains intercellular matrix of cartilage, bone, and dentine; important in collagen synthesis	Scurvy (degeneration of skin, teeth, blood vessels, epithelial hemorrhages)	Relatively nontoxic; possibility of kidney stones

Continued.

107

TABLE 3–6. (cont.)

108

Vitamin	RDA for Healthy Adult Male and Female (mg)†	Dietary Sources	Major Body Functions‡	Deficiency	Excess
Fat-soluble Vitamin A (retinol)	1.0 0.8	Provitamin A (β-carotene) widely distributed in green vegetables; retinol present in milk, butter, cheese, fortified margarine	Constituent of rhodopsin (visual pigment); maintenance of epithelial tissues; role in mucopolysaccharide synthesis	Xerophthalmia (keratinization of ocular tissue), night blindness, permanent blindness	Headache, vomiting, peeling of skin, anorexia, swelling of long bones
Vitamin D	0.075 0.075	Cod-liver oil, eggs, dairy products, fortified milk, and margarine.	Promotes growth and mineralization of bones; increases absorption of calcium	Rickets (bone deformities) in children; osteomalacia in adults	Vomiting, diarrhea, loss of weight, kidney damage
Vitamin E (tocopherol)	10 8	Seeds, green leafy vegetables, margarines, shortenings	Functions as an antioxidant to prevent cell-membrane damage.	Possibly anemia	Relatively nontoxic
Vitamin K (phylloquinone)	0.07–0.14 0.07–0.14	Green leafy vegetables; small amount in cereals, fruits, and meats	Important in blood clotting (involved in formation of active prothrombin)	Conditioned deficiencies associated with severe bleeding; internal hemorrhages	Relatively nontoxic; synthetic forms at high doses may cause jaundice

*Adapted from Scrimshaw NS, Young VR: The requirements of human nutrition. *Sci Am* 1976; 235:50; and *Recommended Dietary Allowances*, revised. Washington, DC, Food and Nutrition Board, National Academy of Sciences–National Research Council, 1980. From the National Dairy Council. Used by permission.
†First values are for males.
‡FAD = flavin adenine dinucleotide; FMN = flavin mononucleotide; NAD = nicotinamide–adenine dinucleotide; NADP = nicotinamide–adenine dinucleotide phosphate.

TABLE 3–7.

Mineral Safety Index*

Mineral	Recommended Adult Intake†	Minimum Toxic Dose	Mineral Safety Index
Calcium	1,200 mg	12,000 mg	10
Phosphorus	1,200 mg	12,000 mg	10
Magnesium	400 mg	6,000 mg	15
Iron	18 mg	100 mg	5.5
Zinc	15 mg	500 mg	33
Copper	3 mg	100 mg	33
		<3 mg‡	<1
Fluoride	4 mg	20 mg	5
		4 mg§	1
Iodine	0.15 μg	2 mg	13
Selenium	0.2 μg	1 mg	5

*From Hathcock JN: Quantitative evaluation of vitamin safety. *Pharm Times,* May 1985. Used by permission.
†Highest of the RDA (except those for pregnancy and lactation) or the U.S. recommended daily allowance, whichever is higher.
‡For people with Wilson's disease.
§Level producing slight fluorosis of dental enamel.

TABLE 3–8.

Vitamin Safety Index*

Vitamin	Recommended Adult Intake†	Minimum Toxic Dose	Vitamin Safety Index
Vitamin A	5,000 IU	25,000 to 50,000 IU	5 to 10
Vitamin D	400 IU	50,000 IU	125
		1,000 to 2,000 IU‡	2.5 to 5
Vitamin E	30 IU	1,200 IU	40
Vitamin C	60 mg	2,000 to 5,000 mg	33 to 83
		1,000 mg§	17
Thiamin (B_1)	1.5 mg	300 mg	200
Riboflavin	1.7 mg	1,000 mg	588
Niacin	20 mg	1,000 mg	50
Pyridoxine (B_6)	2.2 mg	2,000 mg	900
		200 mg‖	90
Folacin	0.4 mg	400 mg	1,000
		15 mg¶	37
Biotin	0.3 mg	50 mg	167
Pantothenic acid	10 mg	10,000 mg	1,000

*Adapted from Hathcock JN: Quantitative evaluation of vitamin safety. *Pharm Times,* May 1985.
†Highest of the individual RDA (except those for pregnancy and lactation) or the U.S. recommended daily allowance, whichever is higher.
‡For infants and also for adults with certain infections or metabolic diseases; 50,000 IU for most adults.
§To produce slightly altered mineral excretion patterns.
‖For antagonism of some drugs; 2,000 mg for most adults.
¶For antagonism of anticonvulsants in epileptics; 400 mg for most adults.

Sound Nutrition

There are several basic rules to review when one is questioning nutritional well-being:

1. *All of the nutrients needed can be obtained by eating a variety of foods.* It is obvious that not all persons have balanced diets. If you are worried about your diet containing enough nutrients, simply write down everything you eat over a 1-week period, then ask your doctor or a registered dietitian about your food choices. If your diet is deficient, learn which foods will improve it. You do not need to go overboard on supplementation. Pill form versus food form will always be a red-hot issue, but a poor diet with vitamin supplementation is still a poor diet.

2. *Body weight is a matter of arithmetic. If you consume more calories than you need, you will gain. To lose weight, you must burn more calories than you take in.* It would be wonderful if there was a pill. Evidently some consumers think there is, and they are the ones who buy diuretics, starch blockers, or ear staples and read and accept the severe restrictions to diet that are proposed by the radicals of the dietary world. Research is underway to develop a weight loss pill, and it may be available in the next century. For now, though, consumers must rely on caloric control, exercise, behavior modification, and good old-fashioned common sense. The unfortunate truth is that no pill can guarantee better health than three balanced meals each day.

3. *Moderation in all things is a principle of healthful eating.* Too much of a good thing is not a good thing. (Imagine overdosing on chocolate chip cookies and then not liking them anymore. Life would have no meaning!) Pay attention to quality, quantity, frequency pattern, and variety for your health's sake. Focusing on a single nutrient is not the best approach, and it may be harmful. The more we understand, the clearer it becomes that going too far in any direction can have unfortunate nutritional consequences. For instance, much of

the debate over cancer and diet is focused on fats; vitamins A, C, and E; the mineral selenium; and fiber. With any of these, only certain amounts in certain forms seem to be helpful.

4. *No proposed remedy should be considered safe or effective until proved by scientific investigation or controlled clinical trials.* The pharmaceutical industry recently jumped on the bandwagon for ω-3 fatty acids. Research indicated that populations with a high ratio of these acids in their diets also had low coronary heart rates. The industry's response was a capsule to be taken several times a day. There probably is no harm in taking this preparation, but one needs to be cautious before accepting general statements about the efficacy of a product. No one wants to die of coronary artery disease, nor did anyone want to die of scurvy. But though there was a 1:1 ratio of effectiveness in the prevention and treatment of scurvy, heart disease is a much more complicated matter. If you cannot eat fish or refuse to change your eating habits but want extra insurance, a supplement of fish oils may be helpful. Again, moderation applies. As with all forms of supplementation, choose one that provides nearly 100% of what is recommended, and check the expiration date.[44]

An example of scientific scrutiny, most applicable to the athlete, is fluid, electrolyte, and carbohydrate replacement. To date, effective carbohydrate feeding during or prior to exertion has been interesting but controversial. Critical variables are the timing of the ingestion and the duration of the event.

Common advice is to "think water" for moderate exercise in moderate temperature. Heavy exercise, high temperature or humidity, or both may warrant electrolyte replacement. A dilute glucose solution (2.5% concentration) ingested during prolonged exercise tends to maintain blood glucose and spare muscle glycogen and will empty efficiently from the stomach. New products made with glucose polymers (at 5%–10% concentration) provide energy for continued muscular exertion without delaying gastric emptying.

Research is beginning to address the question to what extent will absorption of a single nutrient, such as carbohydrate, be changed in a situation of dehydration, hyperthermia and minimal gastrointestinal blood flow? Most studies have been centered on cyclists and may not reflect situations in which severe gastrointestinal disturbances and complaints occur. The data indicate that regurgitations, gastric acid reflux, and vomiting may be related to the composition of the feeding (too high, perhaps, for the individual),[45] and diarrhea and cramping may be related to functional changes in the gut. It may be that this question will be answered outside of the laboratory at the event itself (e.g., athletes are telling us that when carbohydrate intake is the first priority, concentrated drinks and glucose polymers are handled very well during heavy sustained competition).

REFERENCES

1. Nash HL: Elite child-athletes: How much does victory cost? *Phys Sports Med* 1987; 15:129.
2. Messerly J: Children and adolescents: Special concerns in sports. *Sportswatch* 1986; 1:4.
3. Storey M: Personal communication, 1987.
4. Miller T: American Osteopathic Academy of Sports Medicine, 1987.
5. Williams MH: *Nutrition for Fitness and Sport.* Dubuque, Ia, William C Brown Co, 1983.
6. American Academy of Pediatrics: Climatic heat stress and the exercising child. *Phys Sports Med* 1983; 11:155.
7. Bar-or O: Climate and the exercising child—a review. *Int J Appl Physiol* 1980; 48:104.
8. Tufts University: Small children have special iron needs. 1986; 3:7.
9. Peterson MS: Unpublished data, 1986.
10. Anonymous: Wheelchair marathoners: Some metabolic and physiological aspects in the spinal cord-injured participant. *Sports Nutr Rev* 1987; 1:4.
11. Shangold MM: How I manage exercise-related menstrual disturbances. *Phys Sports Med* 1986; 14:113.
12. Loucks AB, Horvath SM: Athletic amenorrhea. *Med Sci Sports Exerc* 1983; 17:56.

13. Monahan T: Treating athletic amenorrhea: A matter of instinct? *Phys Sports Med* 1987; 15:184.

14. Zimmerman DR: Maturation and strenuous training in young female athletes. *Phys Sports Med* 1987; 15:219.

15. Worthington-Roberts B: Nutrition during pregnancy, in *Nutritional Concerns of Women*. Seattle, University of Washington Press, 1987, pp 55–72.

16. Gorski J: Exercise during pregnancy: maternal and fetal responses. A brief review. *Med Sci Sports Exerc* 1985; 17:407.

17. Anonymous: Adolescent pregnancy—counseling considerations. *Nutr MD* 1986; 12:1.

18. Worthington-Roberts B: *Nutrition in Pregnancy and Lactation*. St Louis, CV Mosby Co, 1977.

19. Krause MV, Mahan LD: *Food, Nutrition, and Diet Therapy*. Philadelphia, WB Saunders Co, 1984.

20. Roe DA: Nutritional needs and concerns of American women. *Nutr Newslett* 1986; 49:9.

21. Shangold M, Mirkin M: *The Complete Sports Medicine Book for Women*. New York, Simon & Schuster, 1985.

22. McCrath C: Unpublished data, 1987.

23. Peterson KD: Unpublished data, 1987.

24. Sharkey BJ, Smith MH: Altitude training: Who benefits? *Phys Sports Med* 1984; 12:48.

25. *Mountaineering, The Freedom of the Hills*. Seattle, The Mountaineers, 1982.

26. Potera C: Mountain nutrition: Common sense may prevent cachexia. *Phys Sports Med* 1986; 14:233.

27. Lickteig JA: Dietary adjustments to altitude. *Sports Nutr News* 1985; 3:4.

28. Lickteig JA: Fueling winter sports. *Phys Sports Med* 1986; 14:200.

29. Guyton AC: *Human Physiology and Mechanisms of Disease*. Philadelphia, WB Saunders Co, 1987.

30. Bangs CC: Cold injuries, in *Sports Medicine*. Philadelphia, WB Saunders Co, 1984, pp 323–343.

31. Sutton JR: Heat illness, in *Sports Medicine*. Philadelphia, WB Saunders Co, 1984, pp 307–322.

32. Murphy P: Ultasports are in—in spite of injuries. *Phys Sports Med* 1986; 14:180.

33. Armstrong LE, Hubbard RW, Jones BH, et al: Preparing Alberto Salazar for the heat of the 1984 olympic marathon. *Phys Sports Med* 1986; 14:73.

34. Gisolfi CV: Temperature regulation during exercise: Directions— 1983. *Med Sci Sports Exerc* 1983; 15:15.

35. Gallagher-Allred C, Esselstein LS: *Critique of United Sciences of America.* Columbus Dietetic Association, 1986.
36. Gubernick L: Optimal health for whom? *Forbes* 1986.
37. Taylor WN: Synthetic anabolic-androgenic steroids: A plea for controlled substance status. *Phys Sports Med* 1987; 15:140.
38. Gelernter CQ: Muscle-bound for glory. *Seattle Times* 1987.
39. Groves D: The Rambo Drug. American Health, 1987, pp 43–48.
40. Chausow S: Common controversies for weight lifters. *Sports Nutr News* 1986; 5:1.
41. Worthington-Roberts B: Food faddism. *Medicine* (Baltimore) 1984; 10:7.
42. Raab CA: Vitamin and mineral supplement usage patterns and health beliefs of women. *J Am Diet Assoc* 1987; 87:775.
43. Thomsen PA, Terry RD, Amos RJ: Adolescents' beliefs about and reasons for using vitamin/mineral supplements. *J Am Diet Assoc* 1987; 87:1063.
44. Tufts University: Should you be taking fish oil supplements? 1987; 4:1.
45. Brouns F, Saris WHM, Rehrer NJ: Abdominal complaints and gastrointestinal functions during long-lasting exercise. *Int J Sports Med* 1987; 8:175.

4

Nutritional and Physical Assessment

NUTRITIONAL ASSESSMENT IN THE PHYSICAL EXAMINATION

We can quite easily spot the athlete who has clinical signs of malnutrition due to dietary excess, and it is not difficult to identify nutritional disorders such as pellagra, scurvy, or severe protein or caloric malnutrition. Other nutritional deficits, however, often present a dilemma.

Frequently, only one diagnostic method is used to determine nutritional status; it may be the only protocol where comfort of methodology exists. But the nutritional status of the athlete, let alone the group or team, cannot be assessed by using a single measuring tool, be it medical history, family history, clinical examination, dietary history, or biochemical evaluation. To perform a complete assessment,[1] one must address the following questions:

1. Is there a nutritional problem?
2. What is the magnitude of the problem?

116 *Eat to Compete: A Guide to Sports Nutrition*

3. What are the major nutritional deficits?
4. What segments of the population have already been studied so that we might apply this information to our patient?
5. Is the problem at the dietary, biochemical, or clinical level of recognition?
6. What influence will the superimposition of increased activity, growth, pregnancy, lactation, infection, trauma, and so forth have on the athlete?

It is important to remember when we refer to interpretation of data on the nutritional status of age groups, that is, the *Ten State Nutrition Survey 1968–70*[2] (TSNS), that original data were obtained from persons who are in the lowest quartile of the U.S. socioeconomic scale. Because a large percentage of athletes come from a lower economic background—athletic achievement plays a part in the American dream—the myriad of information from nutritional surveys is useful. Remember, too, that the listed criteria for the recommended dietary allowances (RDAs) meet the nutritional requirements for most healthy people.[3, 4]

There are few surveys or observations of athletes' dietary habits. Those available did not find good eating habits, even over a 4-year term. Even though observable health status in the athletic population encompasses a wide range, we are still working with a select group that, for the most part, is willing to perform tasks that require a large amount of energy. Clinical features that suggest a nutrient imbalance are outlined in Table 4–1. The practitioner should examine these signs as well as an athlete's past dietary practices regarding future health status.

In regard to the TSNS,[5] it is interesting to note that some form of pica was being ingested on a regular basis by a significant portion of the preschool and adolescent population tested, 7% had been diagnosed and were under current treatment for renal disease and allergies, and 3% had had a prior major operation. All of these conditions have potential nutritional implications.

Examination of the pediatric and adolescent medical history of children participating in the Texas nutrition survey reveals anemias, allergies, obesity, high blood pressure, and fractures.[5]

Overall, is the nutrient intake of school-aged through adolescent children adequate? If one compares the mean nutrient intake in the participants in the Texas nutrition survey and the TSNS, it appears that the answer is yes; but if one looks at the percent adequacy of the same data, there is a significant proportion of youngsters eating less than 50% of the RDAs.

How appropriate is relating the information offered in these studies to the athlete of the 1980s and 1990s? These studies were complicated and costly and will probably not be repeated for many years; however, they are all we have at present. It is logical to assume that the athletes examined (despite their higher aspirations of physical fitness) will exhibit some of the trends shown for the national averages, and these trends should be screened.

Is growth retarded among some segments of the population? Biological markers, such as the age of onset of menses or x-ray

TABLE 4–1.

Clinical Features That Suggest a Nutrient Imbalance

Clinical Signs	Possible Nutrient Imbalance	Specific Patients at Risk
Hair		
Dull, dry, brittle	Protein-calorie malnutrition	Undernourished people
	Iodine deficiency	Rare in United States today
	Selenium excess	Food faddists
Hair loss	Vitamin A excess	Patients overtreated for severe acne, food faddists
Eyes		
Night blindness	Vitamin A deficiency	Undernourished people, especially children
Optic neuritis	Vitamin B_{12} deficiency	Vegetarians
Photophobia	Vitamin A or B_{12} deficiency	
Mouth		
Inflamed, burning lips	Vitamin B_1 or B_2 deficiency	Alcoholics, generally undernourished people
Gingivitis	Vitamin A, niacin, or vitamin C deficiency	Alcoholics, elderly poor
Aphthous stomatitis	Folic acid deficiency	Patients receiving cancer chemotherapy
Pale mucosa, depapillated tongue	Iron or vitamin B_6 deficiency	Women of reproductive age, infants, patients with chronic blood loss
Painful tongue	Vitamin B_6 or niacin deficiency	Alcoholics

(Continued.)

TABLE 4–1   (cont.).

Clinical Signs	Possible Nutrient Imbalance	Specific Patients at Risk
Mottled tooth enamel	Fluoride excess	Children
Poorly formed teeth	Vitamin D deficiency	Children, especially those receiving prolonged antibiotic therapy
Skin		
Dehydration	Sodium deficiency	Patients using diuretics or vomiting
Edema	Protein deficiency	Not usual in the United States except for cachectic patients
Pallor	Iron, folic acid, or vitamin B_{12} deficiency	Women of reproductive age, vegetarians, patients with chronic blood loss
Increased yellow-orange pigmentation	Carotine excess	Food faddists
Dry, scaly, or acneiform lesions	Vitamin A or fatty acid deficiency	Dieters
Petechiae	Vitamin C deficiency	The elderly, especially those living alone; alcoholics; infants whose mothers ingested megadoses of vitamin C
Musculoskeletal system		
Weakness, fatigue	Potassium	Patients using thiazides
	Vitamin B_1 deficiency	Dieters, alcoholics
Decreased bone mass	Calcium deficiency	Postmenopausal women, patients with lactose intolerance
	Vitamin D deficiency	Patients confined indoors
Swelling of long bones	Vitamin A excess	Food faddists
Swollen, painful legs	Vitamin C deficiency	The elderly, especially those living alone; alcoholics; infants whose mothers ingested megadoses of vitamin C
Gastrointestinal system		
Bleeding	Vitamin K deficiency	Patients who avoid green, leafy vegetables
Diarrhea, flatulence	Fiber, fruit, or vitamin D excess	
	Niacin deficiency	Dieters, alcoholics
Nausea, cramps	Selenium or zinc excess	Food faddists
Neurologic system		
Ataxia	Vitamin B_{12} deficiency	Vegetarians
Dementia	Niacin deficiency	Alcoholics
Depression	Vitamin B_6 deficiency	Women using oral contraceptives
Irritability	Protein-calorie deficiency	Persons on starvation diets
	Selenium excess	Food faddists
Footdrop and wristdrop	Vitamin B_1 deficiency	Alcoholics

TABLE 4–1 (cont.).

Clinical Signs	Possible Nutrient Imbalance	Specific Patients at Risk
Peripheral neuropathy	Vitamin B$_6$ deficiency	Alcoholics
Tremor	Magnesium deficiency	Alcoholics
Metabolic system		
Obesity	Caloric excess	Common
Anemias	Iron, folic acid, or vitamin B$_{12}$ deficiency	Vegetarians, patients with chronic blood loss
Anergy	Protein deficiency	Patients with infection (rare in ambulatory patients)
Goiter	Iodine deficiency	Residents of "goiter belt" (rare in United States today)
Hypertension	Sodium excess (?)	
Siderosis	Iron excess	Transfused patients
Slow healing	Linoleic acid deficiency Zinc deficiency	Patients on fat-restricted diets
Vascular system		
Flushing, burning, and tingling in neck, face, hands	Niacin excess	Patients overtreated for hyperlipidemia

*From *Patient Care*, June 15, 1986. Used by permission.

assessment for the determination of bone maturation, are usually used. In TSNS there is an assumption of a significant degree of growth delay in Spanish-American children. Comparison of growth grids (e.g., those published by the National Centers for Disease Control) to midparent height probably give an accurate guideline for status of growth. As strange as it may seem, all growth charts and grids conclude that some segments of the population have a mild degree of growth retardation. Because nutrition is related to growth in stature, it should be apparent to the athlete-patient and physician that nutritional guidance is beneficial (Figs 4–1 and 4–2).

How specific and reliable are laboratory (biochemical values) in determination of nutritional deficiency? In many states, a preseason physical examination is mandated every 4 years, or only once during the participant's entire experience with athletics in high school. Since this is such a rapid growth period for youngsters, yearly (or even seasonal) examinations will yield more us-

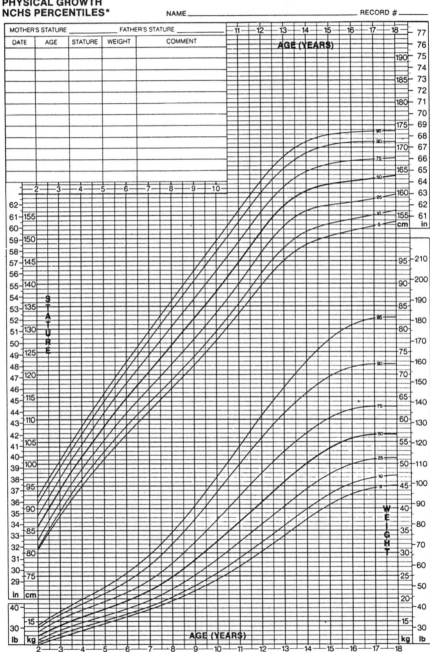

GIRLS: 2 TO 18 YEARS
PHYSICAL GROWTH
NCHS PERCENTILES*

able information. When comparing norms of values, such as iron status, keep in mind that these are presented in ranges and are for the general population.

There are numerous pitfalls on the road to completely accurate reports, according to laboratory technicians. What determines the outcome of values are methods of collection, length of time before analysis, storage and transportation, and fasting status of the patient. What is abnormal for one athlete may be normal for an entire family. And to label an athlete "at risk" usually changes dietary protocol, if not the entire medical protocol (see Appendix 6).

From an overall standpoint, the most informative way to examine the nutritional status of the young athletic population is to combine several variables into a biochemical index. Examining hemoglobin, vitamin A, serum albumin, and urinary thiamin levels and then comparing these to family income might better inform the diagnostician. At any rate, when we look at all of the data from most tables, graphs, studies, or papers, the young child and the adolescent represent an at-risk group, regardless of the factors of sex, ethnic origin, or income level.

Do medical personnel have biases when recording physical findings? Of course. As humans, we respond to the influences. Whether the investigator is obese or thin will influence the readings on the skinfold caliper or slant perspectives when he or she is called on to rate a patient as being overweight or underweight. Consider also the medical specialty. An orthopedic physician will be more interested in surgical intervention than a physical therapist who desires rehabilitation for an injury.

Duplicate findings are rare among clinicians, and as an observer becomes more accustomed to seeing a problem, such as anorexia, interpretations of severity decrease.

Perhaps one of the reasons nutritional assessment and counseling are not often available in the preseason or physical examination is that there are so many interpretations of nutritional and other data. But just as there is an improving standard in

---

FIG 4–1.
Prepubescent physical growth National Center for Health Statistics (NCHS) percentiles for girls. (From Hamill P, et al: Physical growth. National Center for Health Statistics percentiles. *Am J Clin Nutr* 1979; 32:607. Reproduced by permission.)

BOYS: 2 TO 18 YEARS
PHYSICAL GROWTH
NCHS PERCENTILES*

NAME_____ RECORD #_____

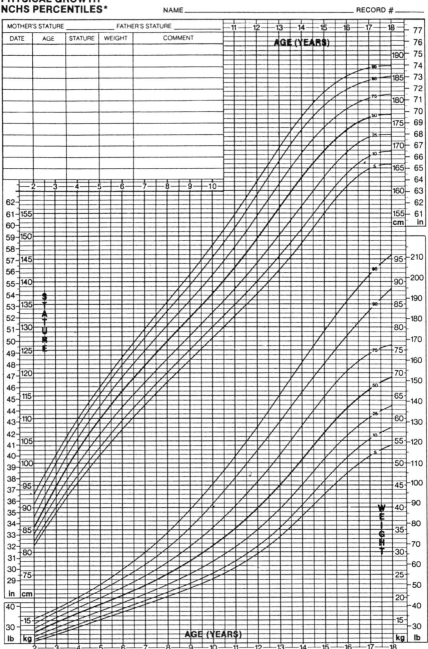

biochemical procedures, there can be standardization in clinical reporting by health personnel. Nutritional assessment within the physical examination is due to become one of the criteria for more accurate and appropriate care for the athlete.

DIETARY HISTORIES

A logical step in evaluating and prescribing diets for athletes is to refer to the 1980 recommended dietary allowances, *Food Values of Portions Commonly Used,*[6] and *Nutrition and Your Health: Dietary Guidelines for Americans.*[7] These references give current and acceptable guidelines and list nutrients generally found in specific food portions. Although they do not give exact requirements for individuals in performance modes, who may need precise adjustments in calories and fluids, they are the standards by which most diets are planned.

The prescribed diet should consider the subject's food preferences, the general pattern of eating throughout the day, and the food sources available. These suggestions can be coordinated with the reference range of nutrient intake, the total calories to be consumed, and the specific food groups from which the nutrients are to be obtained.

Determination of Individual Consumption

Four methods are commonly used to determine individual food consumption: (1) 24-hour recall; (2) food frequency questionnaire; (3) food diary; and (4) weighed food intake.

The easiest method for evaluation is the 24-hour recall. The patient is asked to recall everything eaten within the last 24 hours or the previous day. Although this may be a fairly accurate way to determine food habits of large groups (e.g., an entire team), it is less useful in dealing with an individual. When people are questioned about what they eat, they usually tend to empha-

FIG 4–2.
Physical growth National Center for Health Statistics (NCHS) percentiles for boys 2 to 18 years. (From Hamill P, et al: Physical growth. National Center for Health Statistics percentiles. *Am J Clin Nutr* 1979; 32:607. Reproduced by permission.)

size the good choices and play down the poor ones. Actually, most people cannot remember what they ate over a 5-hour period! Foods least accurately reported are vegetables, eggs, sauces, and some snack items. Often food not actually eaten is added to their lists when patients realize they have not eaten wisely.[8]

The most accurate recall intakes come from the 35- to 44-year-old group. In particular, women with families give the most factual reports. Men report somewhat higher amounts than actually eaten. Younger patients usually need help in determining their true consumption. Food models, pictures, and food games can be helpful here. Because children's attention span is so short, the 24-hour recall may be the most effective determination. This method gives the nutritionist qualitative information as well as data on the variety of foods consumed and the frequency of eating.

A food frequency questionnaire overcomes some of the weaknesses in the recall method. Measurements are made of the number of times food is consumed over a day, week, month, or longer period. The questionnaire is useful in obtaining information on food patterns and availability and food differences between individuals in the same group. Again, this method relies on the patient's memory.[9]

A selective food frequency questionnaire is useful when inquiring about certain suspect foods, such as cholesterol, other fats, sodium, iron, or calcium.

The food diary, record, or history requires the patient to write down everything he or she eats for a certain time period. The nutrient contribution for each food is calculated, and then the total day's intake for each nutrient is totaled and divided by a specified number of days to give an average daily intake. More information can be gained if the patient also notes the time, place, and people with whom he or she eats. Often the exercise pattern is combined with the food record (Table 4–2).

The most accurate estimate of food consumption is obtained by weighing and recording food intake during an experimental period. Unfortunately, this method of gathering data is time-consuming, because it requires weighing equipment as well as food. It also requires considerable discipline on the part of patients and dietary staff (patients often round off values or find other shortcuts).

Actually, a combination of all methods can be used, thus re-

TABLE 4–2.

Keeping a Daily Diet Log*

Fill out a copy of the form below each day, making sure to record everything you eat and drink. Check to see that your name is written in the upper left-hand corner of the sheet in the space provided, and write the date you complete the form in the space at right.

Name: Date:

Time of Day	Location/ Activity	Foods Eaten	Amount	Calories	Mood
Morning:					
Noon:					
Afternoon:					
Evening:					
Bedtime:					
			Total:		

*From *Patient Care*, June 15, 1986. Used by permission.

ducing the range of error expected from any one procedure. For example, a 24-hour recall can determine the usual intake. Information on the patient questionnaire can query frequency, the diet history will provide a basis for future information, and a weighed food intake can be used as a demonstration at some point during therapy (Table 4–3). Any attempt to determine food intake is also a good way to get to know a patient's lifestyle and personality.

Evaluation Methods

The simplest, fastest, yet least accurate, way to evaluate food intake data is to compare it with the four food group plan (Table 4–4). Each of the groups contain foods similar in origin and nutrient content. Nutrients named in the table are representative

TABLE 4–3.
Questionnaire

Name: _____   Birthdate: _____

M   F

1. a. On a typical work/dance day, what time do you usually get up? _____

   b. What time do you first eat or drink? _____

   c.

Time	Place (See Code)*	Typical Food and Beverage (See Code†) Amount		With Whom	Situation

   d. What time on a typical *workday* do you usually go to bed? _____

e. What is the difference in hours between the time you get up and the time you retire? _____

f. How many hours did you spend dancing? _____
   Describe the number of classes, techniques, time of day.

   _____

   _____

   _____

2. a. On a typical *non–work/dance day*, what time do you usually get up? _____

b. What time do you first eat or drink? _____

c.

Time	Place (See Code)*	Typical Food and Beverage (See Code†) Amount	With Whom	Situation

d. What time on a typical *nonworkday* do you usually go to bed? _____

(Continued.)

TABLE 4-3 (cont.).

e. What is the difference in hours between the time you get up and the time you retire? _____

f. What type of work do you try to accomplish on a *non-work/dance day?* _____

_____

_____

3. Do you take vitamin and/or mineral supplements, vitamin C supplements, or iron or calcium pills?

1. No _____

2. Yes _____   If yes:

What kind(s)	What brand(s)	How much/ many each time	How many times per day/wk/mo.	Contain how much iron	What is chemical form of iron	Contain how much vitamin C	Contain what other vitamins and minerals	Liquid or capsule	What kind of coating if tablets

4. a. Have you intentionally tried to gain or lose weight during the last 5 years:

Yes _____   No _____   If yes, how:

_____

b. Present height in stocking feet: _____ (ft & in.) _____ (cm)

c. Present weight: _____ (lb) _____ (kg)

d. Wrist measurement: _____ (in.)

5. What do you usually eat before a performance? _____

   After a performance? _____

6. Describe your favorite meal. _____

7. Describe your favorite snack. _____

8. Has any injury prevented you from dancing in the past 5 years? _____

   Please describe. _____

9. How many years have you danced? _____

10. What are your future plans? _____

11. Are there any questions you would like answered about nutrition? _____

*Place Code: H = home; B = bag lunch; FF = fast food restaurant; R = other restaurant; C = cafeteria; T = tavern or bar; VM = vending machine; Fr = friend's home.

†Beverage code: C = coffee; T = tea; Cc = cocoa; Wa = water; DD = diet drink; SD = soft drink (not diet); FJ = fruit juice; FA = fruitade; M = milk; B = beer; W = wine; L = liquor.

‡Frequency code: 1/W = once/wk; 2/W = twice/wk; 1/M = once/mo.; 2/M = twice/mo.

TABLE 4–4.

The Four Food Group Plan: The Foundation for a Good Diet*

Food Category	Examples	Recommended Daily Servings†
1. Milk and milk products‡	Milk, cheese, ice cream, sour cream, yogurt	2§
2. Meat and high protein‖	Meat, fish, poultry, eggs—with dried beans, peas, nuts, or peanut butter as alternatives	2
3. Vegetables and fruits¶	Dark green or yellow vegetables; citrus fruits or tomatoes	4
4. Cereal and grain food	Enriched breads, cereals, flour, baked goods, or whole-grain products	4

*From National Dairy Council, Rosemont, Ill.
†A basic serving of meat or fish is usually 100 gm, or 3.5 oz, of edible food; 1 cup (8 oz) of milk; 1 oz of cheese; ½ cup of fruit, vegetables, or juice; 1 slice of bread; ½ cup of cooked cereal or 1 cup of ready-to-eat cereal.
‡If large quantities of milk are normally consumed, fortified skimmed milk should be substituted to re- duce the quantity of saturated fats.
§Children, teenagers, and pregnant and nursing women need 4 servings.
‖Fish, chicken, and high-protein vegetables contain significantly less saturated fats than other protein sources.
¶One fruit or vegetable should be rich in vitamin C; at least one every other day rich in vitamin A.

of all the nutrients. The assumption is that if a certain quantity of food is consumed from each group, the diet is adequate. Ten of the designated nutrients are considered *leader nutrients,* which means if the athlete receives adequate amounts of these, the other 40 or so nutrients will also be obtained. Leader nutrients are protein, carbohydrate, fat, vitamins A and C, thiamin, ribo- flavin, niacin, calcium, and iron. Because no single food or food group supplies all the nutrients needed for good health, it is im- portant that a variety of foods from each group be consumed.

Another simple method of evaluation (and planning) uses the exchange lists (see Appendix 7). Foods that are alike are grouped together on the lists. Every food in each category has about the same amount of carbohydrate, protein, fat, and calo- ries. In the amounts given, all of the choices on each list are equal; thus, any food on a list can be exchanged, or traded, for any other food on the same list.

Food Values of Portions Commonly Used presents nutrient values of common portion sizes, according to the most recent data available from the food industry, scientific literature, and the many USDA food composition publications. This information is the basis for most computerized diet analysis systems.

The RDAs are the dietary standards accepted as the guide for planning and evaluating diets and food supplies for population groups and individuals in the United States. They are defined by the Committee on Dietary Allowances of the Food and Nutrition Board as the levels of intake of essential nutrients that are adequate for meeting the known nutritional needs of most healthy persons.

Since these values are very useful in planning diets for individuals and groups, evaluating food supplies and vitamin preparations, and predicting malnutrition, it might be assumed they are "carved in stone." But that is not so. They are simply recommendations for population groups and should be used as references only. Differences in the nutrient requirements of individuals are unknown. The RDAs are estimates that exceed the requirements of most individuals, but intakes below these recommendations are not necessarily inadequate.

Direct application of the RDAs is not without problems. For instance, statements that proclaim megause of vitamin preparations appropriate for the adolescent athlete are unfounded. Consider first the variability of nutritional components in foods and the differences in absorption in a mixed meal pattern. Then add the behavioral, cultural, and socioeconomic factors that affect the family eating pattern. Finally, examine the age categories that match adolescence with probable athletic competition.

Although we may agree that, in general, there is a great variability in nutrient composition of foods, it is very difficult for a family or individual to agree on what extent behavior has on influencing dietary intake. There are also differences of opinion as to when an adolescent first began "growing," as well as different recollections of what the child ate. The experienced parent realizes that breakfasts are sometimes skipped, sack lunches get traded, and parts of home-cooked dinners are often fed to the puppy. In these cases, the determination of nutritional intake by use of the 24-hour recall is inadequate but may, out of necessity, become part of a researcher's scientific data base.[10]

From a physician's standpoint, the preadolescent and adolescent population tends to be relatively healthy and not particularly health conscious. Few, if any, of this group volunteer for nutritional experiments, although several dietary surveys have been performed on this age over the years. Physician shy and too old for the beloved pediatrician, they may come to terms with health and dietary needs only during the back-to-school physical examination or screening. Because there are fairly reasonable data on nutrient requirements for children and adults, simple age and height-weight adjusted figures have been derived for adolescents. It makes sense, as in the case of iron, for example, to increase the RDA from 10 to 18 mg at menarche, realizing that the requirement does not jump overnight or that, in the case of athletes, menarche may not begin until well after athletic competition ceases. Therefore, consider the RDAs as judgment figures with built-in safety factors, know that they will change over time, and know that there will be a great deal of controversy about them, even among the Committee on Dietary Allowances. Remember that some of the essential nutrients do not have established RDA values and that there is the question of unknown nutrient requirements.

The RDA values have their greatest usefulness in planning diets for groups. For the sake of convenience, they are given in average daily figures, which allow flexibility in the span over which they are averaged, to allow for individuals' variable eating patterns. Thus, the megadose, promoted as optimizing nutritional status (the manufacturer's answer to an adolescent's poor eating habits) does not ensure better performance.

Computerized Dietary Analysis

Dietary calculations can be time-consuming and tedious. With computer assistance, though, analysis can be accomplished quickly. Selection of a computerized diet analysis system should include considerations of present and future needs, accuracy, efficiency, and cost effectiveness.

Data Base.—The data base must be accurate, verifiable, and large enough to meet the user's needs. Input nutrient values must be identified or documented and comparable with the RDAs, USDA handbooks 8–1 through 8–5, and include values of supplements and popular fast-food restaurant items. Provisions for routine updates and the addition or deletion of food and recipe items must exist. Another consideration should be whether the system can interact with other systems and can convert to international measurements.

Ease of Use.—Entering food items by code takes time and can be a potential source of error. Systems that allow data entry by food name allow greater accuracy and understanding and decrease entry time.

Printout.—The printout needs to be clear and understandable. A food-by-food nutrient listing; total nutrient summary; or values, options, or recommendations (such as percent of total calories from complex carbohydrate or milligrams of iron) need to be available.

Costs.—This consideration is probably why so few computer programs are available in consulting offices. Overall, the cost will be determined by the system chosen; however, there are several alternatives to weigh: purchasing a complete system, leasing, time-sharing, batching, or accessing a mainframe (e.g., one owned and operated by a university or hospital).

Leasing allows the user to update without repurchasing. Often the hardware can be leased through a software outlet. Time-sharing allows several users independent opportunities for access to the technology. Drawbacks include scheduling time allotment and expense sharing. Some organizations, such as the National Dairy Council, promote batching.

The patient keeps dietary records that are then mailed, analyzed, and returned within a certain time period. Weaknesses of the time-sharing procedure include time lag and misunderstandings when the patient records incorrectly. Another option is to hire a computer technician with nutritional experience who will assist in gathering information, analyzing it, and assisting during the counseling session when data are presented.

Other costs include insurance, maintenance, installation fees, updates of the nutrient data base, optional equipment, and training.

Time Savings.—Accuracy and speed are the chief benefits of computerized analysis.

Although the personal care and response of the counselor can never be replaced with hardware, dietary analysis systems are here to stay.[11]

NUTRITIONAL AND PHYSICAL ASSESSMENT

Within the past decade there has been a tremendous growth of interest in nutritional status in athletes and in the development of methods to assess it. Along with the physical and biochemical status, anthropometry provides a clinically relevant picture. The sports medicine health provider has taken anthropometry many steps beyond the measurement of growth and development of infants, children, adolescents, and pregnant women, bringing it into a field where reliable diet and exercise prescriptions are made.

Height and Weight

Height and weight are still the most common measurements made, but because their significance is not fully appreciated, they are frequently gauged inconsistently and recorded improperly. These dimensions should be growth gridded and kept for reference. For example, attention to growth potential would make the wrestling coach's decision on weight placement much easier.

To determine height, ask the individual to stand erect, without shoes, and look straight ahead. Lower a horizontal bar, rectangular block (or book), or the top of the statiometer to rest flat on the top of the head. Read height to the nearest 1/4 in., or 0.5 cm. To best determine weight, weigh the individual on a beam balance scale that has been calibrated. If possible, weigh him or her before breakfast, wearing lightweight clothing, and after the bladder has been emptied. Record weight to the nearest 1/2 lb, or 500 gm.

Height and weight can then be compared with growth grids or tables. The most commonly used standards are from the Metropolitan Life Insurance Company (Table 4–5). A revised version, which has taken the subject out of shoes and clothing, is found in Table 4–6. There are problems involved in determining appropriate body weight with these tables. Because weight ranges reflect only the weights of insured persons with lowest mortality, they do not show optimal weight for height for individual health.

Frame size determinations are used in some height and weight tables for determination of ideal or desirable weight (Fig 4–3; Tables 4–7 and 4–8).

TABLE 4–5.

Desirable Weight Ranges—Age 25 and Over*†

Height (ft, in.)	Men		Women‡	
	Weight Range	Weight§ MRW = 100	Weight Range	Weight§ MRW = 100
4 9			90–118	100
4 10			92–121	103
4 11			95–124	106
5 0			98–127	109
5 1	105–134	117	101–130	112
5 2	108–137	120	104–134	116
5 3	111–141	123	107–138	120
5 4	114–145	126	110–142	124
5 5	117–149	129	114–146	128
5 6	121–154	133	118–150	132
5 7	125–159	138	122–154	136
5 8	129–163	142	126–159	140
5 9	133–167	146	130–164	144
5 10	137–172	150	134–169	148
5 11	141–177	155		
6 0	145–182	159		
6 1	149–187	164		
6 2	153–192	169		
6 3	157–197	174		

*Revised from 1959 Metropolitan Life Insurance Company data that appeared in Simopoulos AP: Dietary control of hypertension and obesity and body weight standards. *J Am Diet Assoc* 1985; 85:419.
†Weight in pounds, without clothing; height without shoes.
‡For women between the ages of 18 and 25, subtract 1 lb for each year under 25.
§Midpoint of medium frame range used to compute MRW: MRW = [(actual weight)/(midpoint of medium frame range)] × 100.

TABLE 4–6.

Height and Weight Standards for Adults*

Ft.	In.	Small Frame	Medium Frame	Large Frame
		Men (in indoor clothing)†		
5	1	112–120	118–129	126–141
5	2	115–123	121–133	129–144
5	3	118–126	124–136	132–148
5	4	121–129	127–139	135–152
5	5	124–133	130–143	138–156
5	6	128–137	134–147	142–161
5	7	132–141	138–152	147–166
5	8	136–145	142–156	151–170
5	9	140–150	146–160	155–174
5	10	144–154	150–165	159–179
5	11	148–158	154–170	164–184
6	0	152–162	158–175	168–189
6	1	156–167	162–180	173–194
6	2	160–171	167–185	178–199
6	3	164–175	172–190	182–204
		Women (in indoor clothing)†		
4	8	92–98	96–107	104–119
4	9	94–101	98–110	106–122
4	10	96–104	101–113	109–125
4	11	99–107	104–116	112–128
5	0	102–110	107–119	115–131
5	1	105–113	110–122	118–134
5	2	108–116	113–126	121–138
5	3	111–119	116–130	125–142
5	4	114–123	120–135	129–146
5	5	118–127	124–139	133–150
5	6	122–131	128–143	137–154
5	7	126–135	132–147	141–158
5	8	130–140	136–151	145–163
5	9	134–144	140–155	149–168
5	10	138–148	144–159	153–173

*These tables correct the 1959 Metropolitan Life Insurance Company standards to height without shoe heels.
†Clothing is shorts and T-shirt or examination gown.

In the U.S. Health and Nutrition Survey of 1971–1974 (HANES) a classification of body frame size was developed using elbow breadth. Elbow breadth is reported to be a reliable indicator of frame size not affected by obesity or greatly affected by age. This method is used:

Body Frame Type

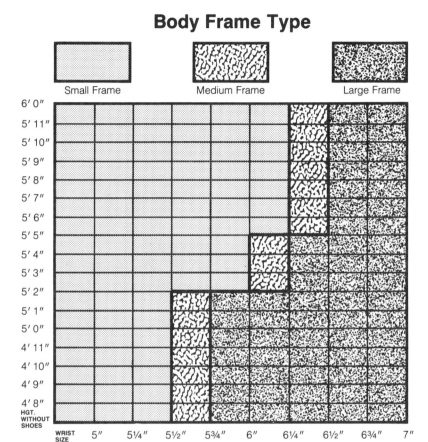

The wrist is measured distal to styloid process of radius and ulna at smallest circumference. Use height without shoes and inches for wrist size to determine frame type from this chart.

FIG 4–3.
Lindner has developed a chart for estimating frame size using wrist circumference and height. (1) select subject's right wrist for measurement. (2) place measuring tape around smallest part of wrist distal to the styloid process of radius and ulna. (3) using height and wrist circumference, refer to body frame type chart. (Redrawn from Lindner P, Linder D: How to Assess Degrees of Fatness. Cambridge, Md, Cambridge Scientific Industries, 1973.)

1. Have subject extend his or her right arm in front and bend the forearm upward at a 90-degree angle. The inside of the wrist should face the body.

TABLE 4–7.

Elbow Breadth for Men With Medium Frame Size*†

Height‡	Height‡ (cm)	Elbow Breadth (in.)	Elbow Breadth (mm)
5 ft 1 in.–5 ft 2 in.	155.0–157.5	2½–2⅞	63.5–73.0
5 ft 3 in.–5 ft 6 in.	160.0–167.6	2⅝–2⅞	66.7–73.0
5 ft 7 in.–5 ft 10 in.	170.2–177.8	2¾–3	69.8–76.2
5 ft 11 in.–6 ft 2 in.	180.3–188.0	2¾–3⅛	69.8–79.4
6 ft 3 in.	190.5	2⅞–3¼	73.0–82.5

*Adapted from the Metropolitan Life Insurance Company, New York.
†Larger values indicate a large frame; smaller values indicate a small frame.
‡Without shoe heels.

TABLE 4–8.

Elbow Breadth for Women With Medium Frame Size*†

Height‡	Height‡ (cm)	Elbow Breadth (in.)	Elbow Breadth (mm)
4 ft 9 in.–4 ft 10 in.	144.8–147.3	2¼–2½	57.1–63.5
4 ft 11 in.–5 ft 2 in.	150.0–157.0	2¼–2½	57.1–63.5
5 ft 3 in.–5 ft 6 in.	160.0–167.6	2⅜–2⅝	60.3–66.7
5 ft 7 in.–5 ft 10 in.	170.1–177.8	2⅜–2⅝	60.3–66.7
5 ft 11 in.	180.3	2½–2¾	63.5–69.8

*Adapted from the Metropolitan Life Insurance Company, New York.
†Larger values indicate a large frame; smaller values indicate a small frame.
‡Without shoe heels.

2. Place thumb and index finger of one hand on the two prominent bones on either side of the subject's elbow, and measure the distance between them (in inches) with a ruler or tape measure.

Body mass index is another method for determining appropriate weight. This index divides weight in kilograms by height in meters squared and correlates well with skinfold measurements. For example, a woman 5 ft 4 in. tall and weighing 110 lb would be considered obese if the index was higher than 24.7 and considered underweight if the index was lower than 19.0. A nomogram for easier calculation is presented in Fig 4–4.

Body Mass Index

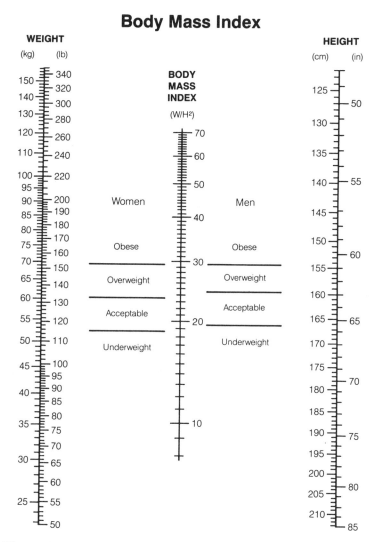

When a rule is aligned at the weight and height values, the point where it intersects the scale in the middle gives the body mass index.

FIG 4–4.

The body weights associated with a body mass index (BMI) of 20 to 25 kg/sq m show little or no increased risk of cardiovascular disease, gallbladder disease, hypertension, or diabetes. When the BMI is less than 20 kg/sq m, individuals have increased risk for respiratory disease, digestive disease, and metabolic complications. Individuals with a BMI of 25 to 30 kg/sq m have low risk, those with a BMI between 30 and 40 kg/sq m have moderate risk, and those with a BMI more than 40 kg/sq m are at high risk. (Redrawn from Bray GA: Complications of obesity. *Ann Intern Med* 1985; 103:1052–1062; 1985; Bray GA: *The Obese Patient.* Philadelphia, WB Saunders Co, 1976.)

Body Composition

Fat is a primary structural component of the human body and is present in every healthy person. Minimal amounts of fat, called *essential fat,* are required for anatomical and physiological functions. Approximately 3% of men's body mass is essential fat; women need the same minimum plus an additional 5% to 9% of sex-specific fat.

At birth, the human body is approximately 12% fat, and this percentage increases and decreases throughout life, depending on maturation and physical activities. Desirable percentages of body fat are approximately 13% to 18% for males and 18% to 24% for females. Certainly there is a wide range of acceptability in these percentages (Table 4–9); this is evident in examining existing ranges of body composition of athletes by sport. In general, it is better to assume that most athletes will perform best if their percentages of fat are within this range of acceptability rather than to assign ideal values.

A number of body fat studies have been done on athletes, and the results give body fat values that differ both between sports and within sports. The body fat values for male and female athletes in various sports are given in Table 4–10.

According to Wilmore, there is not a single value for body fat for all athletes or even for all athletes of a given sex or in a given sport.[12] Minimum body fat levels are 7% for males and 12% for females. As previously mentioned, a general recommendation is 15% to 18% body fat for males and 18% to 24% body fat for females. The well-conditioned male and female athlete will have values slightly lower than these recommendations.

There are three methods commonly used to determine per-

TABLE 4–9.

Percent Body Fat Standards*

	Lean	Healthy	Plump	Fat	Obese
Male	<10	10–14	15–20	21–26	>26
Female	<15	16–20	21–26	27–33	>33

*Adapted from Wilmore JH: *Sensible Fitness.* Champaign, Ill, Human Kinetics Publishing Co, 1986.

TABLE 4–10.

Body Fat Values for Males and Females in
Various Sports

Athletic Group or Sport	Body Fat (%)	
	Males	Females
Baseball	10–15	
Basketball	7–12	18–27
Canoeing	10–14	
Football	8–18	
Gymnastics	3–6	8–18
Ice hockey	12–16	
Jockeys	6–16	
Skiing		
Alpine	10–17	
Cross-country	7–13	18–24
Nordic	8–14	
Ski-jumping	12–16	
Soccer	7–12	
Speed skating	8–14	
Swimming	4–10	12–20
Track and field		
Runners	4–12	8–18
Jumpers/hurdlers		12–22
Discus	12–18	22–28
Shot put	14–20	23–30
Tennis	12–16	
Volleyball		20–23
Weight lifting	6–16	
Wrestling	6–12	

*Adapted from Wilmore JH: *The Wilmore Fitness Program.* New York, Simon & Schuster, 1981, and Wilmore JH: Body composition in sports and exercise: Directions for future research. *Med Sci Sports Exercise* 1983; 15:23–24.

centage of body fat: (1) hydrostatic weighing, (2) skinfold measurement, and (3) electrical impedance. It is well to remember, however, that they are approximations, since they rely on indirect measurements. Actual body fat percentage can be derived only through an autopsy.

The traditional method, hydrostatic weighing,[13] involves being weighed under water. While completely submerged in a tank, subjects are repeatedly weighed, and the results are compared (using a formula) to normal scale weight. Because fat is more buoyant than muscle or bone, body density can be calculated using Archimedes' principle. This may be the most accurate method. There are still controversies about the number of cadavers used as references and the formulas used to determine residual lung volumes and expiratory reserve volumes. Hydrostatic weighing usually is expensive compared with other clinical methods, and accuracy depends largely on the skill of the technician and the cooperation of the subject. This method is referred to extensively in the literature; patients or teams enjoy comparing their results with studies or the often quoted figures of prominent athletes.

Another commonly used technique is the skinfold measurement.[13] The measurement of the thickness of skin in several locations on the body is compared with one of many formulas, or nomographs, and an approximation of the percentage of body fatness is then made. The formulas assume that fat under the skin is proportional to fat stored around body organs. The reliability of this method is probably in direct ratio to the experience of the technician administering it. Because the amount of fat located subcutaneously varies with age and sex, it is important that tables used to evaluate skinfold measurements are age and sex appropriate (Tables 4–11 to 4–13). The apparatus used for skinfold measurement is portable, safe, convenient, low cost, and reproducible.

A third technique involves a recent development, electrical impedance. Electrodes are attached to the foot and hand, and a mild electric current is passed between them. Determination of

TABLE 4–11.

Skinfold Measurement Instruction*

Subscapular:	A fold taken on a diagonal line coming from the vertebral border to 0.4 to 0.8 in. (1–2 cm) from the inferior angle of the scapula (a diagonal fold just below the lowest border of the scapula)
Triceps:	A vertical fold on the posterior midline of the upper arm (over the triceps muscle), halfway between the acromion and olecranon processes, with the elbow in an extended, relaxed position
Biceps:	A vertical fold on the anterior midline of the upper arm (over the biceps muscle)
Iliac crest:	A diagonal fold above the crest of the ilium at the spot where an imaginary line would come down from the anterior axillary line

*From Cambridge Scientific Industries, Cambridge, Md.

TABLE 4–12.

An Example of Skinfold Measurements*

Name <u>Jane Doe</u> Age <u>18</u> Sex <u>F</u>

Measurements

   Present body weight (BW) <u>140 lb</u>   Body fat percentage <u>26.5%</u> (see Table 4–13)

   Triceps <u>17 mm</u>   Total body fat (TBF) <u>37 lb</u> (BW × percent)

   Biceps <u>4 mm</u>   Lean body weight (LBW) <u>103 lb</u> (BW − TBF)

   Subscapular <u>15 mm</u>   Ideal body fat (IBF) <u>18%</u> (18%–24%)

   Iliac crest <u>20 mm</u>   Ideal body weight (IBW) <u>128 lb</u>

   Total <u>56 mm</u>

*If 26.5% TBF weighs 37 lb, 18% TBF will weigh 25 lb. Add 25 lb to 103 lb to calculate approximate IBW.

percentage of fat is based on the rate of electrical resistance. This is a quick, clean, safe, and easy method; however, results vary, depending on the patient's hydration status.[14] The equipment used is very expensive. Although it extrapolates lean body weight by formulas (as does hydrostatic weighing), this method has received a favorable response in research fields.

To identify the percentage of body fat:

1. Select a technique for determining body fat.
2. Set an acceptable range of fat values, depending on age, sex, and sport. Consider the athlete's performance in previous years and his or her growth stages. Allow for individual differences and errors in the techniques used.
3. Measure the athlete, calculate the percent of body fat, and recommend the acceptable range. If the percentage does not seem reasonable, use another formula or method to make the determination.

Then, set up a diet and exercise program to achieve the goals and desired range of percent fat and weight. It is important to allow time to make changes. Once an athlete is losing through a

TABLE 4–13.

Percentage of Body Fat Based on Four Skinfold Measurements*†

Skinfolds (mm)	Males (Age in yr)				Females (Age in yr)			
	17–29	30–39	40–49	50+	16–29	30–39	40–49	50+
15	4.8	—	—	—	10.5	—	—	—
20	8.1	12.2	12.2	12.6	14.1	17.0	19.8	21.4
25	10.5	14.2	15.0	15.6	16.8	19.4	22.2	24.0
30	12.9	16.2	17.7	18.6	19.5	21.8	24.5	26.6
35	14.7	17.7	19.6	20.8	21.5	23.7	26.4	28.5
40	16.4	19.2	21.4	22.9	23.4	25.5	28.2	30.3
45	17.7	20.4	23.0	24.7	25.0	26.9	29.6	31.9
50	19.0	21.5	24.6	26.5	26.5	28.2	31.0	33.4
55	20.1	22.5	25.9	27.9	27.8	29.4	32.1	34.6
60	21.2	23.5	27.1	29.2	29.1	30.6	33.2	35.7
65	22.2	24.3	28.2	30.4	30.2	31.6	34.1	36.7
70	23.1	25.1	29.3	31.6	31.2	32.5	35.0	37.7
75	24.0	25.9	30.3	32.7	32.2	33.4	35.9	38.7
80	24.8	26.6	31.2	33.8	33.1	34.3	36.7	39.6
85	25.5	27.2	32.1	34.8	34.0	35.1	37.5	40.4
90	26.2	27.8	33.0	35.8	34.8	35.8	38.3	41.2
95	26.9	28.4	33.7	36.6	35.6	36.5	39.0	41.9
100	27.6	29.0	34.4	37.4	36.4	37.2	39.7	42.6
105	28.2	29.6	35.1	38.2	37.1	37.9	40.4	43.3
110	28.8	30.1	35.8	39.0	37.8	38.6	41.0	43.9
115	29.4	30.6	36.4	39.7	38.4	39.1	41.5	44.5
120	30.0	31.1	37.0	40.4	39.0	39.6	42.0	45.1
125	30.5	31.5	37.6	41.1	39.6	40.1	42.5	45.7
130	31.0	31.9	38.2	41.8	40.2	40.6	43.0	46.2
135	31.5	32.3	38.7	42.4	40.8	41.1	43.5	46.7
140	32.0	32.7	39.2	43.0	41.3	41.6	44.0	47.2
145	32.5	33.1	39.7	43.6	41.8	42.1	44.5	47.7
150	32.9	33.5	40.2	44.1	42.3	42.6	45.0	48.2
155	33.3	33.9	40.7	44.6	42.8	43.1	45.4	48.7
160	33.7	34.3	41.2	45.1	43.3	43.6	45.8	49.2
165	34.1	34.6	41.6	45.6	43.7	44.0	46.2	49.6
170	34.5	34.8	42.0	46.1	44.1	44.4	46.6	50.0
175	34.9	—	—	—	—	44.8	47.0	50.4
180	35.3	—	—	—	—	45.2	47.4	50.8
185	35.6	—	—	—	—	45.6	47.8	51.2
190	35.9	—	—	—	—	45.9	48.2	51.6
195	—	—	—	—	—	46.2	48.5	52.0
200	—	—	—	—	—	46.5	48.8	52.4
205	—	—	—	—	—	—	49.1	52.7
210	—	—	—	—	—	—	49.4	53.0

*From Durnin JVGA, Wormersley J: Body fat assessed from total body density and its estimation from skinfold thickness: Measurements on 481 men and women aged from 16–72 years. *Br J Nutr* 1974; 32:77.

†Measurements made on the right side of the body using biceps, triceps, subscapular, and suprailiac skinfolds.

program, estimate body fat periodically. Because muscle weighs more than fat, the body weight may not change as much as expected.

The three methods mentioned compare favorably. In a recent class of 140 individuals, fat values varied within a range of 3% to 5%. Greatest variability in results was attributed to actual degree of fatness, amount of obesity, and sex (female). Any instructor or diagnostician should feel comfortable in using any or all of these techniques to inform individuals of body fat status.

There are many other methods: circumference measurements, total body potassium, nuclear magnetic resonance imagery, total body nitrogen, neutron activation analysis, ultrasound, and tritiated water. Each has advantages and disadvantages.[15-22] Two difficulties are cost and the training necessary to make a decision that will still have built-in error.

There are also two other ways, of course. One is the objective, visual appraisal of muscle and fatness. Interestingly enough, most trained technicians have the experience to estimate within 3% to 5% of actual values, reliable enough to meet standards. The other is performance records, which can be used to determine the best body weight for a given athlete.

Methodology for measurement is given in detail in *Exercise Physiology*,[13] *Body Composition Assessments in Youth and Adults*,[23] and *Sports Nutrition: A Guide for the Professional Working With Active People*.[19] Computer software as well as a videotape written by Timothy G. Lohman for measuring body fat for children is available from Human Kinetics Publishers, Champaign, Illinois.

Body fat is very personal data, and I strongly recommend that this information be presented discreetly.

REFERENCES

1. Pre-season exam protocol for the Seattle Mariners, Seattle Pacific University, elite and adolescent athlete. Sports Medicine Clinic, Seattle.
2. Centers for Disease Control: *Ten State Nutritional Survey 1968–70.* DHEW Publication no (HSM) 72-8131. Atlanta, 1972.
3. *Recommended Dietary Allowances,* rev. Washington, DC, Food and

Nutrition Board, National Academy of Sciences–National Research Council, 1980.

4. Herbert V, Olson JA: Recommended dietary intakes of—folate vitamin B-12, iron, vitamin K, C and A—in humans. *Am J Clin Nutr* 1987; 45:661.

5. McGanity WJ: Nutrition survey in Texas. *Tex Med* 1969; 65:40.

6. Pennington JAT, Church HN: *Food Values of Portions Commonly Used*, ed 14. New York, Harper & Row, 1985.

7. *Nutrition and Your Health: Dietary Guidelines for Americans.* Washington DC, US Department of Agriculture and Health and Human Services, 1980.

8. Karvetti R, Knuts L: Validity of the 24-hour dietary recall. *J Am Diet Assoc* 1985; 85:1437.

9. Willet WC, Reynolds RD, Cottrell-Hoehner S, et al: Validation of a semi-quantitative food frequency questionnaire: Comparison with a 1-year diet record. *J Am Diet Assoc* 1987; 87:43.

10. Ferris RP, Frank GC, Webber LS, et al: A group method for obtaining dietary recalls of children. *J Am Diet Assoc* 1985; 85:1315.

11. Krause MV, Mahan K: *Food, Nutrition, and Diet Therapy.* Philadelphia, WB Saunders Co, 1984.

12. Wilmore JH: *The Wilmore Fitness Program.* New York, Simon & Schuster, 1981.

13. McArdle WD, Katch FI, Katch VL: *Exercise Physiology.* Philadelphia, Lea & Febiger, 1986.

14. Van Itallie TB, Segal KR, Yang M, et al: Clinical assessment of body fat content in adults: Potential role of electrical impedance methods, in Roche AF (ed): *Body Composition Assessments in Youth and Adults.* Report of the Sixth Ross Conference on Medical Research, Columbus, Ohio, Ross Laboratories, 1984.

15. Timson BF, Coffman JL: Body composition by hydrostatis weighing at total lung capacity and residual volume. *Med Sci Sports Exerc* 1984; 16:411.

16. Thorland WG, Johnson GO, Tharp GD, et al: Validity of anthropometric equations for the estimation of body density in adolescent athletes. *Med Sci Sports Exerc* 1984; 16:77.

17. Lohman TG, Pollock ML, Brandon LJ, et al: Methodological factors and the prediction of body fat in female athletes. *Med Sci Sports Exerc* 1984; 16:92.

18. Katch FI, Behnke AR: Arm x-ray assessment of percent body fat in men and women. *Med Sci Sports Exerc* 1984; 16:316.

19. Sports and Cardiovascular Nutritionists, American Dietetic Association: *Sports Nutrition: A Guide for the Professional Working With Active People.* Chicago, American Dietetic Association, 1987.

20. Volz PA, Ostrove SM: Evaluation of a portable ultrasonoscope in assessing the body composition of college-age women. *Med Sci Sports Exerc* 1984; 16:102.
21. Hudash G, Albright JP, McAuley E, et al: Cross-sectional thigh components: Computerized tomographic assessment. *Med Sci Sports Exerc* 1985; 17:417.
22. Wilmore JH: Body composition in sport and exercise: Directions for future research. *Med Sci Sports Exerc* 1983; 15:21.
23. Roche AF: *Body Composition Assessments in Youth and Adults.* Report of the Sixth Ross Conference on Medical Research, Columbus, Ohio, Ross Laboratories, 1984.

5

Protocols for Developing Diets and Meal Plans

Diet is important. The athlete's nutrient intake must supply calories to cover basal metabolic requirements, exercise needs, and, in most cases, growth demands. In general, experimental studies conclude that athletes require more fluids, and diet adjustments may need to be made in vitamin and mineral content and in amounts of protein and carbohydrate. A balanced diet, consisting of a wide variety of foods, applies to any phase or condition of an athlete's life: fast growth, injury, chronic or acute illness, pregnancy, lactation, aging, training, or participation.[1]

With these straightforward facts, it would seem a simple matter to construct diets that will meet athletes' nutritional needs, even on an individual basis. (Appendix 2 emphasizes the importance of increasing calories when energy demands rise.) However, that is usually not the case. Most coaches, trainers, and athletes believe that nutrition is important. Yet, examinations of large numbers of athletes' diets reveal that most do not even approach 75% of the recommended dietary allowances (RDAs) for nutrients or calories.[2] It may be the case that even with dietary knowledge, athletic management is so complicated that it is difficult to find the right foods at convenient times. Or, even worse, the accumulated evidence is not reaching the coach and athlete in an understandable form. In surveys conducted to help identify the differences between what is known and what is practiced, results indicate that most elite athletes believe that performance is improved by high-protein diets, that athletes require larger amounts of vitamins than nonathletes, and that nonfood products may provide benefits in performance. This is the very information dietitians have been trying to suppress for many years! Or, it just might be, in the face of all the unknowns regarding performance, that diet may be the scapegoat, and that there will always be a search for the magic food, as there is for the magic training method, that will help athletes win.

If we as health professionals have identified the nutrients that will have positive benefits on performance, and if we also know that not all athletes are following these recommendations, then this alone is rationale for change.[3, 4]

The nutritional status of the athlete is a long-term event, and change in nutritional status is a long-term event. For example, hemoglobin levels do not improve overnight; body fat is not lost instantly; lipid profiles cannot be lowered in 1 day; bone mineralization does not occur in 1 mile's walk. The athlete cannot immediately change nutritional status with a pill, for instance, just as he or she cannot adapt immediately to a specific mode of training. Still, many of the athlete's greatest concerns can be addressed by wise food selection directly before, during, and after the competitive event. Adequate hydration before and during events, a diet that emphasizes carbohydrate, and appropriate precompetition meals are three examples of alterations that will aid in maximizing performance.

Any change in behavior takes longer than we think it will, and athletes do not have much time. In addition, there is the ever-present condition of pressure. There is an incredible amount of suppressed stress in athletics, and food helps us cope with stress. It is difficult to reprogram attitudes, and all learned behavior associated with food is taught at an early age. The initiator of change must often bombard the athlete with facts and advice to break into food behavior patterns. The new information may not take hold, because the acceptance factor of any diet regimen is based on what works and who else is doing it.

To help eliminate the bias of individual testimony, each athlete should think in investigative terms of diet for performance. He or she will need help to interpret research or advice, outline a procedure and follow it, keep records of food intake and activity, and review any changes or benefits that might occur, keeping in mind alternative food behaviors that might also have the same effects. A recommended change may be as simple as increasing fluids during practice.

The sequence of change begins with an internal desire for change. After that comes self-awareness, self-encouragement, and monitoring:

Example: "During spring football, I tire easily toward the end of practice and quite often feel nauseous."

Hypothesis: "I'll feel better during exercise if I drink water every 15 minutes during practice."

Procedure: Weigh on locker room scales before and after practice. Weight loss in pounds equals volume of fluids lost from the body during practice. If weight loss equals 2 lb, that amount of fluid, or approximately 32 oz (2 pints) of water, should be available to drink at intervals during practice. Keeping track of environmental as well as rectal temperature would be useful information, as well as recording practice intensity. If the athlete's exhaustion diminishes, it may have been a straightforward example of dehydration. If exhaustion continues, other causes should be examined. Quality of the diet, no breakfast, anemia, or even psychological factors may be contributing to exhaustion.

Self-awareness must follow desire for change. Diet is an individual matter, and the athlete must be aware that it often takes a trial period of several days (e.g., increasing carbohydrates) to several months (e.g., weight loss) to test the success or failure of change. Athletes may attribute any variation in diet to an increased ability to win. The novelty factor alone can temporarily optimize performance. Hence, it is vital to test and retest in practice situations before relying on any diet modification in competition. Determine the realistic expectations of any change.

Example: "I have been eating a high-carbohydrate meal (breakfast: bran cereal with homogenized milk, wheat toast with butter) before running cross-country, but I always have to stop to go to the bathroom about 30 minutes into competition, and sometimes I cramp up."

Hypothesis: "If I cut down on the fiber content of the preevent meal, I can still keep the carbohydrate content high and I won't cramp."

Procedure: Experiment with other forms of carbohydrate, such as glucose polymers, 5% glucose solutions, baby food cereals, or other refined cereals. Determine the amount of fat eaten in combination with the carbohydrate, and substitute a food with a lower fat content. (An oat cereal with skim milk and one half of a banana will have the same amount of carbohydrate and clear the stomach faster.) Most athletes have similar needs in the same type of competition, but what works for one may not work for another. In this case, if lowering the fat and fiber content does not prevent cramping and the need to have a bowel movement, glucose solutions might help. Otherwise, eating the high-carbohydrate meal the evening before or investigating other causes of cramping, such as the calcium or sodium content of the meal, may help.

Self-encouragement thrives on outside help. Remind the athlete often that logical diet practices are based on scientific examination. Again, pose the question, determine and follow a plan, keep good records, investigate alternatives, and then set up individual strategy.

Example: "There are no fast-food restaurants near the playing field, and I won't have time to take the team to a good restaurant. My kids have been in school all day, and they will be starving by game time."

Hypothesis: "My players rely on the preevent meal to relax, and they need extra calories to play the game."

Procedure: Ask the parents to pack a specific type of sack lunch for each team member, or ask several mothers to supply food for each road trip (turkey sandwiches, oatmeal cookies, and enough lemonade for the bus trip as well as during the game). Stop at the local pizza parlor on the way home.

The fourth component of change consists of monitoring. Watching the care and feeding of the athlete includes being receptive to new ideas, being willing to break tradition and accept the diverse needs of the players, and encouraging players and staff to share information and reactions.

PLAN DEVELOPMENT

During the course of a lifetime, athletes' nutritional status and needs change. Their nutrient needs reflect who they are and what they hope to do with their bodies. The care process, or the plan, involves the assessment of an individual's health status, identifying needs, planning objectives to meet these needs (activities or education), and, finally, evaluating. These are very similar to the steps in any educational process.

Nutritional care for the healthy young athlete may be the assessment of health status and encouragement to continue the good work, plus any additional information that will be helpful for the season ahead, such as the fluid or energy requirements of the sport. One of the reasons for the frequency of food-related problems in athletics is that no one health professional takes complete responsibility for the nutritional care of the athlete until he or she becomes a patient. With so many disciplines involved in nutrition, it might be well to form a team that can capitalize on each member's expertise or to at least document a nutritional care plan or process that will be available to all.

After the physical evaluation, a plan that will be acceptable to the athlete and that will deal with any of the problems identified needs to be formulated. Regardless of time allowances or personnel involved, the plan should be realistic, taking into consideration the educational level of the individual and the economic resources of the family.

IMPLEMENTATION OF INDIVIDUAL NUTRITION CARE

This part of the plan involves a meeting between nutritionist and athlete and includes a discussion of all activities or interventions that will help the athlete: the diet prescription; counseling and education; discussion of food, vitamin, and mineral supplementations; and other advice or additional activities.[5]

The first meeting should include a review of the dietary questionnaire, laboratory findings, and any medical problems related to food intake. The individual diet will be a modification of an adequate diet pattern appropriate for the athlete's age group.[6] Guidelines for selecting and planning menus and nutrient levels are based on the basic food groups and the RDAs. The diet should vary as little as possible from the individual's normal diet, unless it is inadequate. The diet needs to meet the athlete's requirements for essential nutrients. The regimen should take into account the athlete's habits, food preferences, economic status, and religious practices and environmental factors (where meals are eaten and who prepares them).

The diet prescription designates the amounts, frequency, variety, and quality, plus amounts and forms of protein, fat, carbohydrate, minerals and vitamins, and other concerns (e.g., fiber and fluids). In this chapter, the dietary exchange system is used in planning diets, whether the purpose is gaining or losing weight, increasing carbohydrate, or planning the preevent meal.

Energy Requirements

Appetite cannot regulate the required energy demands of athletics. There is no way the hypothalamus can predict the requirements of an endurance event like the Ironman. It is necessary to calculate energy needs to maintain body weight. In some cases, actual measurement for basal, or resting, metabolic rates (BMRs) is useful.

Once a range of ideal body weight has been determined, a daily caloric level that covers BMR, growth requirements, and the additional demands of muscle activity can be set. (The BMR is the least amount of energy required to maintain vital functions at rest and varies with weight, height, sex, age, and environment.) The number of calories expended in addition to the BMR is also dependent on body size and other physical factors. For example, an individual involved in light activity spends an additional 40% of calories; moderate activity, 60%; and heavy activity, 100%. Tables 5–1 to 5–3 are examples of calculating energy demands.

There are minor differences in these calculations. It is well

TABLE 5–1.

Food and Nutrition Board, National Research Council Method*

Activity	Men	Women
Very light	1.5†	1.3
Light	2.9	2.6
Moderate	4.3	4.1
Heavy	8.4	8.0

*Sleeping time $= BMR \times 0.9 \times \dfrac{\text{hours slept}}{24}$

†kcal/kg of body weight/hr.

TABLE 5–2.

U.S. Department of Agriculture Method*

	Sedentary	Moderately Active	Active
Males	16	20	30
Females	15	18	25

*Body weight in pounds $\times$ physical activity factor.

TABLE 5–3.

United Nations Food and Agricultural Organization (FAO) Method

Adjustment	Multiply By
Light activity	0.9
Very active people	1.17
Exceptionally active people	1.34
Ages 40–49	0.95
Ages 50–59	0.90

*For a quick estimate of moderately active adults ages 20 to 40, multiply weight in kilograms $\times$ 46 for men, and weight in kilograms $\times$ 40 for women.

to recall from the discussion on dietary histories that errors can be expected in interpreting caloric levels of prescribed diets. Examples of caloric expenditures such as those shown in Appendix 2, which do not account for variables such as age and sex, body composition, intensity of sport, previous conditioning, or playing surfaces, are estimates. These are simply guidelines and should be adjusted according to whether the individual maintains weight on this level of energy intake or is attempting accuracy in recording diet and activity.

Protein Requirements

After the daily energy requirement is estimated, the protein fraction of the diet is determined. The RDA is based on the assumption that 70% of protein is utilized. The adult requirement is 0.8 gm/kg/day, and for adolescents in fast growth it is 1.2 gm/kg/day. These allowances were established to cover the needs of most healthy people. They are increased for pregnancy and lactation and may be increased in athletics to as much as 2.0 gm/kg/day.

When caloric intake is reduced and energy needs are high, there may be risk of inadequate protein intake, which can be a problem for many dancers, runners, and gymnasts. A diet providing 12% to 15% of calories from protein usually provides adequate protein when a minimum of 1,200 kcal is consumed by women and 1,500 kcal by men.[7]

The protein allowance for a growing athlete is calculated as body weight in kilograms times 1.2 equals grams of protein. For example, 50 kg × 1.2 = 60 gm of protein/day. He or she will need to drink three glasses of milk and eat 5 oz of good-quality protein to meet this requirement.

Dietary Advice

Dietary advice is often given only once, without benefit of follow-up, and something can happen to all of this information between the consultation and the car. Minimum contact is one session with the athlete during the physical examination or after a request by physician or coach, followed by at least one monitoring session where compliance is checked, and that followed by a third visit where results may be charted and reviewed. Unfortunately, there is no secret formula for motivating adolescents and young adults to adopt healthful dietary habits. Many approaches do prove successful on the field and in clinical circumstances, and every health professional finds certain tactics superior to others. Of greatest importance in any setting is the establishment of rapport with the athlete. Unless a relaxed and trusting atmosphere is created for discussion, little successful interchange can take place. Often, concerns involving issues other than diet come up, and the counselor should be prepared to provide guidance.

One must remember, however, that dietitians, exercise physiologists, nurses, physical therapists, coaches, or athletic trainers *do not make diagnoses.* This responsibility comes within the domain of the physician. In sports medicine, physician approval must be given for all prescriptions—diet or exercise.

Weight Loss

Losing weight is tough for an athlete in training. It is hard to diet when there are caloric growth requirements to meet and it is hard to diet when top performance is required. The body works much better on a stream of incoming carbohydrate than on stored fat. Yet, in sports where there are strict weight classifications, where the athlete is overfat, or when those in charge believe that the performance will generate more approval at a lower weight, dieting to lose weight may be inevitable.

There is a difference between being overweight and being overfat. Some athletes may weigh more than height-weight charts recommend, so that technically they are overweight. If the additional weight is from muscle, they are not overfat, and there is no need for them to lose pounds. This situation is positive if the athlete is a developing linebacker in his junior year of high school. But it is negative if the junior in high school wants to compete in wrestling at last year's weight category. To lose weight, he will probably need to lose muscle mass as well as to dehydrate.

Be very careful in determining the weight that is best for the competing athlete. Once it is ascertained, weight can be *contracted* by a group of experts, which should include the team physician, dietitian, coach, and, especially, the parent. Be realistic in deciding if this weight can be attained, and then maintained, during the season. Determinants include the stage of fast growth, genetic capabilities, present weight, the time allowed for weight loss, percentage of body fat available for weight loss, the cooperation of parents or those in charge of the refrigerator, and the nutritional knowledge of the athlete. All too often, athletes lose weight by eliminating food rather than by making wiser food choices.

Growth may be suppressed if adequate calories are not available in the diet. What difference does it make if your athlete wrestles at 135 lb or 142 lb? You have a spot at 135 and a senior at 142! Allow both athletes to gain weight to the next classification. Toward the end of the season they will be wrestling opponents who are desperately maintaining weight by dehydration and starvation, and your athletes will be pinning them in the first round. In dancing and gymnastics, two activities where weight is continually monitored, both technique and endurance are affected when caloric levels are not adequate to protect growth potential.

Many better preseason weight decisions are made when a team member is accompanied to the preseason physical by parents. A brief observation will give clues to the food supply at home and the number of fat cells inherited by your athlete. A nutrition quiz will help screen out problems that may face the coach during the season (Appendix 19). Weight loss is inadvisable if the percentage of body fat is less than 7% for males and 12% for females.

It is possible to safely lose 1 to 2 lb of body fat/week. If the athlete loses weight any faster, it will be a combination of fat, protein, and indispensible body fluids. For each pound of fat lost, 3,500 calories need to be eliminated from the diet. This can be done by restricting calories and increasing exercise. Diet alone is not an effective way to take off fat. Caloric levels below 1,200 for females and 1,500 for males do not supply adequate nutrition for growth, repair, and development. Caloric levels below 1,800 for females and 2,000 for males usually do not supply the energy necessary for training and competition. A rule of thumb is that a minimum of 250 gm of carbohydrate/day are needed for training.[8]

A starved athlete will not want to exercise; glycogen will be depleted in a few days. Fatigue, depression, decreased endurance during exercise, and weakness on exertion will occur. Starvation increases the use of body protein. The goal, even during weight loss, is for optimum nutrition and good health. Weight loss should always be accomplished before the season.

The only alternative may be to increase exercise (though losing weight through exercise alone involves increasing activity, which may be impossible for the athlete who spends 2 to 3 hours/day in training). Because fat is the body's preferred fuel, the athlete will lose fat more readily if exercise is of moderate intensity and long duration. A change in activities, such as swimming for the runner or biking for the swimmer, may offer exercise options.

There are many diets and devices that promise quick weight loss. The weight loss is usually water, but this is an important issue. Athletes have been known to spit, sweat, vomit, and even give blood to achieve what they feel is the perfect competitive weight when time allowances do not allow for a more sensible approach. *Of course, it is far wiser to handle weight loss in a long-term program to assure maximum loss of fat.*

Weight Gain

Gaining weight is the other side of the coin. In many sports, hockey, football, even basketball and track, a few extra pounds can come in mighty handy. Clinical records show fast growth is extended when weight gain procedures have been prescribed, and income tax records show that playing years have been extended when individuals conform to the expectations of professional coaches.

Weight gain, independent of steroid use, can still raise cholesterol and triglyceride levels, raise blood pressure, cause stretch marks, and place the athlete at risk for obesity. In the pre–weight gain physical examination, blood lipid profiles, percentages of body fat, and parental risks of heart attack must be addressed. Weight gain is not advisable if cholesterol levels are more than 200 mg/dl, triglyceride levels are more than 150 mg/dl, body fat is more than 20% of total body weight, or if the athlete is genetically at risk for coronary heart disease. (It is not surprising that many professional athletes have all of these.)

To gain weight, the athlete needs to eat more calories than are used, which means eating more food. This can be fun, but for some athletes in heavy training it may not be easy. An adolescent biking to school, training for crew, and still on the paper route may need 7,500 calories daily to gain 1 lb/week. He or she can increase the caloric intake by substituting high-calorie for low-calorie foods. Some of these are nutrient rich, such as dried fruits, nuts, shakes and malts, pizza, and Dagwood-style sandwiches. The question then is, if a weight gain candidate is eating a nutrient-dense diet that covers all normal requirements, can the extra calories (to add the additional weight) come from any food choices the athlete desires? For instance, it is easier to eat two candy bars for an additional 1,000 calories than to munch through 10 large apples. Cakes, pies, doughnuts, and buttered popcorn may have a place in a weight gain diet, but only in addition to a basic adequate diet.

ESTIMATION OF CALORIC NEEDS

I. To calculate the maintenance level of calories:

A. Determine normal or ideal weight for height and build.

B. Multiply the ideal weight by:
1. 15, if adult/sedentary
2. 20, if adult/active
3. 30, if adolescent/active

C. Add calories of extra expended energy. Figure minutes of activity and cost per minute, or estimate that the caloric cost of running or walking is 100 kcal/mile; biking is 50 kcal/mile; swimming is 200 kcal/mile.

D. This gives the approximate level of energy intake necessary to maintain ideal body weight. For example, woman, 5 ft 4 in., small frame, 19% body fat, age 18 years:
1. Ideal weight   108 lb
2. Adult/active   <u>× 20</u>
                2,160 kcal

3. Running 12 minutes at 5 miles/hour, or:
   1.2 miles   + 120 kcal
4. Desired caloric level is 2,280 kcal/day.

II. To lose weight:

A. To lose 2 lb/week (7–8 lb/month), decrease food intake 500 kcal/day and increase exercise 500 kcal/day (5-mile run).

B. To lose 1 lb/week (4–5 lb/month), decrease food intake 250 kcal/day and increase exercise 250 kcal/day (5-mile bike ride). Note: rapid weight loss may cause irritability, decreased reaction time, decreased concentration, and insomnia. It is advisable to lose only 1 to 2 lb/week, preferably before the competitive season begins.

III. To gain weight:

A. To gain 1 lb/week, increase food intake 500 kcal/day above maintenance needs.

B. To gain 2 lb/week, increase food intake 1,000 kcal/day above maintenance needs. Note: too rapid a gain will usually result in deposition of fat and accumulation of fluid. Optimum muscular development will occur if gradual gain in weight is balanced with a regular exercise program.

These guidelines are estimations. Carefully kept records of diet and exercise will provide a more accurate appraisal for individual goals. Although research is not in total agreement with the effectiveness of weight gain regimens after fast growth, in general, most of the weight gain experienced in the adolescent will be additional muscle. This adds legitimacy to weight gain protocols. The major concern of weight gain in adult populations is the fact that many subjects gain primarily fat tissue. Investigaters have recently proved that fat cell hyperplasia is possible at any time of life and not limited to overeating during birth to 2 years and during adolescence (if caloric levels are high and exercise levels are low). There are other problems associated with weight gain, especially if it is rapid—gastric reflux, beyond the occasional burp; changes in the breath of the athlete, and the problem of heartburn. Stretch marks across the chest, back, and upper leg are common when weight is accelerated. In addition, 8 oz of fluid are required to digest and metabolize 200 calories of food. Because the stomach does not grow when large amounts of food are continually introduced to it, discomfort is inevitable, and the required water is not drunk. This leads to dehydration and, in time, will lead to weight loss. The general recommendation is for weight gain to be gradual and not over twice what the individual in fast growth would expect to gain. (During fast growth, an adolescent can expect to gain from 1 to 2 lb/month.) A weight gain handout may be found in Appendix 4.

The prescription for weight loss for the athlete is to eat less and exercise more. Restricting calories will always decrease metabolic rate, and the dieter will eventually stop losing weight if exercise is not constant. Exercise increases the body's metabolic rate or at least will not allow the metabolic rate to decrease to the point of plateau. When diet is combined with exercise, fat loss will occur more rapidly than if either diet or exercise is used alone.

Endurance activity (aerobic exercise) over strength activity is preferred for fat loss. At the rate of 2,000 kcal/week, the body will maintain protein tissue, selectively lose fat, and readjust the set point, or that point where weight quickly returns when dieting ceases. After the dietary maintenance level has been reestablished, exercise expenditures must remain at the 2,000 kcal/week level for about 1 year. (Approximately 20 miles of walking, 40 miles of biking, or 10 miles of swimming burn 2,000 kcal.) Increased frequency and duration of exercise will cause greater fat loss. Calories need to be adjusted upward gradually, because our bodies tend to recognize former eating patterns as an excuse to regain lost weight. The best recommendation is to set realistic goals that can be followed consistently, ones that will not interfere with training.

For years, several athletic activities have discouraged the advantage of aerobic contribution to weight maintenance. These activities, especially dance, gymnastics, figure skating, and wrestling, have many problems associated with achieving ideal (or competitive) weight. Until there is greater acceptance of aerobic activity in the field of the dance, for instance, dancers will maintain their weight by caloric monitoring alone. Until crew and wrestling forbid quick weight loss opportunities to athletes wanting to qualify at suboptimal weight classifications, there will be a prevalence of food behavior problems in those sports.

At some point in muscular work, a mixture of fat and carbohydrate are used for energy (Fig 5–1). Then, as demands for oxygen increase, as in strenuous physical activity, carbohydrates contribute most of the energy supply. When the literature on nutrition is reviewed, it becomes more apparent that although broad statements can be made about the carbohydrate contribution to work, the results vary between individuals.

Strength

Although muscle composition approximates 70% water, 22% protein, and 8% fat storage, it is difficult to evaluate additional muscle growth. The biopsy technique, which avails the counting of muscle bundles from a tissue sample, is painful and impractical outside of the physiology laboratory. Assuming that this composition is approximate, we can use the following prescription:

1. Calories:
   Adult athlete: expected ideal body weight × 15 + 500 calories = total calories/day
   Growing athlete: expected ideal body weight × 30 + 1,000 calories = total calories/day
2. Protein: 15% to 20% of total calories, or 1.3 to 2.0 gm/kg of ideal body weight.
3. Carbohydrate: 60% of total calories.
4. Exercise: a supervised weight training program of at least 1.5 hours, 3 times/week; aerobic exercise 3 to 4 times/week at 300 calories/session.

FIG 5–1.
In any exercise bout, fuel utilization is determined by intensity and duration of activity. For most individuals, a greater proportion of fat is used at lower exercise intensities, whereas glucose supplies more of the energy at higher levels of work. However, when glycogen is no longer available for glucose conversion, fat will become the predominant fuel. (Redrawn from Peterson JA, 1987.)

Fuel Utilization in a One Hour Exercise Program

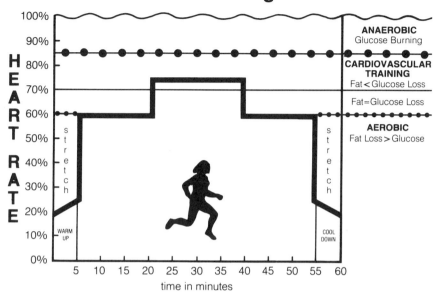

Aerobics in Heart Training Zone
Training at *Low* End of Zone

Increased fat burning capacity in muscles (slow-twitch muscle fibers)
Increased blood circulation in muscles
Increased skeletal strength
Increased skill of exercise
Decreased percent body fat

Aerobics in Heart Training Zone
Training at *High* End of Zone

Increased fat-burning capacity (fast oxidative glycolytic muscle fibers)
Increased blood circulation
Increased heart pumping volume
Decreased resting heart rate
Increased lung volume
Increased blood volume
Increased endurance
Decreased length of exercise

Aerobics Below Heart Training Zone
"Fat Loss Aerobics"

Long Duration, 1 Hour or More/Day
Maximum Percent Fat-Glucose Utilization of Calories
Training threshold: That heart rate or oxygen consumption that improves aerobic fitness level (e.g., your maximum volume of oxygen)
Anaerobic threshold: An exercise intensity higher than the training threshold where exercise becomes predominantly anaerobic and lactic acid increases and exhaustion results. No additional improvements in aerobic capacity or fitness is attained.

After ideal body weight has been reached, percentages of fat can be determined by hydrostatic weighing. If body fat is more than 20% increased aerobic exercise at the low end of the target heart rate is initiated. Otherwise, weight training and diet readjustment are appropriate at this time.

Endurance

The goal is to establish a weight at which performance is best. Usually the body will adjust to that weight after several years of training; however, several problems exist. One is that an efficiency factor is evident. Many elite athletes use fewer calories in training, which are usually compensated for in increased mileage. Another is that, with an increase in the intensity of exercise, the use of protein as a fuel increases. If vegetarianism prevails, or if red meat consumption is lowered, muscle will be used to provide protein, and iron deficiency may also occur:

1. Calories:
   Adult athlete: ideal body weight × 15 + training expenditure = total daily calories
   Growing athlete: ideal body weight × 30 + training expenditure = total daily calories
2. Protein: 1.5 to 2.0 gm/kg of body weight.
3. Carbohydrate: 60% to 65% of total calories.

Change in Altitude (More Than 5,000 Feet)

Increase fluids, avoid excess salt, increase carbohydrate to 70% of calories, and keep protein status at 15% to 20% of calories. Eat smaller meals and eat more frequently. Take time to rest.

Off-Season

Most females gain weight and males lose weight in off-season. For example, a male rower, after 10 months of training and competition, may find sleeping more, eating less, and just relaxing and catching up necessary. The female may sleep more and eat more. It is a good idea to talk over weight expectations before going home for spring break. Write down a few guidelines and be realistic about the changes that occur during off-season. A 5-lb fluctuation is not serious; a 15-lb fluctuation is a disaster. Adolescents will find weight gain much easier during off-season. If this is desirable, as in football, make sensible plans early and become accustomed to the new weight before preseason.

Preseason

Caloric expenditure is as high during this time as during competition or finals. Weight loss often occurs due to dehydration and change of pace. Monitor weight daily. Increase fluids. Adjust calories upward until weight is maintained. Weight loss during practice is probably water and should be replaced on a daily basis by drinking 16 oz (1 pint) of water for each pound of body weight lost.

Competition

Several years' experience ingrains a program that works on an individual basis. Until that comfort level exists, the regimen in Table 5–4 can be adapted to individual needs. Dietary protocol is individual. Record dietary intake on several competitive occasions, and note other issues such as weather conditions, location, emotions (e.g., perceived exertions), and results.

Recommended electrolyte levels in sports drinks are 10 mEq

TABLE 5–4.

Regimen During Competition

Time Period	Training	Dietary Emphasis
Day 5–3	Moderate	Eat high carbohydrate (65% of calories); drink fluids to maintain weight
Day 3–1	Rest or taper	Eat high carbohydrate; drink beyond thirst; avoid alcohol and caffeine
3–5 hr before or previous	Rest	Eat small meal, >500 kcal; drink fluid to toleration; drink no alcohol the night before
1–2 hr before	Rest	Sip fluids slowly, avoid sugary fluids
15 min before		Sip 8–16 oz of fluids
Event		Drink a minimum of 4 oz of fluid every 15 min or 2 miles; also consider water plus 2.5% glucose solution or glucose polymer (7%) *after* event begins; remember that thirst is not an adequate indicator of dehydration

of sodium/L (or 230 mg/L) and 5 mEq of potassium/L (or 195 mg/L).[9]

Carbohydrate toleration is also an individual matter and may be affected by temperature or length and intensity of event. Percentages of carbohydrate in currently available commercial products are listed in Table 5–5.[10]

Caffeine ingestion is also an individual preference. Four to 5 mg/kg of body weight 1 hour prior to exercise may increase free fatty acid availability to the working muscles and be glycogen sparing. Caffeine, however, is also a diuretic and causes increased heart rate and anxiety levels. That, plus the stress of competition, may be detrimental.

Short-Term Taper

The purpose of short-term taper is to resynthesize and store optimum levels of glycogen. Stretching, visualization or other mental preparation, or traveling is done during this time. Carbohydrate portion of total calories is usually about 70%; fluids intake is at least eight glasses of water or juice daily. Weight gain will occur, because water is stored with glycogen at a ratio of 3:1. (If traveling [especially by plane], one should carry a bottle of water to ensure proper hydration before competition.)

Postseason

One should watch for careless eating. A healthful diet is still beneficial. The all too common binge eating that occurs in sports where weight monitoring is usual should be avoided. Writing down food intake is beneficial.

TABLE 5–5.

Percentages of Carbohydrate in Various Commercial Products

Polymer Based	%	Glucose Based	%
Exceed	7.0	Erg	2.5
Max	5.0	Gaterade	5.6
Bodyfuel 450	2.5	Pripps Plus	7.4
Bodyfuel 100	0.2	Supersocco	13.0
Carboplus	18.4		
Carboplex	20.0		

Injury, Illness, or Hospitalization

During these occasions, a physician order will probably take care of nutrient needs. Unfortunately, fat gain and fluid accumulation will often occur. Calories should be adjusted downward to account for inactivity. Body fat percentage should be taken on the first day of illness.

Practice Schedules and Dorm Food

Coordination is the key here, and it is difficult. There is always one sports fan in the kitchen; get him or her on the team, too. If a training table is not available, at least two meals per day should coincide with food availability. The third meal should be a nutritious snack or possibly fast food. Care needs to be taken here, because weight gain may be the outcome. Pooling resources for food caches in the dorm, emergency letters home for oatmeal cookies and fruit, additional funding from the athletic department, or readjustment of training schedules are possibilities.

EVENT PLANNING

Pre-event Meal

The pre-event meal should be considered an important component of the total training program. Pre-event meal considerations include timing, location, size, composition, and availability. A small (>500 kcal but often as high as 1,000 kcal), high-carbohydrate meal, about 3 to 4 hours before competition, eaten in a pleasant situation will be well tolerated by most athletes. Three hours will allow adequate time for digestion and absorption and still prevent hunger. The meal should be composed primarily of carbohydrates and fluids because it will be more easily digested and also because most competition requires carbohydrates for fuel (this meal may spare existing glycogen storage). Protein and fat should be limited because these foods take longer to empty from the stomach. Sandwiches, waffles, pasta, fruit, and other selections from the grain group are all good choices for a pre-event meal. Liquid meals are acceptable alternatives for those who experience gastric discomfort or precompetition anxiety or when schedules do not allow time for the proper digestion of whole foods.[11]

Postevent Feeding

The main purpose of a postevent meal is to rehydrate and replete glycogen in the muscles. Research emphasizes that the first 10 hours after a training session or competitive bout are the most important for recovery. The athlete often experiences intense letdown or fatigue during this time and does not feel like eating or drinking. The physiological response to exercise is increased body temperature and redistribution of the body's blood supply. A cool-down period is recommended, with fluids sipped gradually but consistently. The athlete might eat and drink whatever sounds good! It is not so critical to avoid fat now, so ice cream, pizza, and dessert may be enjoyed.

Carbohydrate Loading

Athletes training for endurance activities, such as crew/rowing, cross-country skiing, distance cycling, running and swimming, marathons, soccer, and tournaments frequently are chronically fatigued. Successive days of training often become more and more difficult. Fatigue is related to the gradual depletion of the body's carbohydrate (glycogen) stores. This depletion may occur independently of the carbohydrate content of the athlete's diet if the total calories and total amount of carbohydrate are not sufficient to fuel exercise and to resynthesize glycogen afterward. Some athletes have found it necessary to increase their daily intake of carbohydrates to 70% of total calories (612 gm or 12 servings of carbohydrate-rich foods for 3,500 calories) to prevent depletion of the body's glycogen stores during hard training.

Resynthesis of muscle glycogen is individual, but it is safe to say that at least 10 hours (often up to 48 hours) are necessary to restore glycogen to preexercise levels. Without a doubt, if the athlete performs heavy exercise on a daily basis, extra carbohydrate must be eaten to permit optimal glycogen resynthesis, and at least 2 days of taper (rest) are necessary to establish levels needed for competition.

Although a full carbohydrate regimen was once prescribed, a miniprocedure (or easy loading) is now recommended.

Few problems exist in adding additional carbohydrates to an athlete's diet. Most carbohydrate foods are enjoyed, quickly digested, and easy to find in the kitchen. Again, weight gain may occur, because water will be stored in the muscles along with the extra carbohydrate. Athletes with diabetes or hypertriglyceridemia or who are trying this technique for the first time should inform their physicians. Although most of the world eats a high-carbohydrate diet (the Far East diet approximates 80% of calories from carbohydrate), those from Omaha may not. It is good to check diet changes with the rest of the family. It is common for the overenthusiastic carbohydrate loader to have flatulence and a distended abdomen after indulging in increased fiber.

Eating a diet high in carbohydrate (about 500–600 gm/day) usually maintains muscle glycogen storage. Table 5–6 gives a food pattern that will synthesize extra glycogen in the muscles.

Super Hydration

At one time athletes thought it was a good idea to limit their water intake. Now it is known that this practice is dangerous and that no athlete can work at top performance in a dehydrated state. In spite of the general acceptance of hydration, most athletes gradually dehydrate during the week before competition and arrive at the event a few pounds lighter. They may be able to work well at low levels of competition, but in the intense moments of the game they often mistake a throbbing heartbeat and slight nausea for excitement instead of indications of dehydration.

Dehydration can best be avoided by drinking plenty of plain, cool water before, during, and after practice and competition. (Thirst is not an indicator of the amount of water the body needs.) Any weight loss should be made up by drinking 2 cups (16 oz) of fluid for every pound lost before another workout begins.

Swimmers sweat and become overheated in water; skiers sweat and become overheated in cold weather; climbers sweat and become overheated at high altitudes. During prolonged exercise, sweat will not evaporate quickly enough to cool down the

TABLE 5–6.

Carbohydrate Loading Diet*

	Calories		
	1,500	1,800	2,100
Breakfast			
Whole-wheat toast	1	2	2
Margarine		1	2
Jam	1	1	1
Fruit: orange, apple, or grape juice, 4 oz	1	1	2
Cereal: Wheat Chex, Rice Krispies, ¾ cup; or Cream of Wheat, oatmeal, ½ cup	1	1	2
Milk, 4 oz	1	1	1
Sugar, 1 level tablespoon		1	1
Subtotal	305 calories	410 calories	460 calories
Snack			
Banana, one medium	½	½	½
Nonfat milk, 8 oz	1	1	1
Subtotal	125 calories	125 calories	125 calories
Lunch			
Whole-wheat bread	2	2	2
Margarine or mayonnaise, 1 teaspoon	1	1	1
Filling: cheese, tuna, peanut butter, 1 oz	2	2	3
Apple, orange, one medium	1		
Salad: Jello, 2 by 2 in.; carrot and raisin, ½ cup; macaroni, mayonnaise, ½ cup		1	1
Nonfat milk, 8 oz	1	1	1
Subtotal	450 calories	565 calories	640 calories
Snack			
Apple, grape, or orange juice, 6 oz		1	1
Subtotal	40 calories	40 calories	40 calories
Dinner			
Fruit: applesauce, cantaloupe, or pear	1	1	1
Soup: cream of pea, bean, one serving		1	1
Vegetable: corn, peas, lima, squash, ½ cup	1	1	1
Entree: pizza, ⅛ small; macaroni and cheese, ¼ cup; spaghetti, meat and tomato, ¼ cup; pot pie (six exchanges)	5	5	6
Tea, coffee, or diet cola	1	1	1
Subtotal	540 calories	580 calories	755 calories

(Continued.)

TABLE 5–6 (cont.).

Snack

Cake: angel or sponge, 2 by 2 in.; sherbet, ⅓ cup; Jello, one serving, ⅕ pkg; banana, ½; Milk, 4 oz	1	2	2
Subtotal	40 calories	80 calories	80 calories

*Exercise: normal to low activity pattern; diet: high carbohydrate, low fat, low protein, six to eight glasses of water. Numbers indicate number of exchanges.

body. Temperature control mechanisms become overwhelmed, and exercise must stop. The body is usually compromised at any temperature above 75°F and relative humidity above 50%.

Predicting those situations and compensating for them by consuming extra fluids provides some protection, because it delays the development of dehydration, increases sweating during exercise, and helps the body adjust core temperature. Although water to toleration is a personal volume, daily amounts of urinary output may be a better indicator that the athlete is well hydrated. Volume should be more than 1.6 quarts, clear or light amber, and odorless. Diuretic stimulation (alcohol, coffee, tea, regular colas, aspirin, or diuretics) should be avoided at least 24 hours before competition. If possible, airline travel should take place well before this time, precompetition exercise should be light and at the coolest time of the day, and clothing should be lightweight to allow sweat to evaporate.[12]

Matching fluid losses (60 oz/hour) with fluid intake during competition is physiologically impossible, because less than 24 oz (or 3 cups) of fluid empties from the stomach during the stress of exercise.

Snacking

Some athletes have such small appetites that they cannot eat as much as they should to support the caloric demands of their sport. Snacking, or eating small amounts between meals, is a sensible approach to cover this energy requirement. And there are other reasons why snacking is sensible: schedules do not fit with mealtimes; more nutrition is needed (i.e., fluids or carbohydrates, iron-rich foods, vitamin C); or home-style cooking is missed in a new environment. Athletes should be encouraged to have nutritious (and delicious) food on hand, keeping in mind food safety, quality, and noncariogenic qualities.

Most of the following foods can be kept for a short time without refrigeration and are available in any grocery store raid:

1. Breads: bagels, rye crackers, pocket bread, and granola.
2. Protein: peanut butter and low-fat cheese spreads.
3. Fruit: all kinds of fruit and individual-size fruit juices.
4. Vegetables: cherry tomatoes, cucumbers, and bell peppers.
5. Dairy (with refrigeration): yogurt, cottage cheese, and all cheeses.
6. From home: oatmeal raisin or peanut butter cookies.

Vending Machines

Vending machines are a special challenge—found everywhere and stocked with expensive, nonnutritive food choices. If one is outside your gym, ask the purveyor to offer better food selections, such as raisins, almonds, peanuts, cheese and crackers, peanut butter and crackers, and apples. If refrigerated machines are available, ask for seltzers and juices, along with pop. If you get no cooperation, offer fruit and freshly popped popcorn after practice or have the machine removed.

On the Road

Any cheerleader or mom will cook her heart out for the team. Too often, it is brownies. Athletes, novice or elite, need more fluids, extra carbohydrates and calories, and additional nourishment. The meal on the road can offer these plus enjoyment and relief from boredom.[13]

The meal in a sack might include a favorite sandwich on variety bread (pack lettuce, tomatoes separately), something crisp and chewy, such as raw vegetables (they will stay crisp in a damp paper towel and in plastic wrap), fruit juice or noncaffeine colas, and favorite cookies. This is not a meal to fuss over; just keep it familiar and keep it healthful. Wrap each food separately, and pack soft foods on top.

When the team is on the road for an extended trip, they will need to consider three meals, plus snacks. Here are some portable suggestions:

1. Snacks: raisins, nonsulfured dried fruits, nuts, healthy gorp, beef jerky, breakfast bars, and sunflower seeds
2. Breakfast: cold cereals, instant hot cereals, peanut butter, packaged hot cocoa, fruit juices, tea, and coffee
3. Lunches and dinners: Cup of Soup, instant lunches, canned soups and stews, Top Ramen, canned meats and fish (chicken, ham, tuna, salmon, Tea Kettle casseroles), instant rice, salami, instant puddings, and freeze-dried meals

Restaurants

Restaurant owners have become so aware of the public's concern with nutrition that the National Restaurant Association has published a guide for incorporating healthful food into recipes and menus! Even fast-food establishments have begun to focus more attention on nutrition. Traditionally, most major chains featured high-salt, high-cholesterol, and other fatty menu items. Now several offer salad bars, whole-grain sandwich buns, plain baked potatoes, and low-fat milk; some have even stopped using beef tallow to fry chicken and fish.

A good combination for the athlete is a salad (easy on the dressing) with a plain hamburger and a half-pint (1 cup) of low-fat milk. This adds up to about 350 calories, with about 35% contributed by fat (more acceptable than a McD.L.T, fries, and a milkshake, which contain 1,300 calories, 45% of which comes from fat, and more than 1,400 mg of sodium). More fast-food chains are test marketing chicken and fish dishes that are baked or broiled rather than fried in fat. And another choice, pizza, is available as thin and crispy, with just 340 calories, only 29% of them from fat. That is just one quarter of a 13-in. pie, so bring a few friends. Add a salad, and the meal is even better balanced.

Mexican and Chinese food may be the answer for dancers, gymnasts, and the calorie-fat conscious athlete. Although they represent only a fraction of the major fast-food chain outlets, ethnic eateries are beginning to attract many of the quick diners. They, for example, were way ahead of other chains in dropping coconut oil or beef fat in cooking.

Even a baseball player cannot survive the fast-food circuit all season long. Meal planning, as difficult as it is on the road (and per diem), must be someone's responsibility.

Again, restaurants offering ethnic cuisine make good dining choices. Chinese- and Japanese-style main dishes, for instance, are almost always comparatively low in fat because the focus is usually on vegetables and rice. A stir-fry dish such as moo goo gai pan, ordered without monosodium glutamate (MSG), served over rice, provides healthful portions of protein, fiber, and vitamins with much less fat and fewer calories than steak and eggs. Italian food, such as pasta, plus a tossed salad, can make a low-calorie, nutrient-dense meal (unfortunately, not fettucine alfredo, which is loaded with cream). Marinara sauce, pola cacciatore, boneless chicken breast served with spinach, and shrimp with white wine all rate high for nutrient density.

Many traditional restaurants are now offering minimeals, such as appetizers and a salad or salad and soup. Or order an appetizer, salad, and entree and split the entree with the coach. Regardless of choices, there is no doubt that restaurants are now offering a wider selection, and it is apparent that "healthy" is now possible. That is not to say that the 12-oz steak; baked potato with butter, sour cream, and bacon; tossed salad with ample blue cheese dressing; asparagus with hollandaise sauce; and garlic toast; followed by pecan pie and ice cream—2,850 calories with 55% coming from fat—will disappear from the menu.[14]

Another restaurant choice is a breakfast meal. And even you know where serves a scrambled egg breakfast with orange juice for 446 calories. Croissant sandwiches or muffins that layer cheese, eggs, and sausages make heavier breakfasts, some with more than 700 calories and more than 2,000 mg of sodium.

Maintaining energy balance and meeting nutrient requirements on the road is a real challenge. Food availability is restricted, and the food budget requires creative, nontraditional eating ideas. But skipping meals is not the way to money management.

A few rules are:

1. Find the restaurants that have a variety of healthful menu items and that will appreciate your athletic talents.
2. For breakfast, eat cereals with low-fat milk or yogurt with fresh fruit. Limit eggs to two and have them poached or soft cooked. Ask for the most wholesome bread choices and skip the doughnuts and pastries.
3. For lunch, salads with low-fat protein such as turkey, chicken, fish, cottage cheese, or beans are filling. Eat lean meat sandwiches such as turkey, chicken, and beef rather than cold cuts. Ask for mayonnaise and butter on the side, vegetable and bean salads for side dishes; soups made with beans, peas, or lentils; and fruit or sherbets for dessert.
4. For dinner, eat vegetables, melon, broth, or shellfish for appetizers; green salads; entrees that are baked, broiled, steamed, poached, or stir-fried. Skip sauces and gravies and ask for vegetables without sauce or butter.
5. Keep fruit in your room, and drink water throughout the day (especially before each meal and during the game). Liquor, wine, or beer add calories, are dehydrating, and do nothing to improve performance.

Time Zone Changes

Before the Trip.—Call the airline to order special diets for team members (low calorie, diabetic, vegetarian, kosher, or no salt). Most companies are cooperative and will allow for changes, such as larger portions, if more than five members of a team are traveling together. Question the host site about food sources and available restaurants, and review the time schedules appropriate for preevent eating. Although the professionals or letter winners on the team may feel comfortable with their own choices, there will always be rookies who will appreciate advice. If possible, conform to the new sleeping schedule several days prior to the trip.

During the Trip.—Set watches ahead to the new time zone, drink as much water as possible, or consume more juices (ask for the whole can). Avoid caffeine, alcohol, and any food item that will cause a change in hydration status, such as chips or nuts.

Caffeine will also disturb napping on the plane or the sleep pattern after arrival.

After the Trip.—Drink water in the airport or canned juices if the water supply is suspect. Many athletes take a day's water supply with them. After check-in, walk around outside. Have a light carbohydrate snack before resting. There are many suggestions available for each condition within performance timeframes, namely, carbohydrate foods for breakfast, proteins in the later part of the day, or consumption of the major meal of the day in the morning instead of the evening. These are individual to each athlete and difficult to manage on the road. A better understanding of capabilities may be obtained by taking measurements of self-rated alertness or mood, heart rate, and simple performance tasks several times a day and determining the best time of day for practice and performance.

Regardless of the routine, some major complaints such as dehydration, fatigue, and bowel changes arise. To readjust, it will usually take the athlete 1 day for each hour of time zone change. Fluids and attention to carbohydrate requirements will help the first; resuming exercise and relaxing will help the second.[15]

School Lunch and Food Service Facilities

Athletes often use food service facilities for training and for precompetition meals. When the diets of athletes eating in off-campus situations are compared with those living and eating on campus, the food service facilities come out on top. Quality and quantity of protein, fat, and carbohydrate as well as other nutrients result in more desirable patterns of dietary intake. Off-campus athletes are influenced by factors such as time, skill in food preparation, food item costs, and restriction on variety. The school lunch provides, at nominal cost, a minimum of one third of the calories, protein, and other nutrients needed by growing athletes. However, it is agreed that with alternative lunch patterns and the availability of fast foods, school lunches have lost some of their appeal.

Recently, a high school in Seattle adopted an all-school, preevent meal as part of its pep rally. Students and fans, including the cooks, wore sweatshirts with logos, ate in the decorated lunchroom, and sent the team off with unparalleled spirit. Fans were invited to meet in the lunchroom after the game for treats, watch the film clips, and listen to the coaches and team members talk about the game. And everyone remembered to thank the cooks!

COUNSELING TECHNIQUES

The preceding chapters have emphasized the increased nutritional demands made by exercise. These requirements include intake of nutrients that are vital for growth and development; increased calories; adequate carbohydrate and protein; and sufficient vitamins and minerals, as well as attention to any individual factors. These considerations provide a framework for nutrition education and guidance.

Again, many variables combine to produce individual needs, whether psychological, physiological, cultural, or economic. Thus, individual nutritional assessment is an integral part of every health examination. Counseling based on that assessment should be an ongoing part of the care of individual athletes. The tools for assessment are outlined in Chapter 4. Approaches for planning an individual (as well as team) program of nutritional care are suggested here.

The rule is to begin where the patient is now. It is essential to learn about the athlete, where he or she is in growth and what his or her needs and expectations are. Counseling includes collecting background data, compiling and analyzing a diet history, and giving basic instruction.[16]

The dietary questionnaire (see Appendix 28) will yield information on former and current living situations, reveal any cultural or ethnic food practices, special diet practices, food dislikes or allergies, medication or supplements, and provide a chance for the athlete to request individual help. It will also show whether he or she has a general understanding of nutritional needs during participation in sports (and growth, pregnancy, rehabilitation, etc.).

Some form of diet history should be obtained. A food frequency chart can be used in a team setting that allows only a 5- to 10-minute interview with each member, or a simple request for a list of favorite (and disliked) foods may be made. When time allows, a 24-hour recall is especially helpful. It shows the patient that keeping good records is important and demonstrates an analysis of diet quality and quantity. It also strengthens the dialogue between athlete and nutritionist. (Even if "but yesterday was an unusual day!" is frequently expressed, more useful information will follow; this is just the beginning.) Other information will also be gained during the recall interview, such as customary eating habits, general preparation of food, usual location of meals, and portion sizes.

Analysis will give an overall view to the patient of his or her diet, as well as giving some tools to use in review of diet quality. If a computer is employed, the recall can be immediately and accurately accessed, and recommendations can be given on the spot. Remember that the goal is for dietary improvement; there is never an excuse for harsh judgments or disapproval. For an informal nutrient calculation, use the *Guide to Good Eating*,[17] and refer to it for general quality assessment. Ask the patient to name the foods he or she likes by group. Several games emphasize quality and variety of foods. These might be played with younger clients. Pictures, food models, and posters are also of assistance. A hand-held computerized program (e.g., Compu-cal) is convenient to use in calculating calories, carbohydrates, proteins, and vitamins and minerals.[18]

Food value tables in standard references or textbook appendices may be used, and totals of each nutrient may be compared with the recommended dietary allowances (RDAs). Reference to the USDA dietary guidelines[19] is a good way to verify statements regarding weight status, carbohydrate and fat intake, and alcohol use. Any areas of obvious deficiency can be addressed immediately (Table 5–7).

A variety of food practices will be revealed by the patient during the interview. Relatively harmless ones (particular food dislikes) can be noted, whereas others, such as megavitamin dosage or high-fat intake, will need correction.

By the time the interview closes, the patient and nutritionist should be able to decide if several further meetings covering diet instruction will be sufficient or if there is a need for counseling on a long-term basis, as in the case of weight or food behavior problems.

TABLE 5–7.
Daily Nutrient Needs of Athletics

Nutrient	Average RDA	Reasons for Nutrient Need	Food Sources
Calories	30 calories/lb for growing athlete 15 calories/lb for fully grown athlete 20 calories/lb for active adult + exercise requirements	Increased BMR, energy needs, protein sparing Problems with overconsumption: weight gain	Carbohydrates, fats, proteins
Protein	1–2 gm/kg of body weight or 12%–15% of calories	Growth, development, cell maintenance, enzymes, hormones, fluid balance, antibodies Problems with overeating: diarrhea, weight gain, kidney problems	Milk, cheeses, egg, meat, grains, legumes, nuts
Carbohydrate	50%–55% of calories to 70% of calories (550 gm/1 week before competition)	Promote glycogen storage, energy	Grains, fruits, vegetables
Water	8–10 cups/day, weigh preexercise and postexercise; replace weight loss	Prevent dehydration, carry oxygen to muscle cell, excrete waste Problems with overconsumption: water intoxication	Water, juices, milk, fruits, vegetables
Minerals Calcium	800–1,500 mg	Bone formation, maintenance of healthy bones, muscular contraction Problems with overconsumption: kidney stones	Milk and dairy products, whole grains, leafy vegetables, canned salmon, fortified foods
Phosphorus	800–1,200 mg	Bone formation	Egg yolk, milk, cheese, lean meats

(Continued.)

TABLE 5-7 (cont.).

Nutrient	Average RDA	Reasons for Nutrient Need	Food Sources
Iron	10–18 mg	Increased circulating blood volume, increased hemoglobin Problems with overeating: stomachache	Liver and other red meats, egg, whole or enriched grains, legumes, dried fruits, oysters
Iodine	150 µg	Increased BMR, increased thyroxine production	Iodized salt
Magnesium	300–400 mg	Coenzyme in energy and protein metabolism, enzyme activator, tissue growth, cell metabolism, muscle action	Nuts, cocoa, seafood, whole grains, legumes
Zinc	15 mg	Wound healing, taste, immune reactions, RNA and DNA synthesis	Oysters, milk, egg yolk
Vitamins*			
A	5,000 IU	Essential for cell development; hence, tissue growth, sight, resistance to infection, bone and tooth development	Butter, cream, fortified margarine, green and yellow vegetables
D	400 IU	Bone growth, absorption of calcium and phosphorus, mineralization of bone tissue	Fortified milk, fortified margarine, fish liver oils
E	30 IU	Tissue growth, cell wall integrity, red blood cell integrity	Vegetable oils, leafy vegetables, cereals, meat, egg yolk, butter
C	60 mg	Tissue formation and integrity, cement substance in connective and vascular tissues, increase in iron absorption, wound healing, resistance to infection	Citrus fruits, berries, melons, tomatoes, chili peppers, green leafy vegetables, broccoli, potatoes

Nutrient	RDA	Function / Problems	Food Sources
Folic acid	400 µg	Prevention of megaloblastic anemia in high-risk patients, increased heme production for hemoglobin, production of cell nucleus material. Problems with overconsumption: may obscure pernicious anemia	Liver, green leafy vegetables, legumes
Niacin	14–18 mg	Coenzyme in energy metabolism, helps utilize carbohydrate for energy. Problems with overconsumption: flushing, headaches, cramps	Liver, meat, poultry, beans and peas, enriched grains
Riboflavin	1.3–1.7 mg	Coenzyme in energy metabolism, healthy skin, and good vision	Milk, yogurt, cottage cheese, liver, enriched grains
Thiamine	1.0–1.5 mg	Coenzyme for energy metabolism, normal appetite nervous system	Pork, beef, liver, whole or enriched grains, legumes, nuts
B_6 (pyridoxine)	1.8–2.0 mg	Coenzyme for energy metabolism	Whole grains, liver, meat, poultry, fish, leafy vegetables, legumes,
B_{12}	3.0 gm	Coenzymes in protein metabolism, especially vital cell proteins such as nucleic acid, formation of red blood cells	Milk and milk products, eggs, meat, poultry, fish, shellfish, cheese

*The 1980 RDA tables do not include vitamin A and D values in IU, but these are included to correspond with supplement and food labelling.

The patient should gain understanding of and receive information on the following:

1. Daily caloric requirements
2. Foods that are high in carbohydrates and high in fiber
3. Foods that are high in protein but low in fat
4. What is meant by a balanced diet
5. Fluid requirements for athletics (Table 5–8)
6. Supplementation
7. Specialized needs (e.g., anemia, weight gain)
8. A sample diet or food plan
9. Follow-up schedules for counseling

The rationale for the interview, or an explanation of laboratory findings (see Appendix 6) may also be given. Handouts are especially helpful at this time. The patient is usually asked to gather specific information and read handouts before the next

TABLE 5–8.

Recommended Fluid Availability and Intake for a Strenuous 90-Minute Athletic Practice

Weight Loss		Min Between Water Break	Fluid per Break	
lb	kg		oz	ml
8	3.6	*		
7.5	3.4	*		
7	3.2	10	8–10	266
6.5	3.0	10	8–9	251
6	2.7	10	8–9	251
5.5	2.5	15	10–12	325
5	2.3	15	10–11	311
4.5	2.1	15	9–10	281
4	1.8	15	8–9	251
3.5	1.6	20	10–11	311
3	1.4	20	9–10	281
2.5	1.1	20	7–8	222
2	0.9	30	8	237
1.5	0.7	30	6	177
1	0.5	45	6	177
0.5	0.2	60	6	177

*No practice recommended.

visit and to complete a 7-day dietary history form (or a 3-day form that includes two weekend days and one weekday). The nutritionist will complete chart notes, review findings, and reestablish requirements for the patient.

Perhaps at no other time in a person's life will he or she be so motivated to accept a change. A positive, personalized approach by the nutritionist will build on these feelings of enthusiasm and anticipation and help develop a desire for learning. What is more important is that what is learned during a successful contact will be carried into other life stages and will likely affect others' attitudes toward nutrition.

During the second visit, food records are reviewed and analyzed, and behaviors that fulfilled the dietary recommendations of the initial visit are reinforced. The nutritional needs of both growth status and athletics should be restated, and any practices that are solutions to problems need to be reemphasized. Simple phrases, such as "You are doing a good job following your diet," are nice assurances.

If little progress has been made, reiterate the relationship between diet and the goal. Show positive concern for habit change. Ask the patient to identify instances of habits that detract, and note in writing those that need to be altered.

Questions that must be addressed are:

1. What are the problems that limit appropriate food behavior?
2. What factors in the living situation need to change?
3. Are there personal reasons for food choices?
4. Is this a problem that may require help from coach, school nurse, parent, physician, or a psychologist?
5. Will group support be a benefit or will extensive, more repetitive counseling be effective?

Then:

1. Help the patient identify situations in which eating a particular food or taking part in a certain practice fails to meet the nutritional demands of athletics.

2. Review how change will help the patient meet the anticipated goals.
3. Define the problems, such as limiting factors, personal reasons, misunderstandings, or psychological or emotional needs. Request from the patient information on finances, time allowances, and schedules.
4. Explore every possible solution to the problems, or investigate an alternative solution.

As an example of the extreme, several years ago I was working wih an Olympic-class hurdler who was anemic and needed to gain weight. Adequate food did not seem to be the problem. She understood her diet but was still unable to gain. Almost since birth she had been a foster child, and her guardian was reluctant to allow her to attend athletic camp or to receive medical attention. She later married her coach, who encouraged her to enter a hospital for a complete medical examination. There it was discovered that she was a host to intestinal parasites. After treatment and during observation (for 6 months) she gained more than 20 lb.

Whatever the situation is, it is necessary to identify needs and limitations and the patient's ability to make changes. In most cases, basic guidance, education, and encouragement suffice to meet needs. If a definite risk exists, careful and supportive counseling is called for and may well determine the health outcome.

Follow-up evaluation needs to be part of the continuing plan of care. Ongoing awareness and concern for nutrition should be a focus of every health examination and should be renewed at the beginning of each season or change in sport. The alert nutritionist will show interest in maintaining counseling and helping with any new problems.

Broader methods of counseling are used when entire teams are addressed. The nutritionist usually discusses the special needs of a sport at the coach's request, such as weight maintenance, special fluid needs, and preevent meals. Individual requests for help often arise from such meetings.

There are currently several physicians[20] who answer general interest questions through syndicated columns[21]; nutritionists,[22] too, often speak via local newspapers, magazines, and newsletters that deal with the athletic population. Community health educators are others who provide information by way of programs and materials for schools and the general public. (Names and addresses may be found in Appendix 1.)

PHYSICIAN RECOMMENDATIONS FOR NUTRITION AND DIAGNOSIS-RELATED CARE

"Would you help this athlete with nutrition?" That request, or variations of it, is heard routinely by dietitians.

Within the past decade, there has been a decided shift of responsibility for giving nutritional advice to those who take part in sports. Although the physician still dispenses diet recommendations with his or her prescriptions, today that task and follow-up consultation fall more often to the dietitian. And rightly so. As more and more is learned about diet and nutrition, it has become apparent that this expanding body of knowledge should be applied by those who have specific training and experience. Because the influence of nutrition on the health and performance of the athlete is tremendously important, the role of the dietitian—a member of the athlete's helping team—is a stellar one.

This section contains combined proposals for currently acceptable nutritional guidelines.[23, 24] It offers no dietary penicillin, because there is none. Aside from sending a boat load of runners to sea without a lemon, controlled scientific studies of nutrient deficiencies, in any phase of life, are unethical. Conclusions must be based on interpretations of data. The physician's responsibility is to consider each patient individually, to evaluate his or her nutritional status, examine life-style and eating habits, and to design the best protective and therapeutic program possible.

Following is dietary protocol for advising and evaluating athletes and other physically active patients. The information is based on entries taken from the pages of a practicing dietitian's notebooks.

Alcohol Abuse

Alcohol abuse is the most common form of drug abuse. About 100 million adults in the United States drink, and it is estimated that 9 million of them are alcoholics. Not just a few of these are athletes. Alcohol is a toxin; is ulcerogenic; decreases absorption of fats, fat-soluble vitamins, thiamine, folic acid, and vitamin B_{12}; and inhibits glycogen metabolism.

Objectives.—Fluid and electrolyte imbalances and nutritional deficiencies (anemia, malnutrition, hypoglycemia, liver damage, etc.) need to be corrected, and a nutrient-dense diet must be accepted.

Dietary Recommendations.—Emphasize high amounts of protein (1.5–2.0 gm/kg of body weight, or 100–150 gm/day), high amounts of carbohydrate (300–500 gm), and low to moderate amounts of fat (25% to 30% of calories). Include potassium-rich foods such as potatoes, carrots, broccoli, brussels sprouts, cauliflower, spinach, bananas, cantaloupe, grapes, and most fruit juices. Supplement with a therapeutic vitamin B complex, especially folacin. Check diet for good sources of vitamins A, D, E, and K and zinc. Stimulate appetite with appealing and familiar foods. Avoid alcohol.

Patient Education.—Review cookbooks, mention the acceptability of nonalcoholic beverages, and work with the dormitory cooks; try anything that will help the patient in preparation of nutrient-dense meals. Review basic nutrition for the particular age group. Review vitamin and mineral supplementation requirements. Explain and document that alcohol cannot be used for muscular work and that it may interfere with oxygen utilization and transport. RDA levels of zinc or cyproheptadine (Periactin) may stimulate appetite.

Review and Monitor.—Check height and weight; glucose, cholesterol, triglyceride, hemoglobin, transferrin, potassium, and uric acid levels; hematocrit; dietary history; and other drug use.

Other Considerations.—Give immediate feedback to other health care team members, coach, and parents. Check on driving record.

Food Allergies

An allergy results from hypersensitivity to an antigen of a food source. Allergic reactions are caused by the release of histamine and serotonin. The most common symptoms of food allergies are anaphylaxis, diarrhea, nausea, vomiting, cramping, abdominal distention and pain, edema, eczema, rhinitis, and asthma. Behavioral changes are also common.

Objectives.—Avoid or exclude offending allergens. If they are unknown, begin a dietary history that includes a description of symptoms from their onset to the present. Eliminate suspected foods and keep a record of symptoms and all foods eaten for 2 weeks. Also record medications. If offending foods are not obvious, use the skin scratch test or the radioallergosorbent test (RAST). These tests frequently give false-negative or false-positive results, however, so keep a daily food and symptom record to confirm the results of these tests. Devise as adequate a diet as possible and consider supplementation. (Avoid "natural" supplements, due to the likelihood of concentration of all ingredients.) Advise the patient to drink ample water to relieve dryness of the mucous membranes caused by medications.

Dietary Recommendations.—Read the labels of all foods served to the patient, check all menus, and monitor all food preparation methods to exclude contact with the allergen. Monitor diet quality. Diet should provide sufficient calories for growth requirements and athletic training.

Patient Education.—Encourage the patient or parent to keep a food diary and to read all labels. Provide reading material on common allergens for the family, and give as much support as possible to the patient. This is a tough time. All members of the athletic team should be aware of the allergies of the player. Most allergy patients need help in ordering restaurant food and may need to carry sack lunches on road trips.

The following are common allergens that may have long-term nutritional consequences:

1. Milk. Check for deficiencies in protein, milk protein, riboflavin, vitamin A, and calcium. Casein is used in many food products.
2. Eggs. Check for iron content of diet. Egg albumin is used in frozen dinners and many other food mixes.
3. Wheat. Check for B vitamins and iron. Read labels on packaged soups and sauces.
4. Citrus fruits. Check for deficiencies in vitamin C.
5. Corn. Check labels for cornstarch, corn syrup, corn oil, baking powder, frozen yogurt.
6. Molds. Use a diet that is low in mushrooms, cheeses, sour cream, bacon, jams and jellies, and spices.

Review and Monitor.—Study general growth trend and recent changes, chronic complaints of gastrointestinal stress, rashes, hemoglobin levels, and hematocrit.

Other Considerations.—It is important to get help from a physician who is competent, experienced, and successful with allergy diagnosis and treatment. Also, it costs little to assess the patient's nutrient needs. Any patient who switches from a high-sugar, high-refined food, nutrient-poor diet (which is fairly common among high school athletes) to one consisting of nourishing, wholesome foods will feel better. Many athletes are affected by pollens and molds. Symptoms are sneezing, watery eyes, fatigue, headache, coughing, congestion, and itching. If the onset of environmental allergies is accompanied by food allergies, the patient usually experiences irritability, loss of appetite, and depression.

Amenorrhea

Primary amenorrhea is a failure to begin menstruation. Secondary amenorrhea is complete cessation of the menstrual cycle (at least 3 months' duration). Both conditions are associated with low estrogen levels, low body weight, low body fat, intense physical training, and high stress. It is frequently seen in dancers, swimmers, gymnasts, ice skaters, and long-distance runners or in any other sport where there is a high-energy demand. The situation is compounded by growth needs.

Objectives.—Determine the duration of amenorrhea, and chart related conditions such as stress fractures and food-related problems. Estimate caloric expenditure in exercise. Provide a nutritionally balanced, individualized diet pattern that can allow for 8 oz to 1 lb of weight gain weekly.

Dietary Recommendations.—Calculate the patient's ideal body weight. Determine caloric requirements by adding metabolic energy requirements, athletic expenditure, and any other extra caloric needs such as growth or vigorous work. Emphasize high-protein and high-calcium intake, with frequent feedings.

Education.—Help the patient plan meals in her regular environment, emphasize the connection between amenorrhea and osteoporosis, and explain the importance of weight-bearing exercise on all parts of the body.

Review and Monitor.—Check height and weight, ideal body weight, usual weight, recent changes in weight, estrogen count, hemoglobin level and hematocrit, and onset of menses.

Other Considerations.—Advise a complete gynecological examination. Review dietary recommendations with the coach and parent. Examine any available x-rays for possible osteoporosis.

Premenstrual Syndrome

The duration of premenstrual syndrome (PMS) varies widely. It may last any length of time before the menstrual period and is characterized by intense mood swings, irritability, breast tenderness, and bloating.

Objective.—Instruct the patient regarding diet changes that may help to relieve symptoms.

Dietary Recommendations.—Suggest low-fat foods, fewer snacks like potato chips and chocolate bars, elimination of most sources of caffeine and alcohol, a decrease in salt, and an increase in fiber. Increase fluids and avoid diuretics.

Patient Education.—Explain that improving the diet may have something to do with reducing the symptoms but is not a guarantee of relief. Certainly it is better than submitting to cravings for high-fat, high-calorie junk foods and avoiding the temptation to replace meals with desserts.

Review and Monitor.—Check weight gain during menstrual cycle, diet history, and salt intake.

Other Considerations.—Activities such as walking and biking have been reported to give relief. Since the average woman may have as many as 400 menstrual periods during her lifetime, it is wise to be careful about the quality of her diet.

Folic Acid Anemia

Folic acid is required for the synthesis of DNA and RNA and maturation of red and white blood cells. Folic acid deficiency is usually caused by inadequate diet, alcoholism, oral contraceptive use, or pregnancy.

Objectives.—Increase folic acid in the diet and improve the diet so that it provides all nutrients needed to make red blood cells. Check for any malabsorption syndromes.

Dietary Recommendations.—Give diet instructions for adequate folic acid, proteins, iron, vitamin C, and vitamin B_{12} (fresh fruits and vegetables, fish, legumes, whole grains, and meats).

Patient Education.—The athlete should understand the basics of formation of red blood cells, nutrient requirements, absorption enhancers, and correct diet planning.

Review and Monitor.—Check serum folate, hemoglobin, and transferrin levels, hematocrit; and complete blood cell count. Inquire about other drug use. Oral contraceptives, folic acid antagonists, and anticonvulsants interfere with the body's use of folic acid. Supplementation of folic acid, as in prenatal vitamins, works better than diet alone.

Iron Deficiency Anemia

Anemia can result from inadequate dietary intake (or impaired absorption) of iron, from loss of blood, from repeated pregnancies, or during accelerated growth (which occurs in puberty, pregnancy, and lactation). There are small losses from sweat, feces, and urine. Approximately 90% of the body's iron stores are recycled. Loss of iron from menstruation is approximately 30 mg/month. Some form of pica behavior is seen in one half of the patients with anemia.

Objectives.—Prescribe a diet adequate for iron requirements; examine the need for supplements; monitor ice chewing, crunching of Lifesavers, lettuce, or celery, gum or tobacco chewing, or any other type of pica behavior.

Dietary Recommendations.—Include some food with high heme values in each meal, such as liver, eggs, kidney, all forms of beef, oysters, and sardines. Eat liberal amounts of dried fruits, whole-grain products, molasses, iron-fortified cereals (1 cup of Cream of Wheat contains 18 mg of iron), and increase intake of ascorbic acid–rich foods at each meal to enhance iron absorption (e.g., oranges, grapefruit, tomatoes, broccoli, cabbage, baked potatoes, and strawberries). Screen the diet for excessive fiber, coffee, and tea (which reduce iron absorption). Encourage cooking in cast iron cookware. Legumes are an important iron source for vegetarians.

Patient Education.—Suggest that those engaged in strenuous activity and competition should have greater awareness of their iron status. Explain that hemoglobin is made from amino acids, iron, and copper, whereas red blood cells require vitamin B_{12}, folacin, and amino acids. Acid foods enhance iron absorption;

tannins, phytates, phosphates, and oxalates inhibit absorption. Iron needs are 18 mg/day for women and 10 mg/day for men. Iron deficiency is a major health problem. Supplementations may cause constipation, stomach ache, or both; increase their use slowly (stool color will change).

Review and Monitor.—Check weight, red blood cell count (small, microcytic, hypochromic), transferrin and ferritin levels, complete blood cell count, differential white blood cell count, and menstrual losses.

Other Considerations.—Investigate complaints of fatigue, inability to carry out training demands, pale skin, lack of appetite, antacid use, hyperactivity, and reduced attentiveness. Inquire about birth order.

Sickle Cell Anemia

Sickle cell anemia is a familial, hereditary, hemolytic anemia. It is most common in black athletes. Cells are crescent shaped. Iron stores are frequently in excess.

Objectives.—Improve the patient's ability to participate in activities. Encourage him or her to accept a nutritionally sound, individualized diet.

Dietary Recommendations.—Determine if there is or is not an iron deficiency. If iron stores are high, avoid those foods that are high in iron or highly fortified. Ascorbic acid foods should be eaten alone. Diet, regardless of iron stores, should be high in folate (400 µg) and zinc (15–30 mg) and may need supplementation of these minerals.

Patient Education.—Encourage the patient to plan meals that are high in folic acid, good-quality protein, zinc, and vitamin E.

Review and Monitor.—Evaluate height and weight, growth grids from age 1, urinary zinc and transferrin levels, and complete blood cell count.

Other Considerations.—Check for abdominal pain, hepatitis, gallstones, renal function, failure to thrive, and release of iron from the liver.

Sports Anemia

Sports anemia is a condition in which there is an increased destruction of erythrocytes, decreased hemoglobin levels as a result of an acute stress response to exercise, increased uptake of iron in muscle, and greater plasma volume. Possible causes include subnormal iron stores, poor iron absorption, high iron loss due to sweat, high trauma rate, hematuria, and poor diet. Also implicated are increased erythrocyte osmotic fragility, causing reduced red blood cell survival time, and a possible shift in the oxygen dissociation curve. It has not been determined if this nonclinical anemic state is harmful to the athlete.

Objectives.—Determine if the patient is iron deficient. Calculate a diet with at least 18 mg of iron/day for females and 10 mg of iron/day for males.

Dietary Recommendations.—The diet prescription should emphasize the variety and quality of foods as well as foods high in iron content and those containing enough energy to cover total caloric needs. Prescribe iron supplementation if appropriate.

Patient Education.—Explain the relationship between hemoglobin levels and oxygen-carrying capacity (reduced working capacity). All individuals at risk for anemia should have periodic iron status evaluations. Hemoglobin levels may fluctuate but do not vary significantly until iron stores are inadequate. All athletes should make only gradual changes in their training programs.

Review and Monitor.—Check former diet, recent dietary evaluations; body weight, iron content in diet, amount of menstrual flow, approximate sweat rate, serum ferritin level, percent of transferrin saturation, hemoglobin level, red blood cell count, hematocrit, and mean cell hemoglobin level.

Other Considerations.—Do not overlook cushioning in running shoes, duration of training schedules, vegetarian diets, weakness or fatigue, and other forms of anemia.

Anorexia Nervosa

Anorexia nervosa is a condition where the patient exhibits distorted body image, fear of obesity, weight loss of at least 25% of ideal body weight, refusal to maintain normal weight, amenorrhea of 3 months or longer, and absence of other illnesses that might induce weight loss. Patients have low BMRs, edema, hypercarotenemia, disturbance in hair growth, cold intolerance, dry skin, and loss in bone mass. Anorexics remain highly active; they deny hunger yet are often very interested in food preparation.

Objectives.—Determine realistic goals for the patient: (1) no further weight loss, (2) maintenance of weight, and (3) gradual weight gain. Obtain a diet history to assess original and present diet. Consider any other food-related problems such as bulimia or use of diuretics. Average length of corrective therapy is 2 years.

Dietary Recommendations.—Refeeding should take place gradually and with careful monitoring. Nutrient requirements are determined on actual weight, not on ideal body weight. Obtain a food preference list. Serve attractive meals in small amounts frequently throughout the day. Gradually increase caloric levels.

Nutritional care in the beginning of treatment is geared to providing information, helping the anorectic to change his or her ideas regarding food, and ensuring survival. Fat and milk may need to be restricted in severe cases since many patients have stopped making the enzymes necessary to digest them. Highly nourishing liquids may be given if the patient refuses food. Parenteral or nasogastric feedings are reserved for life-threatening states and are usually unnecessary.

Patient Education.—Continually encourage the patient to follow a balanced diet and to share low-calorie, nutrient-dense recipes. Patient may become constipated or bloated in refeeding as rehydration and glycogen storage gradually begins. He or she will need help in eating out, eating with others, weighing, recognizing hunger, and achieving satisfaction with weight gain and fit of clothing. Explain that the overall goals of treatment are to restore normal body weight and resolve the psychiatric and social components of the illness.

Review and Monitor.—Check present weight; weight changes; cholesterol, glucose, and hemoglobin levels; hematocrit; changes in growth; and menstrual history.

Other Considerations.—No single treatment for anorexia has been established as being superior. Behavior modification, individual and family counseling, diet counseling, and nutritional support have all proved successful. The highest athletic populations with anorexia are ballet dancers, gymnasts, and runners. Psychotherapy is necessary to turn the focus away from food to the underlying social problems. The average length of time before patient submits to therapy is close to 5 years.

Bulimia

Bulimia involves chronic binge eating, which is rapid consumption of large amounts of food in a short time, accompanied by a pattern of vomiting, abuse of laxatives and diuretics, and weight fluctuations. Medical consequences indicate electrolyte abnormalities, glandular swelling, gastric distention, tooth erosion, and rectal bleeding (from laxative overuse). Bulimics usually recognize that they are out of control, and compulsive (as indicated by high rates of stealing, substance abuse, and suicide).

Objectives.—Help the patient to assess the relationship between weight and food, accept reasonable weight for height, give up vomiting or purging, understand the importance of a good diet in reaching goals, and adapt a more physiologically normal diet pattern.

Dietary Recommendations.—Have the patient set his or her own weight goal, and provide a nutritionally balanced diet from favorite foods. Avoid foods that the patient vomited most frequently (cookies, breads, cereals, pies, etc.).

Patient Education.—The patient will need help in taking responsibility for eating habits and will benefit from the support of a faithful friend. Counseling must be on a frequent basis until vomiting subsides. The breakthrough will occur when the patient realizes that vomiting or laxatives will not aid in weight loss. Although these habits are often seen as a part of the syndrome of anorexia nervosa, these symptoms are recognized as a separate illness.

Review and Monitor.—Assess dental health; irritations to the throat; swollen glands; swollen and bloodshot eyes; edema; electrolyte balance; insulin, glucose, and triglyceride levels; quality of diet; growth grids; and weight changes.

Other Considerations.—Since bulimics frequently teach each other new methods of purging, group therapy has not proved successful. Aspiration of vomitus and mouth infections are frequently seen. Dancers and wrestlers often binge and purge during the dance or athletic season. The counselor needs to ask direct questions, to firmly contract with the patient: "Do you feel fat, binge/purge, fast, use laxatives, think a lot about food, have irregular periods, believe that your eating habits are abnormal?" Patient charting should be more detailed for young people who are extremely thin, are not growing, or who have recently lost weight during growth. Symptoms are not always apparent, because unlike the anorexic, the bulimic will usually be close to normal weight. All members of the health team need to be aware of the serious consequences of this eating problem.

Bronchitis

Bronchitis is caused by inflammation of the air passages. The acute form may follow a cold or other upper respiratory tract infection, producing sore throat, nasal discharge, fever, cough, and back and muscle pain. The chronic form is often a result of cigarette smoking, air pollution, or exposure to items such as dirty mats in gymnastics and wrestling.

Objectives.—Normalize body temperature, prevent dehydration, and allow rest.

Dietary Recommendations.—Provide instructions for a well-balanced diet. Sufficient calories will increase BMR and ventilatory drive. The optimum proportions of fat, protein, and carbohydrate for the treatment of bronchitis, or any other respiratory problem, has not been determined. Increase the intake of fluids and ascorbic acid; avoid milk if it promotes the formation of mucus. Avoid drinking stimulant beverages (i.e., coffee, tea) with medications (e.g., theophylline). Bronchodilators may cause gastric irritation.

Patient Education.—Explain that malnutrition decreases the ability of the lungs to exchange gases, remove secretions and foreign matter from the body, and resist infection. The fact that all of these functions are restored by proper diet and hydration emphasizes the importance of good nutritional status in patients with respiratory compromise.

Review and Monitor.—Look at the caloric content of the diet, growth, ideal body weight, hemoglobin level and hematocrit, edema, urine volume, and the total white blood cell count.

Other Considerations.—Screen for general health habits such as rest, quality of sleep, stress levels, and intense training levels.

Burns

Simple redness, as in sunburn, occurs with a first-degree burn. In a second-degree burn, redness and blistering occur. This is often seen in crew regattas, all-week track festivals, sailing, hiking, and mountain expeditions. Third-degree burns, where skin and tissue destruction occurs, have been reported in mountain and cross-country experiences, hydroplane races, Ironman, and biking competitions.

Objectives.—Although the main objective is prevention, the second is to relieve pain and restore fluid and electrolyte balance—to prevent shock and avoid renal shutdown from decreased plasma volume and reduced cardiac output. Any type of burn elevates basal metabolism. Infection is extremely common.

Dietary Recommendations.—On-site first aid treatment may require immediate use of intraveneous fluids to prevent gastric distention and paralytic ileus. Follow-up treatment should advise high-calorie, high-protein foods, with five or six small meals/day plus snacks. Protein intake should be 2 gm/kg of ideal body weight. Weigh every 24 hours. Caloric intake should be 40 to 60 kcal/kg every 24 hours. (The maximum calorie load the body can handle is near 100% above the resting metabolism rate). Provide extra fluid (this may amount to a volume equal to 12% of the total preburn weight and depends on the extent of burning), and encourage the consumption of apricot, grapefruit, or orange juices for potassium. Supplement the diet with 500 mg of ascorbic acid, RDA levels for zinc calcium and iron, and two to three times the RDA for vitamin B complex.

Some dressings (e.g., silver nitrate) leach sodium, potassium, magnesium, calcium, and B vitamins from the body. The burn patient may need added salt. Pain medications often suppress appetite. Regular meals need to be encouraged.

Patient Education.—Every athlete has probably experienced mild to severe sunburn, but this condition is not to be ignored, especially because it usually occurs in situations where dehydration, cramping, exhaustion, and glycogen depletion are common. Prevention is the key, and, perhaps, experience with the ensuing pain provides the best lesson. Many athletes do not allow recovery time between competitions, and this compounds the hazard. If the patient is hospitalized, as may be the case in automobile racing, the previous recommendations also are appropriate. Fat is a helpful way to supply extra calories. A firm and persistent approach to total calorie requirements is necessary.

Enlist a family member to help monitor caloric and protein intake.

Review and Monitor.—Be aware of preburn weight, current fluid intake and urinary output, hemoglobin level and hematocrit, and electrolyte levels.

Other Considerations.—The diet should include favorite foods (screen for allergies and dislikes), but remember, this is not a time for junk food. The severity of dehydration is affected by weight lost and percentage of body burned. The patient should be assisted with feeding, and a record should be kept of intake. Keep mealtimes pleasant, without interruption for laboratory tests or physician visits.

Insulin-Dependent Diabetes Mellitus

Diabetes mellitus is a disorder of carbohydrate metabolism. Type 1, or insulin-dependent diabetes mellitis (IDDM), generally occurs in young individuals. In this condition, the pancreas lacks the ability to make sufficient amounts of insulin, and there is a rapid onset of symptoms (thirst, frequent urination, tiredness, and weight loss). It is difficult to control, and there are wide blood glucose swings and insulin reactions.

Objectives.—Diabetes can be controlled by diet, exercise, and insulin. Consistency is the key to management. Encourage regular mealtimes plus interval feedings. For athletes, it may be necessary to make two plans, one for exercise days and one for nonexercise days. Achieve and maintain ideal body weight.

Dietary Recommendations.—Develop a meal pattern according to the type of insulin, frequency of injection, and physical activity. Determine calories by multiplying the ideal body weight by 10. Add 100 to 200 calories for growth requirements (subtract 100 to 200 calories if the patient is short or elderly). Add 30% for light activity and 50% to 75% for moderate to heavy activity. If weight loss is necessary, subtract 500 to 750 calories. (Some diabetics may need even less to lose weight.) Monitor weight, and adjust energy intake depending on weight change. Protein should account for 12% to 20% of calories; carbohydrates should comprise 50% to 60% percent, and fat should be less than 35% (individualize the diet to fit the patient's life-style and present eating habits). Increase intake of complex carbohydrates from legumes (dried beans, peas, and lentils), and pastas. Include adequate fiber and potassium; encourage reduction of sodium, cholesterol, and saturated fats; and avoid large amounts of concentrated sweets.

Patient Education.—Teach the use of the exchange lists, and encourage the patient to keep a dietary history. Promote regular mealtimes and snacks, the importance of self-care, emergency feedings during illness or stress, how to dine away from home, and instructions on how to read labels. Emphasize that good nutrition for the diabetic is a well-balanced diet that everyone should follow.

Review and Monitor.—Carefully watch ideal body weight, growth, fasting glucose levels, blood glucose monitoring values (urine glucose and ketones if patient is not routinely doing blood glucose tests), cholesterol levels, triglyceride levels, electrolyte values, the hemoglobin A_{Ic} test, and dietary histories.

Other Considerations.—During heavy exercise, it is necessary to replenish glucose. (Swimmers need orange juice mid-training; runners need snacks along the way.) Individuals need to monitor their glucose needs daily, keep sugar cubes or hard candy in their pockets (something small, convenient, and concentrated) if practice is hard and sustained, have a snack before practice, and have a source of carbohydrate halfway through the workout. For the average athlete, increase food intake accordingly; anticipate sudden changes in activity that may drastically lower blood glucose levels or decrease insulin dosage. Instead of carbohydrate loading before activity, extra carbohydrates should be consumed during exercise. Glucose monitoring during exercise will help determine energy needs, as during intense exercise in cold temperatures. The abdomen is the best injection site if insulin's effects need to be delayed. Exercise should be done with a friend who is aware of states of confusion, weakness, tiredness, unconsciousness, and even convulsions. Solitary exercise or activities such as scuba diving, free-falling, and mountain climbing (where patient is isolated) should be avoided.

It is advisable to quantify exercise and prescribe it in the same way as insulin and diet. For assistance, send for *Diabetes and Exercise: How to Get Started*. It may be obtained by sending $2.50 to International Diabetes Center, 5000 West 39th Street, Minneapolis, MN 55416.

Non-Insulin-Dependent Diabetes Mellitus

Non-insulin-dependent diabetes mellitus (NIDDM) generally occurs in later life and most often in older, overweight individuals. It is different from IDDM in that the pancreas produces insulin, often more than needed, but the body's cells lack receptor sites to receive it. Non-insulin-dependent diabetes mellitus develops slowly, with mild symptoms. Treatment involves diet *control,* exercise, oral medication, and, in some severe cases, insulin injections.

Objectives.—Achieve and maintain ideal body weight. Prescribe a diet that is well balanced and includes the correct number of calories based on age and on activity and weight changes required. Aim for behavior modification and planned activities. Prevent or predict complications (hypertension, hyperlipidemia, retinopathy, nephropathy, and neuropathy). Blood glucose levels that are under or less than 130%, and 80% normal urine results, are desired.

Dietary Recommendations.—Prescribe three meals/day, with small snacks. Determine caloric level by formula listed in IDDM. Avoid concentrated sugars; use more complex carbohydrates. Limit cholesterol to less than 300 mg daily, limit saturated fats, and limit sodium to 3 gm/day. Maintain a liberal fiber intake (at least 30 gm/day). Avoid alcohol.

Patient Education.—Consider use of food diaries, and emphasize regular mealtimes and exercise. When diabetics are out of control, their bodies mobilize fat for energy. The amount of cholesterol and triglycerides in their blood rises. Impaired circulation is responsible for an increased risk of amputation. Emphasize self-care, glucose monitoring, instructions on illness, stress, and label reading. Discourage alcohol use.

Review and Monitor.—Follow the same procedures as in IDDM, and stress weight control. Achieving and maintaining a healthy weight, in addition to partaking in some form of aerobic exercise to increase heart and lung capacity, will make all the difference in the world.

Other Considerations.—Of utmost importance is *control.*

Simple Depression

Quality nutrition is an adjunct to good physical health. Deficient intake of many essential nutrients over a long period of time can result in damage to the nervous system and consequent changes in behavior. Although psychiatric and behavioral effects of water-soluble vitamins have been documented, controlled trials in humans reveal various results, and most megavitamin therapy is classified as anecdotal.

Objectives.—Provide and instruct for an adequate nutritional intake, monitor weight weekly, and determine if weight loss is caused by inadequate calories. Assess eating habits and problems that may include loneliness; difficulty in shopping or food preparation; boredom; poor sleep habits; drug or alcohol abuse; or troubles with school, coach, family, or peer group.

Dietary Recommendations.—Prescribe a diet that is high in a variety of foods, good-quality proteins, and that has a high-calcium content. Monitor levels of iron, thiamin, riboflavin, niacin, and vitamins B_6 and B_{12}. A tyramine-restricted diet (for patients given monoamine oxidase drugs) excludes aged cheese, beer, wine, ale, pickled herring, chicken livers, yeast, coffee, bean pods, figs, sausage, salami, eggplant, pepperoni, commercial gravies, meat extracts, yeast concentrates, bouillon cubes, and chocolate.

Patient Education.—Encourage simple, creative menu planning. Advise at least one meal/week in a good restaurant and company to dinner (or breakfast or lunch) once weekly. Promote water intake. Monitor binge eating; high-salt, high-fat snacking; and fast-food eating. Urge the patient to think of the pleasantries of dining, such as candles, flowers, music, family, and friends.

Constipation

This condition occurs when fecal mass remains in the colon longer than the normal 24 to 72 hours after meal ingestion. It is often associated with intestinal gas and upper gastrointestinal pain during competition. Sometimes constipation is followed by explosive diarrhea.

Objectives.—For atonic constipation (reduced bowel motility), provide bulk to stimulate peristalsis (movement of the digestive tract). Spastic constipation (narrowing of the colon, with small ribbon-like stools) caused by obstruction, anxiety, and stress is helped by resting the gut. Both conditions are very common in athletics, especially when weight management or dehydration are problems. Anticipating situations when constipation is likely to be a problem is effective prevention.

Dietary Recommendations.—For atonic constipation, increase fiber with additional whole grains, fruits, and vegetables; add a bran muffin to breakfast and a salad to lunch and dinner. Increase fluid. Establish normal bowel movements by allowing time in the morning. Often hot water or coffee, followed by abdominal stretching, is sufficient to start peristalsis. Spastic constipation is often relieved by resting the gut, consuming high-calorie, high-protein liquid supplements, avoiding high fiber, using a stool softener during the 2 days before competition, and resolving anxiety and arousal related to competition and training (control of mood shifts).

Patient Education.—Communicate that constipation is not abnormal during stress. Medicines containing high levels of iron or calcium may be causes. Check ingredients of supplements. Check laxatives for sodium levels; some are very high. Plant fibers such as Metamucil must be taken with at least 8 oz of fluid/teaspoon. Diet may produce relief but cannot cure the condition. Fiber may help but should be introduced to the diet slowly. There may be a need to increase water to 10 glasses/day.

Review and Monitor.—Watch for anxiety and stressful conditions, gastrointestinal distress, diet changes, and recent weight changes.

Other Considerations.—A normal bowel routine is needed, but daily fecal evacuation is not needed by everyone. (The need for colonic therapy can be best advised by a physician.)

Diarrhea

Diarrhea is a symptom of many disorders in which there is increased peristalsis with decreased transit time through the gut. Reduced reabsorption of water and watery stools result. The diarrhea may be functional, from irritation or stress, or organic, from intestinal lesions.

Objectives.—Prevent dehydration, alter stool consistency, rest the gut, and try to predict situations where this condition might occur.

Dietary Recommendations.—Abstain from food for 24 hours; give intravenous fluids if necessary and electrolytes and oral fluids as allowed. Parenteral nutrition may be needed for intractable diarrhea. Prolonged diarrhea may cause temporary lactose intolerance, so that milk may not be tolerated. As stools are formed, gradually introduce small amounts of food. Minimal residue foods are well tolerated. Start with broth, tea, toast, bland foods, or diet as tolerated. Fluid volume should not greatly exceed need, because excessive fluid may be a cause of continued diarrhea. Kaopectate has no side effects. Lomotil may cause bloating, constipation, dry mouth, or nausea.

Patient Education.—Describe dehydration and the necessity of both salt and water. Cleanliness and petroleum jelly (Vasoline) may alleviate a sore rectum.

Other Considerations.—Other members of the family may contract diarrhea if the cause is from contamination or influenza. Encourage fluid intake, bland food, and pectins (e.g., in applesauce and bananas) before diarrhea starts.

Traveler's Diarrhea

Commentary.—Dysentery, or inflammation of the bowel, results from poor sanitation; diarrhea, a gastrointestinal bacterial infection, is caused by contaminated food or water.

Objectives.—Reduce irritation, and prevent dehydration.

Dietary Recommendations.—Consume clear liquids (chicken soup, boullion, Diet 7-Up) until diarrhea stops. Add fruit juices and bananas, and then introduce low-fiber foods.

Patient Education.—Advice is most effective when given before the trip. Use only cooked foods and bottled water, juices, and beverages. Brush teeth with bottled water. Avoid fresh fruits and vegetables that have been washed with contaminated water. Avoid ice cubes from contaminated water. Do not eat foods from street carts, or buy from suspicious vendors. When camping, boil water for 10 minutes, and add 1 tablespoon of chlorine bleach to each gallon of water when washing food.

Review and Monitor.—Check weight loss, fluid intake, urinary output (clear or light amber), and electrolyte balance.

Other Considerations.—Carry a 1-day supply of local water and some baby food (applesauce, bananas). Bring Kaopectate, diphenoxylate with atropine sulfate (Lomotil), and small bars of soap. (Many public rest rooms are not supplied with soap, toilet paper, or towels.) Consult your physician on the advisability of carrying tetracyclines.

Food Poisoning

All uncooked foods are contaminated with bacteria, molds, and other microbes. Although most are harmless in the amounts usually consumed or in the home environment when good sanitation is practiced, some microorganisms can cause severe, sudden illness either as a result of reproduction within the host *(Salmonella, Shigella)* or from the toxins they release (botulism). Most bacterial food poisoning is due to improper food handling or inadequate hand washing, cooking, refrigeration, or storage. Some cases can be prevented by avoiding foods during certain seasons (shellfish), destroying contaminated foods, and choosing foods wisely when traveling.

Objectives.—Identify food poisoning in patient; hospitalize if necessary; correct dehydration.

Diet Recommendations.—Withhold food until vomiting, diarrhea, and cramping subside. Give intravenous fluids and electrolytes if needed. (See the section on diarrhea.)

Patient Education.—Prevention of food poisoning may be possible by selecting restaurants wisely and handling food properly.

Review and Monitor.—Assess weight loss, white blood cell count, and intake and output.

Other Considerations.—It is not uncommon for food poisoning to affect the whole team at once, and its consequences can be devastating. Probable occurrence will be at district or state meets, international competition, and meals offered picnic or buffet style in hot weather.

Suspect foods are cream sauces, fish, turkey, or chicken, reheated foods, or foods that have not been cooked to at least 180°F. If you are traveling with the team, bring your laboratory coat and thermometer, and introduce yourself to the food service personnel.

Gastritis

Gastritis is an inflammation of the stomach and intestinal lining, caused by alcohol, food allergy, food poisoning, intestinal virus, cathartics, or other drugs. Complaints include nausea, vomiting, intestinal rumbles, diarrhea, and, often, fever.

Objectives.—Allow the stomach to rest; permit fluids.

Dietary Recommendations.—For acute gastritis, do not allow any food for 24 to 48 hours. Allow crushed ice for thirst, and then progress to soft or bland foods. Do not allow any alcohol or hot beverages. For chronic gastritis, give small frequent feedings of bland foods. Progress gradually to larger amounts and varieties of foods as tolerated. Restrict fatty, highly seasoned food, and alcohol and caffeine. Encourage the patient to chew solid foods well. If solids are not well tolerated, encourage high-calorie, high-protein liquid supplements.

Patient Education.—Encourage a well-balanced diet. Use the diet history to teach about offending foods. Discourage use of gastric stimulants, such as pepper, chili powder, alcohol, caffeine, decaffeinated coffee, aspirin, smoking, chewing tobacco, and individual food intolerances. Provide repetitive dietary instructions. Urge check-ins each day.

Review and Monitor.—Observe weight changes, electrolyte balances, daily dietary intake, duration of inflammation, and use of prescription or over-the-counter drugs.

Other Considerations.—Other causes of gastritis may be high levels of stress or poor eating habits, such as skipping breakfast (but having coffee and donuts) or eating various combinations of hot, fatty, spicy, and nonnutritive food. Check the protein quality of the diet, and screen for ulcers. Gastritis is a common complaint of athletes who continually restrict food and consume high amounts of caffeine. Antacids can cause constipation.

Heartburn, or Hiatal Hernia

Hiatal hernia is caused by a protrusion of part of the stomach above the diaphragm muscle (which separates the chest from the abdomen), resulting in the enlargment of the diaphragm opening through which the esophagus passes to join the stomach. There may be no symptoms, or there may be pain, swallowing difficulties, and frequent and objectionable burping.

Objectives.—Normalize reflux into esophagus; achieve ideal body weight; improve posture; reduce gastric acidity, if possible; avoid large meals eaten quickly; and avoid meals eaten before bedtime. Design an individual diet that reflects the patient's needs.

Dietary Recommendations.—Prescribe small, frequent feedings of soft or bland foods; avoidance of nighttime eating; an increase in protein and decrease in fat; and a decrease of irritating foods (citrus fruits, spicy or greasy foods). Limit coffee, alcohol, peppermint, and spearmint. Antacid overuse will increase body levels of sodium and may provide too much calcium, which will diminish levels of magnesium and phosphorus.

Patient Education.—Discuss dietary goals with the individual. Screen for bulimia, weight gain, intense stress, and pregnancy. Have patient maintain an upright position for at least one hour after eating.

Review and Monitor.—Check ideal body weight; glucose, gastrin, cholesterol, and triglyceride levels; and recent weight gain.

Other Considerations.—The condition is prevalent in weight lifters, body builders, and other sports where weight gain is a factor. Forced weight gain should never exceed 2 lb/week, even in adolescence. Esophagitis in wrestlers usually occurs toward the end of the season when they are vomiting to maintain competitive weight. Check for blood in vomitus.

Ulcer

An eroded lesion in the gastric mucosa or intestinal mucosa is termed an ulcer. A gastric ulcer is located in the stomach; a peptic ulcer is located in the duodenum.

Objectives.—Dietary treatment should consider the patient as a whole and should provide essential nutrients and acid-reducing features.

Dietary Recommendations.—Advise frequent and regular meals; sufficient calories to maintain ideal body weight; increased consumption of complex carbohydrates and fiber; restricted intake of fat, sugar, alcohol and caffeine, and other foods that may cause gastric distress (e.g., pepper and garlic). If there is doubt of nutritional adequacy, protein, vitamin, and iron supplements should be added.

Patient Education.—Complete healing takes from 14 to 100 days. Discuss predisposing factors, namely, faulty dietary habits, excessive smoking or use of chewing tobacco, overuse of aspirin, high consumption of coffee and cola drinks, rushed meals and irregular meals, and inadequate sleep and rest. Emotional conflicts, psychological stress, nervous strain, or trauma can cause a disturbance of the nerves that control the blood supply to the stomach.

Review and Monitor.—Check height and weight; red blood cell count; hematocrit; hemoglobin, transferrin, cholesterol, and triglyceride levels; nutritional adequacy of the diet; and the patient's pain profile.

Other Considerations.—Antacids should be taken between meals before bed, or both. Cimetidine (Tagamet) should be taken with food (it may cause diarrhea or constipation). Decaffeinated coffee increases gastric secretion. There is no proof that a strict bland diet increases the healing rate or prevents the recurrence of peptic ulcer. Often bedtime or night eating will cause discomfort.

Gout

Gout is a hereditary, abnormal metabolism of purines that causes a form of acute arthritis (inflamed joints), usually in the knees and feet. Elevated levels of serum uric acid lead to deposits of uric acid crystals. It is frequently associated with large consumption of protein, calories, alcohol, high-fat food, and chronic dehydration.

Objectives.—Achieve and maintain ideal body weight, increase excretion of urates, and force fluids. Assess incidence of hypertension, coronary heart disease, and diabetes.

Dietary Recommendations.—Increase carbohydrates and decrease fat; limit or exclude purine yielding foods, such as liver and other organ meats, shellfish, anchovies, smoked meats, sardines, and meat extracts (found in sauces and gravies and in frozen dinners and soups); exclude alcoholic beverages (especially beer and wine); yeasts; large quantities of legumes; and increase fluids to 8 to 10 glasses/24 hours. Fruits, vegetables, low-fat dairy products, and cereals may be consumed as desired. Discourage fasting.

Patient Education.—Review other episodes and question whether they are related to drinking, eating, severe dieting, ketosis, or intense exercise. Review purine-yielding foods, and omit those from the diet. Drugs that block renal absorption of urates, such as probenecid (Benemid), require a large intake of fluids. Indomethacin (Indocin) or adrenocorticotropic hormone (ACTH) may require a restricted sodium intake.

Review and Monitor.—Observe weight changes, ideal body weight, pattern of attacks, serum uric acid level, urate crystals in urine, cholesterol levels, triglyceride levels, fluid intake, and alcohol use.

Other Considerations.—The disease resembles arthritis and is extremely painful but also can be diagnosed as muscular pain or strain after prolonged athletic exertion, such as bike racing. It usually occurs after the age of 30. The first attack may last for only a few days and may be treated as an overuse injury. Occasionally, an attack follows surgery or high levels of stress. With advancement of the disease, attacks become more frequent and prolonged.

Fever

Fever may be acute, as with influenza, or chronic, as with infection. Bacterial infections cause severe and prolonged loss of nitrogen. Mild viral invasion, such as that in chickenpox, will produce negative nitrogen balance even when the patient is receiving adequate protein for ideal body weight.

Objectives.—Return patient to a positive nitrogen balance, rehydrate, meet increased nutrient needs caused by the hypermetabolic state, and replenish glycogen stores.

Dietary Recommendations.—Determine normal BMR, and then add 7% of the BMR for each degree Fahrenheit (13% for each degree Celsius) of elevation of temperature above normal. Adjust calories upward if there is blood poisoning or restlessness or if the fever is associated with any other complicating factors (e.g., in bone fractures). During the first few days of fever, supply 1.0 gm of good-quality protein/kg of ideal body weight (meat, fish, poultry, eggs, milk, cheese, and soups and broths made from protein sources). As fever subsides, increase protein to 2.0 gm/kg of ideal body weight and calories to 35 to 45 calories/kg of ideal body weight.

Patient should consume 350 gm of carbohydrates to spare protein and restore glycogen, often 3 to 4 quarts (16 cups) of fluid/day are needed. Fevers increase the need for vitamin B complex, ascorbic acid, and vitamin A. As energy needs increase, thiamin, riboflavin, and niacin requirements increase.

Antibiotics should be taken with water on an empty stomach. They may cause diarrhea and nausea. Penicillin should not be taken with acidic foods or fluids (e.g., fruit juices). Tetracycline should be taken with water on an empty stomach. Do not give with milk or 2 hours before or after use of calcium-containing foods. Supply salty broths and fruit juices to replenish minerals.

Patient Education.—Stress self-care. Many of the best athletes are the worst patients. If a temperature is more than 100°F, training should stop, the situation should be assessed promptly, and dietary recommendations should be followed. Training cannot be resumed at the same level, because the patient will probably be in negative protein balance and will have a depleted store of glycogen. Special attention must be given to food selection because appetite is poor when one has a fever. Foods should be appealing and easily digested, be good sources of protein, and have concentrated food value (e.g., high-protein soups, cereals, baked or mashed potatoes, ice cream, custards, and high-calorie beverages such as hot chocolate and eggnogs).

Review and Monitor.—Check initial body weight, weight loss, temperature, volume of fluid input and output, and electrolyte balance.

Other Considerations.—Look at medications, and calculate protein intake. (To increase the daily protein and energy intake in 500-kcal steps, refer to Appendices 14 and 15.)

Heat Injury Syndromes

Water is absolutely essential for all body processes and is of particular concern to the athlete. It regulates body temperature, helps to carry nutrients and oxygen to the working muscles, and is necessary for the excretion of the waste products of metabolism. Because of higher activity levels, an athlete needs to drink considerably more water than a nonathlete.

Objectives.—The objective is to prevent dehydration leading to heat cramps, heat exhaustion, heat stroke, nausea, and injury due to fatigue.

Heat Cramps.—Heat (muscle) cramps are painful, involuntary contractions of muscles caused by dehydration (5% reduction in body weight), imbalances of body electrolytes, inadequate blood supply, and low intake of calcium.

Dietary Recommendations.—Be sure of adequate fluid replacement; adjust the diet to include bananas, citrus fruits, and green leafy vegetables; and add calcium foods or a supplement.

Heat Exhaustion.—Heat exhaustion is characterized by headache, nausea, chills, unsteadiness, and fatigue. The athlete may become dizzy and lightheaded when he or she stops exercising or may suddenly collapse, due to a sudden drop in blood pressure. Rectal temperature should be less than 105° F. Anything above this level is heat stroke. Pulse may be rapid but weak. Skin is usually cool and pale. Sweating is active.

Dietary Recommendations.—Predict situations where maximum dehydration will occur, namely, high temperature and high humidity, heavy and lengthy competition, and heavy uniforms and equipment. Drink fluids before and during training and competition.

Heat Stroke.—Heat stroke (sunstroke) is characterized by a flushed, hot face, headache, weakness, and dizziness. It may be followed by unconsciousness. It is also characterized by a rectal temperature of 105° F, 7% body weight loss, warm skin, and rapid, pounding pulse.

This condition is an emergency, and immediate medical referral is necessary. On-site first aid treatment requires immediate use of intravenous fluids. Reduction of the athlete's core temperature is vital. Apply wet, cold towels to the body. Never force fluids on an unconscious person. After the patient is stabilized, determine weight loss and replace it during the next 24 to 36 hours by slow hydration (patient should continuously sip small amounts of cool, diluted fluids).

Nausea and fatigue are symptoms of heat stroke but are also warning signals.

Patient Education.—Review safety guidelines for water intake:

1. Two hours before the event or workout, drink up to 32 oz of fluid.
2. Fifteen minutes before the event, drink up to 16 oz of fluid.
3. Each 15 to 30 minutes during the event, drink up to 10 oz of fluid.
4. After the event, replace sweat loss (16 oz of fluid for each pound of weight loss).

Review and Monitor.—Check weight, weight loss during practice and competition, fluid intake and output, total calories.

Other Considerations.—Eight ounces of fluid are needed for the digestion of every 200 calories of food. Water can come from fruits, vegetables, juices, and milk. Coffee, tea, cola, and alcoholic beverages are not considered fluid replacements because their caffeine or alcohol content causes fluid loss. To be readily absorbed, fluids need to be cool (40° F), contain a low concentration of glucose (2.5 gm/100 ml), and be consumed in small volumes (2 oz/drink). Athletes should become accustomed to this amount of fluid during training so that they do not experience discomfort during competition.

In normal circumstances, sodium losses through sweat are not a problem and can be handled by eating lightly salted food at mealtimes. Of special concern is the athlete on a weight loss diet. Initial weight lost will be water. Blood volume is then decreased, and the patient is unable to closely monitor body temperature during exercise. Adding small amounts of carbohydrate to the diet will result in sodium and water retention.

Water intoxication (hyponatremia) can occur in long-term competition, as during the Tour de France, Ironman, or lengthy events when electrolytes are inadequately monitored. When plain water is drunk in large quantities, the resulting dilution may cause diarrhea, edema, and exhaustion. It is not appropriate to give this athlete extra water, yet during emergencies, it is difficult to differentiate between this condition and other heat problems. When the activity lasts more than 3 hours, the pre-event meal must supply extra potassium and sodium. Extra servings of lightly salted vegetables and plenty of fruit are recommended.

Dehydration and glycogen depletion can limit exercise performance. Consuming dilute solutions of carbohydrate with/without electrolytes (for example, a 5% to 6% solution of glucose polymer) can enhance performance in long distance activities such as triathlons and marathons or in events involving multiple heats of competition throughout the day.

Athletes who must maintain strict body weight often are tempted to force dehydration for quick weight loss. This is done by spitting, forceful vomiting, or other unhealthful practices. The American College of Sports Medicine and all ethical health practitioners have gone on record against these methods of weight change. The general recommendation for the athlete is to be aware of fluid needs, prevent dehydration whenever possible, and always avoid intentional weight loss.

Hypertension

Hypertension results from a sustained increase in arterial diastolic pressure, systolic pressure, or both. Normal pressure includes systolic-diastolic measurements of 120/80 mm Hg or less.

Measurements from 140/90 to 160/95 mm Hg are considered borderline, and some dietary intervention will be helpful. Blood pressures above 160/95 mm Hg are frankly hypertensive. The condition is a major risk factor for coronary heart disease, renal failure, peripheral vascular disease, and stroke. It affects nearly 20% of the U.S. population and is more common in blacks. Anything that increases the volume of blood flow, decreases the diameter of peripheral arterioles, or strengthens the contractions of vascular smooth muscle will raise blood pressure. Influences include heredity, race, cigarette smoking, stress, and diet. Symptoms include frequent headaches, impaired vision, shortness of breath, chest pain, dizziness, failing memory, or gastrointestinal distress.

Objectives.—Control blood pressure, achieve ideal body weight, regulate sodium in the diet (for those predisposed to hypertension), and reduce pressure-raising factors.

Dietary Recommendations.—Gradually lower the intake of sodium. (Practical intake provides 2 to 4 gm of sodium daily. Be cautious, because sodium restriction decreases blood volume.) Restrict calories if necessary, and increase protein quality but not to excess. Diet should include adequate amounts of calcium and electrolytes, especially potassium. Limit caffeine-containing beverages to two or three servings/day.

Patient Education.—Explain the mechanisms whereby diet affects blood pressure: altering renal excretion of salt and water (sodium, potassium, protein), exchange of ions in arteriolar smooth muscle (chloride, calcium, magnesium), the balance of hormones that control salt and water excretion or smooth muscle contraction (calories, caffeine, fiber), and direct toxic mechanisms (alcohol). Encourage the patient; it may take 4 to 6 weeks to respond. (Some individuals do not respond to diet therapy.)

Review and Monitor.—Assess changes in diet history; weight; intake and output; calcium, cholesterol, and triglycerides levels; and blood pressure.

Other Considerations.—Be aware of environmental situations that will raise blood pressure (e.g., stress), high sodium content of commercial electrolyte drinks, and the use of diuretics. Aldactone is potassium sparing; thiazides deplete potassium, and supplementation is required. By increasing complex carbohydrates, consuming moderate amounts of caffeine and alcohol, moderating salt, increasing calcium and potassium, and maintaining physical activity, the patient may be able to avoid drug therapy and will decrease other chronic disease factors associated with hypertension.

Hyperlipidemias

Hyperlipidemia, or elevated blood lipids, may be caused by a high-fat diet accompanied by other factors or by inborn errors of lipid metabolism that cause abnormal elevations in levels of serum lipoproteins, cholesterol, and triglycerides. Patients with these conditions deposit lipids around tendons, under the skin, and in the cornea. Because they also deposit lipids in arteries, the incidence of premature coronary heart disease is rather high. Among people in developed societies, atherosclerotic placques or lesions appear in infancy, are well established in childhood, and cause significant arterial occlusion by early adulthood. Symptomatic disease usually takes several decades to develop but is hastened by radical weight gain regimens or steroid abuse.

Objectives.—Lower serum lipids, achieve and maintain ideal body weight, and observe prudent heart diet guidelines. See reference in Appendixes 9 and 22.

Dietary Recommendations.—Lower dietary fat to less than 30% of total calories (saturated fats to 10%, unsaturated fats to 10%, monounsaturated fats to 10%). Limit cholesterol to 300 mg or less/day. Limit calories if weight reduction is necessary. Limit coffee, alcohol, sodium, and animal fat. Increase fiber from fruits, vegetables, legumes, and grains; increase fish consumption. Diet should include adequate vitamin C.

Patient Education.—Encourage the use of foods that have no cholesterol (plant origin). Review a prudent diet and sources of polyunsaturated fats. Advise the reading of labels.

Review and Monitor.—Keep track of body weight; cholesterol, triglyceride, hemoglobin levels; hematocrit, blood pressure; and quality of the diet.

Other Considerations.—Iron may be low, because animal proteins are usually limited.

Hypoglycemia

Hypoglycemia, or low blood glucose (40–50 mg/dl) often produces hunger, trembling, weakness, headaches, dizziness, and distorted vision 2 to 4 hours after a meal. It has frequently been reported in athletes who are attempting weight loss or who are exercising beyond normal limits. Fasting hypoglycemia is rare. It may be due to a tumor of the pancreatic islet beta cells, other endocrine tumors, overadministration of insulin, liver damage, starvation, or cancer. Treatment consists of removal of the tumor or correction of the underlying medical problem. Reactive hypoglycemia may be one of the earliest stages of diabetes, characterized by a delay in insulin secretion. Late arriving insulin causes an excessively large drop in serum glucose between 3 to 4 hours after food intake. Symptoms are relieved with carbohydrate intake.

Objectives.—Maintain normal blood glucose levels, and prevent quick absorption of carbohydrates.

Dietary Recommendations.—Adjust caloric content based on patient's normal requirements: protein content, 20%; carbohydrate, 50% to 55%, and fat content, 25% to 30%. Dietary pattern should include three small meals and three snacks daily. Omit most concentrated sweets, such as sugar; sweetened desserts; jellies, jams, and syrups; sweetened fruits, and soft drinks. Restrict alcohol, and omit caffeine.

Patient Education.—Explain gluconeogenesis and epinephrine stimulation. Patient should keep snacks available, eat regularly, and avoid large meals.

Review and Monitor.—Check ideal body weight, blood glucose after oral glucose tolerance test, or mixed meal tolerance test.

Other Considerations.—Continued exercise will reduce blood sugar. In competition lasting more than 2 hours, blood glucose levels may be sustained by sipping small amounts of dilute carbohydrate solutions every 15 minutes, or every 2 miles. Avoid large amounts of high-glucose drinks before exercise, because carbohydrate intake will stimulate so much insulin production that too much blood glucose is driven into the cells, leaving the blood glucose low.

Infectious Mononucleosis

Infectious mononucleosis (mono) is an acute, infectious disease that produces swollen glands. Symptoms are fatigue, malaise, headache, chills, sore throat, fever, abdominal pain, jaundice, stiff neck, chest pain, breathing difficulties, and coughing.

Objectives.—Restore fluid balance and glycogen stores, and regain weight.

Dietary Recommendations.—Encourage small, frequent feedings of high-protein, high-calorie foods. Consider the use of liquids or supplementation when swallowing is difficult.

Patient Education.—Advise the patient to avoid spreading the infection. Rehabilitation may take longer than expected. Exercise will be important in restoring nitrogen balance, but full physical training will be difficult. Competition is not advised for several months.

Review and Monitor.—Check ideal body weight for age. Give instructions dealing with the quality of diet. Monitor hemoglobin levels, hematacrit, transferrin values, and chart daily body temperature.

Other Considerations.—Recommend a complete physical after recovery. Ask coach to review training procedures and competitive expectations. Patient needs firm guidelines on general health habits (sleep, diet, hygiene).

Lactase Deficiency

When lactase is missing, lactose, or milk sugar, is unable to be hydrolyzed into galactose and glucose. Lactose then remains in the gut, drawing water into the intestines, and causing bloating and cramping. Bacteria ferments the undigested lactose and generates lactic acid, carbon dioxide, and hydrogen gas. The result is flatulence, cramps, and diarrhea. Lactase deficiency is diagnosed from a history of gastrointestinal symptoms that occur after milk ingestion or from a lactose tolerance test.

Objectives.—Decrease or omit lactose from the diet. Check for "actual" tolerance by monitoring food intake. (Most patients can tolerate 1/2 cup of milk per meal.) Patient needs a healthful diet that includes adequate calcium.

Dietary Recommendations.—Ice cream and other milk products containing lactose should be avoided or restricted. Read labels of prepared foods and watch for fillers, whey solids, and milk solids. Lactose-free foods include Ensure, Isomil, and Mocha Mix, as well as most carbonated drinks, coffee, fruit juices, breads and rolls made without milk, most pastas, eggs, nondairy creamers, nut butters, most fruits and vegetables, clear soups, most meat products, kosher foods, and desserts made with water (e.g., fruit ices and gelatins). Lact-aid drops can be used in milk to hydrolyze lactose. This product is available by special order (Sugar-Lo, PO Box 1017, Atlantic City, NJ 08404) or in grocery stores. Cultured milk products such as yogurt, kefir milk, kefir cheese, lactaid milk, and acidophilous milk can be tolerated.

Patient Education.—Learning self-monitoring and using appropriate recipes are the most effective ways to prevent problems associated with lactose intolerance. Calcium supplementation may be necessary if total dietary intake is less than 800 mg/day.

Review and Monitor.—Assess growth (in children), height and weight, hemoglobin levels and hematocrit, and the lactose-free diet. Frequency of symptoms need to be recorded.

Other Considerations.—If the symptoms do not disappear after strict adherence to a lactose-free diet, another diagnosis should be sought.

Malaise

Malaise is vague feelings of discomfort and exhaustion, often coupled with an inability to concentrate.

Objectives.—The patient needs rest or a change of scenery (which might include a different climate).

Dietary Recommendations.—Increase fluids, and eat favorite comfort foods (e.g., chicken soup, hot cocoa, or pizza). But don't overload on junk foods.

Patient Education.—The priority list puts the well-being of the patient first (*moderate* exercise, simple, attractive meals), term papers and job requirements second.

Review and Monitor.—Check body temperature, sleeping habits, intensity of training, and general diet.

Other Considerations.—These feelings of discomfort usually accompany overtraining or uncontrolled stress.

Osteoporosis

Osteoporosis is defined as loss of bone density and is characterized by porous and brittle bones. It is most common in women after menopause, yet everyone begins losing bone calcium between the ages of 55 and 60. Recently, more cases of juvenile and premenopausal osteoporosis have been reported. Women who train intensely and reduce body weight and fat to a point were secondary amenorrhea exists lose estrogen's protective effect on bone and exhibit an early decrease in bone mass.

Objectives.—Increase dietary calcium and lessen the risk of spontaneous fractures.

Dietary Recommendations.—Increase dietary calcium to 1,500 mg/day (through the consumption of low-fat dairy products, leafy green vegetables, sardines, and canned salmon), and avoid large amounts of alcohol, caffeine, tobacco, fiber, or protein. Instant dry milk may be added to many foods. Supplementation of calcium and vitamin D will probably be necessary.

Patient Education.—Identify all the sources of dietary calcium that the patient enjoys, and plan a daily eating pattern.

Establish an ideal body weight for competition, slightly higher than present, if menstrual history reveals amenorrhea.

Review and Monitor.—Check height, weight, and weight changes. Review stress patterns. Continue to assess progression of disease, diet compliance, and calcium supplementation. Record and review urinary calcium, direct measures of bone mass (photon absorptiometry, computerized tomography, and x-ray). Recommend earlier screenings for those at high risk.

Other Considerations.—Encourage systematic activity involving all muscle groups; investigate other hormone imbalances (i.e., insulin, steroids and thyroid) and use drug screens for corticosteroids, thyroid preparations, tetracyclines, and other medications that induce calcium loss; screen for pituitary or ovarian dysfunction, intrauterine adhesions, history of eating disorders, and previous history of exercise.

Overweight (Overfat)

Overweight is defined as a body weight that is 10% or more above ideal body weight, or a triceps skinfold thickness equal to, or greater than, 18 mm in adult men or 25 mm in adult women. Obesity is defined as a body weight 20% or more above ideal body weight, or a triceps skinfold thickness equal to, or greater than, 25 mm in adult men or 30 mm in adult women. In athletics and physical performance, these terms take on a greater significance. Percentages of body fat are usually related to performance and aesthetics as well as to health. Causes of overweight are usually related to a caloric imbalance. (In cases such as football, it is often intentional.)

Objectives.—Determine ideal body weight and the ratio of fat to lean tissue. Prescribe a diet and exercise program that will induce a weight loss.

Dietary Recommendations.—Provide a nutritionally balanced, individualized diet pattern that will prevent loss of body protein and avoid other complications of starvation (behavioral changes, anemia, loss of hair, etc). Decrease fat calories to less than 25% of total calories. Protein calories should follow the RDAs appropriate to the patient's age and physiological state; carbohydrate calories should represent about 60% of total calories. Smaller, more frequent meals will encourage compliance. Increase water intake to six to eight glasses/day. Avoid alcohol and empty calories when possible. (Examples of improved food behaviors are found in Appendix 5.) Anorectic drugs may cause excitability, gastrointestinal distress, dry mouth, unpleasant breath, dizziness, diarrhea, and anorexia.

Patient Education.—Instruct the patient on maintaining a nutritionally sound diet, such as use of shopping lists and menus, recipes, tips on restaurant dining, trips and vacations, portion control, snacking, and food preparation methods. Initiate behavior modification through food diaries, recording of activity, and control of food cues.

Review and Monitor.—Check exercise and weight changes. Assess risk factors, hemoglobin levels and hematocrit, signs of malnutrition, dehydration, and uric acid, triglyceride, and cholesterol levels. Collect diet histories.

Other Considerations.—Recognize the weight level at which an athlete should be told to reduce; calculate a realistic weight reduction before competition begins. The condition may require long-term reinforcement, follow-ups, psychotherapy, and support personnel. If weight gain is intentional, consider the problems associated with carrying additional fat cells after athletics.

Surgery

Metabolic effects after surgery are related to the extent of the operation, prior nutritional state of the patient, and the relationship of the surgery to the patient's ability to digest and absorb nutrients.

Objectives.—*Preoperative.*—The patient should be in the best possible nutritional state. (Emergency surgery, of course, does not allow time for preliminary treatment.) Proper nourishment should be emphasized so the patient's body may prepare for stress, wound healing, blood loss, and dehydration. Screen for malnutrition, vomiting, diarrhea, or prolonged bleeding.

Postoperative.—Replace protein and glycogen stores, and correct electrolyte and fluid imbalances.

Dietary Recommendations.—*Preoperative.*—Advise a high-protein, high-calorie diet. If the patient needs to lose weight, use a low-fat, low-calorie diet. Check vitamins C and K and hydration. Food by mouth is not allowed for at least 6 hours before surgery. An elemental liquid diet with minimal residue can be used preoperatively.

Postoperative.—In general, intravenous glucose and electrolytes are administered preoperatively, during surgery, and postoperatively. Clear liquids may be followed by full liquids. Return the patient to normal feeding as tolerated. Although some surgeons are specific about postoperative diet orders, there are general principles applicable to all patients (i.e., estimate or measure actual energy demands). Energy increase varies with the extent of injury. For no complications, increase calories 10%; for fractures or trauma, increase 10% to 25%. Protein recommendations are from 1.0 to 2.0 gm/kg of usual body weight. Ensure adequate vitamins C, A, K, and B complex and zinc. Fluids can be given by mouth when patient has recovered from anesthesia. Many patients meet their energy and protein needs with the standard hospital diet. Those with small appetites or increased nutritional needs may require supplements or alterations.

Patient Education.—Immobilization often causes unwanted side effects, such as constipation, depression, or anxiety. Encourage increased fluid intake, consumption of favorite foods, and family support. Patients should eat and drink slowly to prevent gas formation; they can suck on ice or sip carbonated beverages to alleviate nausea from anesthetics.

Review and Monitor.—Check height and weight, percentage of body fat; hemoglobin levels and hematocrit, intake and output, serum albumin, and other information as ordered.

Other Considerations.—Vegetarians should be instructed to include more protein in their diets. All other medications should be controlled. Check for antacids, laxatives, megavitamins, food dislikes, and allegies.

Other Health Conditions

Other health conditions, such as hemorrhoids or heart attacks, may be food related; however, in these cases first aid for the athlete is the primary concern. Any professional who works with athletes should know treatment protocol for hemorrhage, poisoning, shock, and complications from animal and insect bites.

REFERENCES

1. Nelson RA: Nutrition and physical performance. *Phys Sports Med* 1982; 10:55.
2. Loosli AR, Benson J, Gillien DM, et al: Nutrition habits and knowledge in competitive adolescent female gymnasts. *Phys Sports Med* 1986; 14:118.
3. Wilmore JH: Nutrition and the athlete. *Sports Med Digest,* 1986; pp 2–16.
4. Fox EL (ed): Nutrient utilization during exercise. Columbus, Ohio, Ross Laboratories, May 1983, pp 1–138.
5. Vickery CE, Hodges PAM: Counseling strategies for dietary management: Expanded possibilities for effecting behavior change. *J Am Diet Assoc* 1986; 86:924.
6. Stare FJ, Whelan EM: Proper nutrition for the adolescent. *Female Patient,* May 1979.
7. Lemon PWR, Yarasheski KE, Dolny DG: The importance of protein for athletes. *J Sports Med* 1984; 1:474.
8. Town GP, Wheeler KB: Nutritional concerns for the endurance athlete. *Diet Curr* 1986; 13:2.
9. Brouns FJPH, Saris WHM, Ten Hoor F: Dietary problems in the case of strenuous exertion. *J Sports Med* 1986; 26:306.
10. Reynolds G: Drink, don't dry. *Runner's World,* June 1987, pp 41 45.
11. Duda M: Use whatever works for the pregame meal. *Phys Sports Med* 1985; 13:29.

12. Nelson RA: Preventing and treating dehydration. *Phys Sports Med* 1985; 113:176.
13. Clark N: Eating nutritiously on the road. *Phys Sports Med* 1985; 13:133.
14. Young EA, Sims O, Bingham C: Fast foods 1986: Nutrient analyses. *Diet Curr* 1986; 13:1.
15. Winget CM, DeRoshia CW, Holley DC: Circadian rhythms and athletic performance. *Med Sci Sports Exerc* 1985; 17:498.
16. Snetselaar LG: *Nutrition Counseling Skills*. Rockville, Md, Aspen Systems, 1983.
17. *Guide to Good Eating*. Rosemont, Ill, National Dairy Council.
18. Mattson C: Compu-cal. 9545 Delphi Road SW, Olympia, WA 98502.
19. *Nutrition and Your Health: Dietary Guidelines for Americans*. Washington, DC, US Department of Agriculture and Health and Human Services, 1980.
20. Sheehan G: The diet-exercise connection. *Phys Sports Med* 1985; 13:45.
21. Olson RE: A contemporary approach toward healthful diets. *Contemp Nutr* 1981; 6:5.
22. Clark N: Increasing dietary iron. *Phys Sports Med* 1985; 13:131.
23. Nestle M: *Nutrition in Clinical Practice*. Greenbrae, Calif, Jones Medical Publications, 1985.
24. Krause MV, Mahan LK: *Food, Nutrition, and Diet Therapy*. Philadelphia, WB Saunders Co, 1984.

When It's Time to Ask for Help

The locker room and dressing room are open to few besides coach, trainer, physician, and athlete. This is where preparation for competition and performance takes place, and time spent here may be seasonal or year-round. The athletes who gather here expect care and encouragement. They want to talk, be listened to, and be told as much as possible. Their peers are here, and they feel comfortable. There is no communications problem, but there may be an accuracy problem when nutritional information is given by teammates who share what has worked for them. Testimonials are more frequent than references to dietary texts, and problem solving is only a token effort. As one wrestling coach related, "When I don't know the answer to their questions, I just give them a vitamin C tablet."

Nutritional information is better accepted from the trainer or coach than from a physician or dietitian. The coach is there at the right time and the right place, but since the field of nutrition is changing rapidly, he or she needs to keep current. Perhaps take a course in nutrition, visit a dietitian, read recommended journals or texts, and take the information back to the players. The athlete in the locker room does not want volumes of information but needs clear, understandable, workable guidelines. Bulletin boards with tear-off information can offer the basics. When there is time, the athlete can receive individualization. If there are serious problems, intervention should take place immediately, right where it is first identified.[1-3]

TARGETS FOR NUTRITIONAL INTERVENTION

1. Individuals in the midst of adolescent growth spurts
2. Those exhibiting health complications, such as influenza, bronchitis, or allergies
3. Those who are underweight or overweight
4. Those who have poor nutritional status, lack education, or have no communication skills
5. Those who lack parental involvement
6. Those who exhibit addictive behaviors

The Adolescent Growth Spurt.—Undernourishment delays or suppresses the adolescent growth spurt. Most commonly, coaches work with adolescents or preadolescents. When sports activities have specific weight requirements, such as a light weight to qualify for a class of wrestling, malnutrition is common. We know that nutrition can determine cell multiplication in the newborn. This is also true during the adolescent growth spurt. Although we realize that there is an individual *maximum growth event,* we do not know the exact protein and caloric requirements, for instance, on a specific basis. The range of the recommended dietary allowances (RDAs) covers the 98th percentile individual and his or her growth spurt, yet surveys repeatedly show that lightweights are not eating correctly for growth requirements. Coaches need to monitor athletes' height and weight during successive competitive seasons. The average American male increases in height from 4 ft 8 in. at age 10 to 5 ft 9.6 in. at age 18 (a change of almost 14 in.); the average female height increases from 4 ft 7.2 in. at age 10 to 5 ft 4.8 in. at age 18 (a change of almost 10 in.). The references male at age 10 weighs 71.7 lb and the female 118.8 lb. (This is a change of weight of 67 lb for the male and 49 lb for the female.) Although this information does not begin to relate how growth takes place, it defines the distance of growth curves and indicates when growth usually occurs. If it appears to be delayed, the athlete's dietary habits need to be questioned (followed with a telephone call to the parents, school nurse, or team physician).

Health Complications.—As has been noted, athletic competition can aggravate an existing health situation (e.g., allergies) or be the cause of others (e.g., anemias). Nutritional status is often the main factor in recovery. And even if coaching responsibilities go along with being the principal and school bus driver, the coach still must be accountable to the athlete; no one has more contact or sees the athlete undressed as often as the coach.

Underweight and Overweight.—Some weights are associated with certain activities, such as lower weights for dancers, but there are definite limits. The guideline for intervention is 10% below or over the range for ideal body weight for height, as established by the 1959 Metropolitan Life Insurance tables.

Poverty, Poor Nutritional Status, and Lack of Education or Communication Skills.—Significant malnutrition exists in the adolescent population all over the world. Aside from the fact that certain adult diseases have nutritional roots in childhood, inadequate dietary intake (regardless of the cause) is the principal factor in malnutrition. There will always be some doubt that manipulation of the diet—with the exceptions of carbohydrate, fluids, and calories—can improve performance, but there is no doubt that less than an adequate diet results in poor performance. Those athletes unable to meet their dietary needs must be helped. Contacts in parents' clubs, church organizations, school lunch programs, booster clubs, and other team members can often be effective channels to assistance. However, if a team member is the source of misinformation, and in some cases this can be detrimental to team performance, he or she should be reeducated, or a respected outside resource who can relate to the team should be called in. To give an example: Several years ago, the Phoenix Suns asked a sports nutritionist to be present at the preseason physical examinations. Although she answered general dietary questions and offered other reliable information, the main purpose for her being there was to dispel the fabrications spread by one of the team members who had become a food faddist. He had been bringing nonpasteurized milk and fertile eggs to practice, had boycotted several pregame meals, and had organized his own organic food co-op. As the nutritionist interviewed each player, she reassured him about the quality of the team's food supply, offered information and handouts about appropriate food supplementation, gave recipes for preevent and postevent meals, and addressed their special nutritional needs and concerns. Her efforts effectively stemmed the team's problem. Follow-up information was given throughout the season by the athletic trainer.

Parent Involvement.—Too much involvement is better than none at all. The adolescent athlete needs his or her parent for transportation, food, reassurance, money and love, and as a number one fan. It is difficult for a coach to demand discipline from team members who do not have money, wheels, or love. Car pools and surrogate cookie bakers can take some pressure off, but quality time on the playing field is limited if parents do not support their children's athletic events.

Addictive Behavior.—Confrontation in the locker room is often critical to success in dealing with situations such as food behavior problems. Trainers and coaches probably feel inadequate in dealing with bulimia, anorexia, binge eating, sex addiction, or other disorders that are common in performance field, yet most athletes will confide in them. For example, the physician may be treating a sore throat, not realizing it has been caused by repeated vomiting in response to a demand for weight loss, perhaps by the one person the athlete is able to share a confidence with without being judged.[1–3]

Sometimes we wonder if athletics causes addictions or if the addict turns to athletics as a means of escape. Being an "athlete" will not, of course, solve personal problems. It only momentarily relieves the loneliness. If we use athletics as a substitute for nurturance, love, power, or anger, it is no longer the wonderful connection between ourselves and our bodies. It becomes, instead, a commodity that is used to avoid intimacy, to mask needs, and to substitute for love.

It is not unusual to see a father pacing on the sidelines, "coaching" his son and "coaching" the coach; or to observe a mother, year after year, drinking coffee in her car parked in the swimming pool parking lot. Are these parents doing this for their children or to solve their own addictions?

Misinterpretation of the goals of sports often leaves athlete and family frustrated and empty because desires are never fulfilled:

Several years ago, one of the top cross-country runners in the country participated in an extensive physiological profile at the Junior Nationals in Lincoln, Nebraska. She was casually told that although her body fat was 12% of her total weight, she might run better if she would bring it down even lower. She was 5 ft 4 in. tall and weighed 105 lb. After 6 weeks of drinking two diet colas daily and not eating, she visited her physician. Her performance had deteriorated badly. She weighed in at 85 pounds and measured 11% total body fat. She lost her college scholarship and was unable to compete in the state track and field events her senior year.

A young dancer came to live with a medical family after she had unsuccessfully tried to deal with bulimia on her own. Under close supervision, she was able to prepare and eat individual and group meals and not vomit. Then an insult from a dance instructor made her feel angry, hopeless, and also powerless to deal with the basic tools the family was trying to teach her—trust and self-assurance. When they left for a weekend, she ate everything edible in the house. She felt completely out of balance, unable to achieve any pleasure or satisfaction from eating but helpless to stop. She vomited until the blood vessels in her eyes broke. She wanted the family to be angry with her, and when they offered continued support and love, she was confused. She was not able to completely accept others' support.

About half of all dancers eat correctly: they eat when they are hungry; they eat what they want to eat; they love life and enjoy the sensations food gives them; they can leave favorite foods on their plate; and they love dance, but it is not their entire world. They have sacrificed for

*dance but have made plans for "after dance," and they will not need to
"recover" from dance.*

One of our children's favorite friends is a famous basketball
player. Although they have seen him many times "at his job,"
they have also seen him with his family, with his friends, and in
church. He has always seemed very alive to his senses and not
controlled by them. He has gained what many in sports look for:
internal personal power. He has accepted with grace what he
cannot have and will share truly intimate experiences with an
entire arena of fans. Although he "has it made," he has never
allowed himself or his family to become a commodity for trade.
He has many plans for "after basketball."

People often approach athletics with a hidden agenda, mis-
takenly believing that power, people, and money (and substance
abuse) will make them happy. They anticipate a rewarding experience but often end up with athletics being part, and often
the only part, of their personality. They forget several things.
When the seasons are long, they will lose some and win some.
And they overlook the fact that the dance or athletic career will
not last a long time. Even worse, someone will always jump
higher or run faster, and they will be forgotten.

Part of their hidden agenda is suppressing the present and
the enjoyment that is possible from each day. They may say to
themselves, for example, "When I have the perfect figure, I'll
have all the good parts"; "when I develop my long shot, I'll be
happy." Their minds are never quiet, and even if they achieve
some goals, the pursuit goes on. "When I weigh 100 lb I'll run
better; when I weigh 95 lb, I'll run even better."

When the season is over, athletics are viewed in a different
light. It is only a little while in the athlete's life, an important
time, but so short. Enjoy it, learn from it, revel in its ups and
downs, and reap all its rewards. At the same time, never lose
sight of the fact that you are a separate person, living your own
life. You will miss sports terribly at first but will get over that
and go on.

> Now you will not swell the rout
> Of lads that wore their honors out,
> Runners whom renown outran

And the name died before the man.
So set, before its echoes fade,
The fleet foot on the sill of shade,
And hold to the low lintel up
The still-defended challenge cup.
                              A.E. Houseman

Each year at halftime during homecoming football games, lettered alumni athletes descend onto playing fields. They sing their school fight songs, and when they return to their seats, they always seem surprised by the teary-eyed greetings from those in the stands. The seasons were not all good, but the memories are grand!

When athletes talk about their problems, they usually talk about abuse of food, substance, and sex. These addictions stem from early life experiences and programming and may be masked until the intensity of athletics bring them out. One addiction may be covered with another. In the recovery process, one is often given up while another emerges.

It is normal to have addictions, and it is normal to talk about them. We all want to indulge in Christmas goodies, for instance, and not get fat; we all want to have wonderful bodies but not to run three or four times/week to achieve aerobic fitness. When the world is not treating us well, we return to our comfort foods, and they make us feel better. As we mature, we gain insight from our experiences. We cannot eat everything in sight because we will get fat, and that will make it even more difficult to have that wonderful body. We have bad days, but there will be other days. The little addictions that make us feel better will be kept in check because we do not want them to become life threatening.[4]

But sometimes athletes do not become mature; they do not have to. Someone identifies them as a potential star about the time they are 12 years old, and from that moment on, the athlete part of their personality is dominant. Someone makes decisions about how they will spend their time and money, and they never have to learn such day-by-day drudgeries as balancing a checkbook, making plane reservations or, even worse, making friends. (They have lots of them already; there are five on the basketball team, 11 on the football team, and so on.) And, for a long time, this works. They do not have to try to be popular because all they have to do is make a basket, catch a football, or make a turn en pointe, and everyone likes them. An athlete does not need to remember names because everyone knows his or hers. To be an elite athlete takes so much time that part of the personality may start ailing. When this happens, the athlete's world becomes smaller and smaller, and eventually so do problem-solving abilities. Not all, but many, athletes do dumb things with money, food, sex, drugs, and relationships.

A gymnast, for example, begins to feel overweight when one of her peers calls her "fat" during practice (she is 5 ft 2 in. and weighs 100 lb). She cannot escape the feeling that she would be a better gymnast if she weighed less. Therefore, she does not eat all day and enjoys a sensation of power. She skips dinner, too, then runs several miles. During study hours she begins to feel very hungry. There is a convenience store across from campus that sells cookies (it also sells juice, fruit, milk, etc.). Maybe just a few cookies would be a nice reward for not eating all day. "No," she tells herself, "I can't stop at a few; I'll eat the entire bag." But the longer she dwells on the cookies, the more enticing the idea seems. Then she realizes she is out of hair spray and must go to the store anyway. She passes the cookies on her way to the sundries shelf and ends up leaving the store with the hair spray and about 2,000 calories, disguised as a little reward. She eats one or two on the way back to the dorm, several more as she walks up the stairs, then quickly finishes the bag before she sees her roommate. For a few minutes she is very happy. Then she becomes disgusted. She does not have many alternatives at this point. She can return to her room, vow never to let cookies get in the way again, and learn from the experience. Or, she can drink a big glass of water, wait a few minutes, and then vomit up the entire package of cookies. She vomits, then feels angry, empty, and very alone. But until she makes the decision to ask for help, this closed loop pattern of dealing with stress will continue.

Sex, too, can be a commodity in athletics—far different from the bartering nature of most sexual addiction. It can become a substitute for achievement. If he or she cannot have love and respect, they will take sex instead. A woman may not make the team at the trials, but if she sleeps with the coach, she will somehow get on the team. She probably will not look that good during competition, but every team has injured players or those with off-days. The coach spends lots of time with her, so the other team members believe she must be good. But, gradually, they come to understand the situation, and the resentment starts to build. He is their coach, too. They need his time, talents, observations, and encouragement. Meanwhile, the coach feels very powerful. He does not understand that the athlete is not in love with him; she is using him, destroying the team's confidence and his abilities to teach and recruit. If he is coaching on a national level, excuses will be made for the situation (with the rationale that this behavior is expected in the tense world of competition). But think about the team in a few years. Will the players go down at halftime with joy in their hearts? Think about the school. Will it be able to recruit and provide an opportunity for development in a team? Think about the coach's family. Will they still be around after they realize that a young athlete is competing for their time with husband and father?

Is it okay to fall in love? Yes, when it wakes us up to an experience that may lead to greater growth. No, when it gets us hooked on a high, and we become addicted to sex, people, or both. We need to remember that often all we are doing is attempting to resolve our problems through athletics. In *On Golden Pond*, the father coached his daughter on the swim team. She could never dive as well as he could because he would not let her know how good she was. When she finally does a back flip and wants his approval, it does not come. She has to be satisfied that she could do it for herself; she does not need to please him. When the high is punctured by rejection, the result can be a painful fall that may lead to other addictive behaviors (e.g., food problems follow sex; drug use follows food).

The muses must have had a good laugh when they designated chocolate, sex, running, and falling in love as catalysts to release endorphins from the brain to create, temporarily, feelings of comfort and well-being.[4]

When addictions control athletics, there is no real enjoyment, high-energy levels, or humor, openness, and warmth. If assistance is not available on the team, it will have to be looked for elsewhere. There is always help. The good team—and team member—can always have a comeback season!

WHEN WORKING WITH PEOPLE DOES NOT WORK

Individuals return to situations in which they have been successful. After a few failures, it usually becomes clear to us that we are not suited to an endeavor or we do not have sufficient talent in that area. So we move on to other things. We need positive feedback not only from others but from ourselves. Athletes are good examples of this. Physically, it makes more sense for a tall, lean individual to play basketball and for a shorter person, with a lower center of gravity, to be a gymnast. For the basketball player, it is just more fun if all the work is worthwhile and the ball goes through the hoop. Sometimes we fit the job, and sometimes we have to change a lot to fit the job (e.g., a freshman may wrestle easily at 115 lb, but a junior may need to change his entire life-style to make that weight).

Distinctive personality traits are often associated with particular sports. It takes a certain type of individual to be a boxer or a high jumper. Likewise, each team has its leaders and its characters (witness the team jester). As the team and its members jell, success can be determined by psychological preparation not only for competition but for training.

In large training camps, the personalities of teams are obvious. Let us say that you walk into the cafeteria. The wrestlers are eating together; the weight lifters are off in a corner; the archery team usually stays together; and the soccer team has found all the pretty girls. A grandmother would say, "Oh, those rowers are such nice boys!" But she may privately judge the weight lifters as "animals." For health advisors, it is easier to give advice to a team of "nice boys" than it is to a group that may not appeal to the speaker (or vice versa). Most dietitians are called on for their expertise in weight management. The principles of weight gain are about the same for the recovering anorexic dancer as they are for the lineman with a professional future in mind. Likewise, the advice for weight loss is identical for runner and soccer player, but the message is received on different channels. Not only is the reception different, the process of examination and application are different. And the timing, extent of acceptance, and action are also different.

This is not to say, for instance, that every first baseman will interpret dietary advice the same way when confronted with the need for iron supplementation. However, recall the pitchers who have walked into your office. It does not make any difference if they are right handed, are left handed, or have only one finger on their pitching hand; they all tend to be intelligent, clear thinkers, good predictors, leaders, independent, like to take on responsibility, and love the fact that they have been given authority to carry things through. Power and challenge are basic ingredients for their satisfaction. These are what make them pitchers, quarterbacks, or volleyball team captains.

When this type of person needs to lose weight or make other dietary adjustments, try giving him or her a clearly communicated set of directions. When they make a mistake or misjudgment, call them on it immediately. Such staunch individuals appreciate this. At the same time, create an atmosphere for involvement, giving unique assignments, such as choosing the restaurants when the team is on the road or helping others with problem identification. This type of person commands admiration yet frequently has little tact and will be unhappy if your game plan does not have immediate results. He or she will want to get the job done and move on to other challenges. Do not philosophize about the many ways to reach the goal. The shortest distance between two points is a straight line.

I recently counseled an older weight lifter who had always run and skied well. He was a retired engineer who had owned his own company. He possessed self-confidence and had skills in dealing with others, planned his time well, and was creative yet practical. He worked out when the weight room was full and enjoyed having his friends note his improvement. But he was tired, was anemic, had lost weight, and was very concerned about cholesterol. He was impatient and had tried using large quantities of bran, very low-protein diets, and all types of supplements. He found himself in the difficult position of admitting his own limitations. He needed to slow down and relax, gain weight, and eat more protein, but he wanted proof of every health decision. In reality, he was afraid of being perceived as an "old softie." He became bored when he did not clearly understand the relationships between diet and endurance. Including megadoses of vitamins with his oatbran made more sense to him than being trapped by the dietary exchange system. He tried every way he could to prove that dietitians do not know a thing about free radicals and such, but he gradually succumbed to meal planning, grocery shopping, and cooking!

Have you ever started a lecture, only to find that there is an individual in the audience who self-admittedly knows more than you do? It is uncomfortable when he or she adds comments to your statements or suddenly cites from the literature about your topic. This person needs recognition from the group and to demonstrate competence. Although you may be tempted to dismiss the "expert" as a loudmouth or nuisance and move on, it might be more productive to delegate some responsibilities that he or she can carry out. These need to be stimulating. Some projects could be grading papers, setting up visual aids, and giving reviews. These persons love to sell their points of view, and as team organizers and communicators they have no peers. Be explicit with your protocols, or they will do their own thing and just might charge you for it. For example, one of my interns could not stand to sit in class and listen quietly. Every time I spoke he would smile, nod, or give questioning glances. I assigned him the task of giving a lecture on food. He spent hours collecting visuals and writing his presentation and ended up doing an excellent job. Later, I watched him while I lectured, and he was far less judgmental. At the end of the course, class members evaluated us on our presentations. He, like myself, was anxious as he awaited comments that he hoped would be positive.

The kids from California are poised and outgoing, talented and enthusiastic. These individuals create a pleasant and friendly climate for an interview. They seem overly concerned with relationships, are name droppers, and spend time collecting contacts. They will come to you to look good and may not really listen to advice. It is not uncommon to spend an entire appointment listening to these patients. I sometimes wish there were pills to give to this type of person: a "happy" pill, a weight loss pill, a quick energy pill, a "beautiful" pill. They want a quick fix. If they return for a second visit (and most of them do not), they will need close supervision, factual data, firm objectives, and, perhaps, opportunities to motivate others or sell themselves as models of good nutrition.

In my field there are problems with planning, time control, routine, and data collection. We do not know exactly when or how changes are made on an individual basis in our patients. Until some documentation takes place, it is difficult to be specific, make a diagnosis, or give suggestions.

Several years ago I worked on weight loss with a unit of police officers. All of the men rode squad cars during the night shift and sat and ate during their breaks. They were not overly worried about their expanding waistlines, but the department's doctor was concerned. All complained of low back pain.

As a group, these men were objective and fact oriented. They demonstrated a powerful drive to attain results. Once they accepted the message (determination of ideal body weight, caloric level of diet, necessary caloric expenditure in exercise), they became extremely motivated and actually seemed to resent close supervision. They were very interested in getting past the diagnosis rather than working through their feelings, excuses, or behavior patterns. They trusted their own skills in monitoring weight changes and kept their own records. Contests were held between individuals on rates of loss. Their biggest problem was that they tended to set standards that were unrealistic for some of them.

Because the art of compromise was not appreciated by them, I decided to base my lectures on their entries to the "question box," such as, "Why can't I lose weight as fast as some of the others?" My tactic worked fairly well.

These men wanted to know only what they wanted to know. In fact, several months after our initial contact, one officer knocked on my door and came into my office. He took off his uniform, piece by piece, uncovering a new uniform that fitted his "ideal" body. He was pleased, but I did not ever see him again.

Other groups require more individual attention and encouragement. One such group, part of a class on ideal body weight, is an example. For several years these women have attended class together, bonded by their continuing relationships. They like to feel ownership in the class, refer it to their friends, and seem to welcome each lecture, although they have heard it before. They are delightful women. They bring notebooks, keep graphs, turn in their homework, and love to talk about their experiences. One makes coffee; others always stay after class to clean up.

This year they will graduate; they have run out of opportunities to take the class for credit. We are planning to hold a retreat. We will meet at the office, have a general health evaluation, take a walk along the canal, and then return to the office to snack and watch videos and discuss eating habits. We will probably talk a long time. Next morning we will stretch, go for another walk, and complete our seminar by establishing new diet and exercise routines for fall and the holiday season, and by realistically examining our goals.

Some patients need well-established standards and definite structure in their nutritional programs. They want to know what you expect and how they will be evaluated. Usually they are members of a team or club or want to be identified with the personalities of an organization. This type of patient could be Joe Average, who tries to gain muscle mass and ends up adding fat tissue, or someone who has lost 100 lb and cannot yet feel good about it. Often, they try to build security by being as competent as possible.

A formerly obese young man found his new slender body as unacceptable as his overweight one (too much loose skin, and not enough muscle). Determined to make a change, he joined a health club and was attracted immediately to the muscle builders. He decided to come to me for dietary counseling to gain weight. (Technically, it is possible for some individuals to gain muscle weight when they are in a lifting program in coordination with a diet that provides extra calories and sufficient protein.) He gained 10 lb in 2 months, and although his skinfold measurements remained the same for triceps, biceps, and subscapular, his iliac crest measurement increased 9 mm (not much, by any means). He ultimately chose to lose 5 lb and concentrate on lifting, having agreed to give up protein powders, garlic, ginseng, and laxatives. He trusted me but believed the plan did not work because some of his weight gain was fat. A more practical approach would have been to advise lifting for 6 months to 1 year, then a gradual weight gain of 1 to 2 lb/month.[5]

CLINICAL MYOPIA

How can we acquire the perceptual skills that will allow us to make crucial connections among food, health, and performance? How can we speed up the unfolding of an idea into actualization?

Somehow, those with the theories and those who are involved in practice seem to remain out of touch with each other, even with our academies, societies, licensure, and periodical reviews. Sometimes we accept an idea too quickly; sometimes we wait too long before putting new information to use.

Experience is often a curse as well as a blessing, and the passing years build a comfort zone into our questions and methodology. Our students and interns shock us into the reality that times do change, that there are no "dumb" questions, that to get answers to some of our quandaries on patient care we need to turn to outsiders who may have a clearer vision of the problem (e.g., engineering has recently been credited with impressive medical advances). New ideas need champions or they die; old ideas and questions also need champions.

The following is a wish list for changes and new procedures. These are broad personal statements. I invite you to investigate new reference points of your own that will define nutrient requirements for the athlete.

1. It would be useful to list additional categories in the recommended dietary allowances. So much happens to adolescents between age 9 and age 19. Wouldn't it be practical to have a biyearly recommendation? It is recognized that this is a period of tremendous variation, but there is an increased need for all nutrients at some point, and to lump an 11-year-old into the same category as a 14-year-old does not help us understand the relationships of growth, sex maturation, and

caloric and protein requirements. It would also be advantageous to enlarge the age groupings for both males and females (many lifetime events occur between the ages of 23 and 50). For instance, one use of protein during the adolescent growth spurt is for additional protein mass, but at what point in development does protein become only the supplier of maintenance factors and calories? Will more protein in the diet increase protein tissue turnover until the age of, say, 30 years?

2. We need a strong research statement regarding megavitamin dosage that is specific to athletes. Just about the time when a sound eating pattern begins to make sense to an individual in diet therapy, along comes a commercial product whose claims (based on whatever is news) are difficult to knock down, especially when testimonials from famous athletes are used to advertise it. How much is enough? How much is too much? How much is too minimal? These are questions that are difficult to answer, and it is important to consider alternatives that are safe. If, for instance, a cyclist expends 6,000 kcal/day, he or she may need more thiamin. Half of this could be from normal intake during meals, the rest from nutrient-dense snacks. Gulping large quantities of B complex pills "to be on the safe side" would be unnecessary.

3. International standards for collecting and recording dietary information, using the best procedures available, should be set up immediately. Too many controversies have risen over methodology, just when every country is becoming interested in the nutritional needs of athletes.

4. The school lunch and breakfast programs (as well as training tables) should compete favorably with the fast-food industry. Why can't we have neon lights, deli bars, interesting food, music, and sound nutrition, too?

5. The food industry needs to promote more nutritious snacks. Teenagers need alternatives to diet soda and french fries.

6. We need a listing of social events that influence the dietary intake of the adolescent. We can attempt to control all

the aspects of nutritional evaluation. However, when working with adolescents, one aspect that is resistant to control is that frustrating, wonderful drive known as "peer group pressure."

Medical Examination Forms

Intergenerational medical examination forms, which would follow athletes during their careers, would be of long-term benefit. They could help every professional who treats the athlete. In addition, if a player's children enter athletics, the historical biochemical, anthropometric, and growth velocity data could be invaluable, perhaps helping to predict high-risk conditions (e.g., anorexia, diabetes, drug and alcohol addiction, or the potential for obesity).

Physiology

1. If we intend to make nutritional recommendations based on body composition, improved standards of collecting and interpreting data must be available. There must be a better correlation between body mass index, for example, and skinfold measurements. We need more analyses of cadavers from late childhood through old age, from both sexes, and from all races. It would be helpful to have a nomograph of all body composition changes from the prepubertal to the aging athlete for both sexes.

2. We need clearer statements regarding energy requirements for sports. Especially perplexing is the question of energy efficiency on an individual basis.

REFERENCES

1. Dummer GM, Rosen LW, Heusner WW: Pathogenic weight-control behaviors of young competitive swimmers. *Phys Sports Med* 1987; 15:75.
2. Rosen LW, McKeag DB, Hourgh DO, et al: Pathogenic weight-control behavior in female athletes. *Phys Sports Med* 1986; 14:79.
3. Satter EM: Childhood eating disorders. *J Am Diet Assoc* 1986; 86:357.
4. Kasl CE: Unpublished data, 1987.

5. Peterson MS: Case reports based on work at The Sports Medicine Clinic, Seattle; The Bellevue Athletic Club, Bellevue, Washington.

SUGGESTED READING

Boskind-White M, White W: *Bulimarexia: The Binge/Purge Cycle.* New York, WW Norton & Co, 1983.
Bruch H: *The Golden Cage.* Cambridge, Harvard University Press, 1978.
Bruch H: Eating disturbances in adolescence, in *The American Handbook of Psychiatry.* New York, Basic Books, 1974.
Crisp AH: *Anorexia Nervosa. Let Me Be.* New York, Academic Press, 1980.
Kasl CD: *Women, Sex, and Addiction: Lost in the Search for Love and Power.* Boston, Houghton-Mifflin, 1988.
Murphy P: Stress and the athlete: Coping with exercise. *Phys Sports Med* 1986; 14:141.

Appendixes

APPENDIX A: NUTRITION RESOURCE LIST

Name and Address	City	Department	State	Zip Code
AEB/UEP Egg Nutrition Center 2501 M St NW	Washington		DC	20037
American Allergy Publications PO Box 640	Menlo Park		CA	94026
American College of Nutrition 100 Manhattan Ave, no 1606	Union City		NJ	07087
American College of Sports Medicine PO Box 1440	Indianapolis		IN	46206
American Diabetes Association 2 Park Ave	New York		NY	10016
American Dietetic Association PO Box 10960	Chicago	Sales Order Dept	IL	60610-0960
American Heart Association 7320 Greenville Ave	Dallas		TX	75231
American Heart Association 7320 Greenville Ave	Dallas	Publication no 51-054-A and no 62-023-A	TX	75231
American Home Economics Association 2010 Massachusetts Ave NW	Washington		DC	20036
American Institute of Nutrition 9650 Rockville Pike	Bethesda		MD	20014
American Medical Association 535 N Dearborn St	Chicago	Nutrition Information Section	IL	60610
American Public Health Association 1015 Fifteenth St NW	Washington		DC	20005

American Society for Clinical Nutrition 9650 Rockville Pike	Bethesda	MD	20014
Anorexia Nervosa Information Office of Research Reporting NICHD NIH Rm 2A 32 Bldg 9000 Rockville Pike	Bethesda	MD	20205
Anorexic Information Father Flanagans Boys Home	Boys Town	Boys Town Communications and Public Service	NE	68010
Arthritis Information Clearinghouse PO Box 9782	Arlington	VA	22209
Athletes Against Drug Abuse 2434 N Greenview	Chicago	IL	60614
Book Department-Review and Herald Publishing Company 55 W Oak Ridge Dr	Hagerstown	MD	21704
Campbells Institute for Health and Fitness Campbell Place	Camden	Campbell Soup Co	NJ	08101
Center for Health Promotion and Education Bldg 3 no SSB 33A 1600 Clifton Rd	Atlanta	Centers for Disease Control	GA	30333
Center for Science in Public Interest 1755 "S" St NW	Washington	DC	20009
Clearinghouse on the Handicapped 400 Maryland Ave SW	Washington	Switzer Bldg Rm 3119	DC	20202

(Continued.)

APPENDIX A (cont.)

Name and Address	City	Department	State	Zip Code
Cling Peach Advisory Board PO Box 7111	San Francisco		CA	94120
Communication Resources/ Distribution 1420 Eckles Ave	St. Paul	3 Coffey Hall University of Minnesota	MN	55108
CompCare Publications 2415 Annapolis Ln	Minneapolis		MN	55441
Consumer Information Center	Pueblo		CO	81009
Dept Social & Health Services ET-24	Olympia	Health Promotion Section	WA	98504
Food and Drug Administration 5600 Fishers Ln (HFE-88)	Rockville	Office of Consumer Affairs— Public Inquiries	MD	20857
Food and Nutrition Information Center	Beltsville	National Agricultural Library Bldg no 304	MD	20017-2299
Food Fight 1515 Webster St no 401	Oakland	Citizens Policy Center	CA	94612
Foods for Health Program Bldg 31 Rm 4A21	Bethesda	NHLBI Information Office	MD	20205
General Mills PO Box 113	Minneapolis		MN	55440
Health Education Services 10000 Culver Blvd Dept N5	Culver City	Division of Social Studies School Service	CA	90232-0802
How To Be Slimmer Trimmer & Happier Rt 2 Box D 301	Hettinger	Diamond Books	ND	58639

Organization / Address	City		State	ZIP
International Diabetes Center 5000 W 39th St	Minneapolis		MN	55416
Kraft—The Consumer's Right to Know Box 802	South Holland	Dept WJ	IL	60473
Little Brown and Co Medical Division 34 Beacon St	Boston	Pediatric and Adolescent Sports Medicine	MA	02106
March of Dimes Birth Defects Foundation 1275 Mamaroneck Ave	White Plains	National Headquarters	NY	10605
National Clearinghouse for Alcohol Information PO Box 2345	Rockville		MD	20852
National Council Against Health Fraud Box 1276	Loma Linda		CA	92354
National Dairy Promotion & Research Board 211 Wilson Blvd Suite 600	Arlington		VA	22201
National Diabetes Information Box NDIC	Bethesda	Clearinghouse	MD	20205
National Health Information Clearinghouse PO Box 1133	Washington		DC	20013-1133
Nutra Sport Publishing PO Box 5902	Whittier		CA	90607
Nutrition Graphics PO Box 1527	Corvallis		OR	97339
Nutrition Tips 12200 Preston Rd	Dallas	The Cooper Clinic Aerobics Center	TX	75230

(Continued.)

APPENDIX A   (cont.)

Name and Address	City	Department	State	Zip Code
Nutrition Today Society PO Box 1829	Annapolis		MD	21404
Office on Smoking and Health 5600 Fishers Ln Prk Bldg no 116	Rockville	Technical Information Center	MD	20857
Overeaters Anonymous 2190 190th St	Torrance		CA	90504
Pacific Kitchens Division 190 Queen Anne Ave N	Seattle	Evans Food Group	WA	98109
Pam Bagett RD 310 S 5th St	Enid		OK	73701
Physical Fitness/Sports Medicine (Pub) US Government Printing Office	Washington	Superintendent of Documents	DC	20402
Positive Eating Patterns PO Box 6071	Kokomo		IN	46902
Practitioners Guide to Obesity Prevention 23391 Park Sorrento no 65	Calabasas	Inside-Out Nutrition Consultants	CA	91302
President's Council on Physical Fitness 450 Fifth St NW	Washington	Fitness and Sports	DC	20001
Public Inquiries and Reports Branch Bldg 31 Rm 4A21	Bethesda	National Heart Lung and Blood Institute	MD	20205
Referral Service Phone 1-800-252-6465		Alcohol and Drug Related		

Referral Service Phone 1-800-548-8700	National Federation of Parents for Drug Free Youth			
Referral Service Phone 1-800-554-5437	Narcotics Education Inc			
Referral Service Phone 1-800-662-4357	National Institute on Drug Abuse			
Referral Service and Treatment (Drugs, ETOH) Phone 1-800-722-0100	Naples Research and Counseling Center			
Ross Laboratories 625 Cleveland Ave	Director of Professional Services	Columbus	OH	43216
Society for Nutrition Education 1736 Franklin St		Oakland	CA	94612
Sports Nutrition News PO Box 986		Evanston	IL	60204
Sportsmedicine Department c/o Teach'em Inc 160 E Illinois St		Chicago	IL	60611
The American Alliance for Health 1900 Association Dr	Physical Education Recreation and Dance	Reston	VA	22091
The Bob Hope Institute 528 18th Ave	International Heart Research Institute	Seattle	WA	98122
The Nutrition Co PO Box 11102		Tallahassee	FL	32302
The Potato Board 1385 S Colorado Blvd no 512		Denver	CO	80222

(Continued.)

APPENDIX A (cont.)

Name and Address	City	Department	State	Zip Code
Tufts University Diet and Nutrition Letter 475 Park Ave South	New York		NY	10016
UC Berkeley Wellness Letter PO Box 10935	Des Moines	Subscription Dept	IA	50340-0935
United Fresh Fruit and Vegetable Association 727 N Washington St	Alexandria		VA	22314
Vitamin Information Bureau 383 Madison Ave	New York		NY	10017
Vitamin Nutrition Information Service 340 Kingsland Ave	Nutley	Hoffmann-LaRoche	NJ	07110
Vitamins—Weight Loss— Recommendations 9846 S 48th Way No 2	Phoenix	President Arizona Dietetic Association	AR	85044
Washington-Idaho Dry Pea & Lentil Comm PO Box 8566	Moscow		ID	83843

Activity	kcal/min/kg	kg 50 lb 110	53 117	56 123	59 130	62 137	65 143	68 150	71 157	74 163	77 170	80 176	83 183	86 190	89 196	92 203	95 209	98 216
Archery	0.065	3.3	3.4	3.6	3.8	4.0	4.2	4.4	4.6	4.8	5.0	5.2	5.4	5.6	5.8	6.0	6.2	6.4
Badminton	0.097	4.9	5.1	5.4	5.7	6.0	6.3	6.6	6.9	7.2	7.5	7.8	8.1	8.3	8.6	8.9	9.2	9.5
Bakery, general (F)	0.035	1.8	1.9	2.0	2.1	2.2	2.3	2.4	2.5	2.6	2.7	2.8	2.9	3.0	3.1	3.2	3.3	3.4
Basketball	0.138	6.9	7.3	7.7	8.1	8.6	9.0	9.4	9.8	10.2	10.6	11.0	11.5	11.9	12.3	12.7	13.1	13.5
Billiards	0.042	2.1	2.2	2.4	2.5	2.6	2.7	2.9	3.0	3.1	3.2	3.4	3.5	3.6	3.7	3.9	4.0	4.1
Bookbinding	0.038	1.9	2.0	2.1	2.2	2.4	2.5	2.6	2.7	2.8	2.9	3.0	3.2	3.3	3.4	3.5	3.6	3.7
Boxing																		
In ring	0.222	6.9	7.3	7.7	8.1	8.6	9.0	9.4	9.8	10.2	10.6	11.0	11.5	11.9	12.3	12.7	13.1	13.5
Sparring	0.138	11.1	11.8	12.4	13.1	13.8	14.4	15.1	15.8	16.4	17.1	17.8	18.4	19.1	19.8	20.4	21.1	21.8
Canoeing																		
Leisure	0.044	2.2	2.3	2.5	2.6	2.7	2.9	3.0	3.1	3.3	3.4	3.5	3.7	3.8	3.9	4.0	4.2	4.3
Racing	0.103	5.2	5.5	5.8	6.1	6.4	6.7	7.0	7.3	7.6	7.9	8.2	8.5	8.9	9.2	9.5	9.8	10.1
Card playing	0.025	1.3	1.3	1.4	1.5	1.6	1.6	1.7	1.8	1.9	1.9	2.0	2.1	2.2	2.2	2.3	2.4	2.5
Carpentry, general	0.052	2.6	2.8	2.9	3.1	3.2	3.4	3.5	3.7	3.8	4.0	4.2	4.3	4.5	4.6	4.8	4.9	5.1
Carpet sweeping (F)	0.045	2.3	2.4	2.5	2.7	2.8	2.9	3.1	3.2	3.3	3.5	3.6	3.7	3.9	4.0	4.1	4.3	4.4
Carpet sweeping (M)	0.048	2.4	2.5	2.7	2.8	3.0	3.1	3.3	3.4	3.6	3.7	3.8	4.0	4.1	4.3	4.4	4.6	4.7
Circuit training																		
Hydra-Fitness	0.132	6.6	7.0	7.4	7.8	8.2	8.6	9.0	9.4	9.7	10.2	10.5	10.9	11.4	11.7	12.1	12.5	12.9
Universal	0.116	5.8	6.2	6.5	6.9	7.2	7.5	7.9	8.3	8.6	8.9	9.3	9.6	10.0	10.3	10.7	11.0	11.4
Nautilus	0.092	4.6	4.9	5.2	5.5	5.8	6.0	6.3	6.6	6.8	7.1	7.4	7.7	8.0	8.2	8.5	8.8	9.1
Free weights	0.086	4.3	4.5	4.8	5.0	5.3	5.5	5.8	6.1	6.3	6.6	6.8	7.1	7.4	7.6	7.9	8.1	8.4
Cleaning (F)	0.062	3.1	3.3	3.5	3.7	3.8	4.0	4.2	4.4	4.6	4.8	5.0	5.1	5.3	5.5	5.7	5.9	6.1
Cleaning (M)	0.058	2.9	3.1	3.2	3.4	3.6	3.8	3.9	4.1	4.3	4.5	4.6	4.8	5.0	5.2	5.3	5.5	5.7
Climbing hills																		
With no load	0.121	6.1	6.4	6.8	7.1	7.5	7.9	8.2	8.6	9.0	9.3	9.7	10.0	10.4	10.8	11.1	11.5	11.9
With 5-kg load	0.129	6.5	6.8	7.2	7.6	8.0	8.4	8.8	9.2	9.5	9.9	10.3	10.7	11.1	11.5	11.9	12.3	12.6
With 10-kg lad	0.140	7.0	7.4	7.8	8.3	8.7	9.1	9.5	9.9	10.4	10.8	11.2	11.6	12.0	12.5	12.9	13.3	13.7
With 20-kg load	0.147	7.4	7.8	8.2	8.7	9.1	9.6	10.0	10.4	10.9	11.3	11.8	12.2	12.6	13.1	13.5	14.0	14.4

(Continued.)

253

APPENDIX B (cont.)

Activity	kcal/min/kg	50	53	56	59	62	65	68	71	74	77	80	83	86	89	92	95	98
(kg / lb)		110	117	123	130	137	143	150	157	163	170	176	183	190	196	203	209	216
Coal mining																		
Drilling coal, rock	0.094	4.7	5.0	5.3	5.5	5.8	6.1	6.4	6.7	7.0	7.2	7.5	7.8	8.1	8.4	8.6	8.9	9.2
Erecting supports	0.088	4.4	4.7	4.9	5.2	5.5	5.7	6.0	6.2	6.5	6.8	7.0	7.3	7.6	7.8	8.1	8.4	8.6
Shoveling coal	0.108	5.4	5.7	6.0	6.4	6.7	7.0	7.3	7.7	8.0	8.3	8.6	9.0	9.3	9.6	9.9	10.3	10.6
Cooking (F)	0.045	2.3	2.4	2.5	2.7	2.8	2.9	3.1	3.2	3.3	3.5	3.6	3.7	3.9	4.0	4.1	4.3	4.4
Cooking (M)	0.048	2.4	2.5	2.7	2.8	3.0	3.1	3.3	3.4	3.6	3.7	3.8	4.0	4.1	4.3	4.4	4.6	4.7
Cricket																		
Batting	0.083	4.2	4.4	4.6	4.9	5.1	5.4	5.6	5.9	6.1	6.4	6.6	6.9	7.1	7.4	7.6	7.9	8.1
Bowling	0.090	4.5	4.8	5.0	5.3	5.6	5.9	6.1	6.4	6.7	6.9	7.2	7.5	7.7	8.0	8.3	8.6	8.8
Croquet	0.059	3.0	3.1	3.3	3.5	3.7	3.8	4.0	4.2	4.4	4.5	4.7	4.9	5.1	5.3	5.4	5.6	5.8
Cycling																		
Leisure, 5.5 miles/hr	0.064	3.2	3.4	3.6	3.8	4.0	4.2	4.4	4.5	4.7	4.9	5.1	5.3	5.5	5.7	5.9	6.1	6.3
Leisure, 9.4 miles/hr	0.100	5.0	5.3	5.6	5.9	6.2	6.5	6.8	7.1	7.4	7.7	8.0	8.3	8.6	8.9	9.2	9.5	9.8
Racing	0.169	8.5	9.0	9.5	10.0	10.5	11.0	11.5	12.0	12.5	13.0	13.5	14.0	14.5	15.0	15.5	16.1	16.6
Dancing (F)																		
Aerobic, medium	0.103	5.2	5.5	5.8	6.1	6.4	6.7	7.0	7.3	7.6	7.9	8.2	8.5	8.9	9.2	9.5	9.8	10.1
Aerobic, intense	0.135	6.7	7.1	7.5	7.9	8.3	8.7	9.2	9.6	10.0	10.4	10.8	11.2	11.6	12.0	12.4	12.8	13.2
Ballroom	0.051	2.6	2.7	2.9	3.0	3.2	3.3	3.5	3.6	3.8	3.9	4.1	4.2	4.4	4.5	4.7	4.8	5.0
Choreographed	0.168	8.4	8.9	9.4	9.9	10.4	10.9	11.4	11.9	12.4	12.9	13.4	13.9	14.4	15.0	15.5	16.0	16.5
"Twist," "wiggle"		5.2	5.5	5.8	6.1	6.4	6.7	7.0	7.3	7.6	7.9	8.2	8.5	8.9	9.2	9.5	9.8	10.1
Digging trenches	0.145	7.3	7.7	8.1	8.6	9.0	9.4	9.9	10.3	10.7	11.2	11.6	12.0	12.5	12.9	13.3	13.8	14.2
Drawing (standing)	0.036	1.8	1.9	2.0	2.1	2.2	2.3	2.4	2.6	2.7	2.8	2.9	3.0	3.1	3.2	3.3	3.4	3.5
Eating (sitting)	0.023	1.2	1.2	1.3	1.4	1.4	1.5	1.6	1.6	1.7	1.8	1.8	1.9	2.0	2.0	2.1	2.2	2.3
Electrical work	0.058	2.9	3.1	3.2	3.4	3.6	3.8	3.9	4.1	4.3	4.5	4.6	4.8	5.0	5.2	5.3	5.5	5.7
Farming																		
Barn cleaning	0.135	6.8	7.2	7.6	8.0	8.4	8.8	9.2	9.6	10.0	10.4	10.8	11.2	11.6	12.0	12.4	12.8	13.2
Driving harvester	0.040	2.0	2.1	2.2	2.4	2.5	2.6	2.7	2.8	3.0	3.1	3.2	3.3	3.4	3.6	3.7	3.8	3.9
Driving tractor	0.037	1.9	2.0	2.1	2.2	2.3	2.4	2.5	2.6	2.7	2.8	3.0	3.1	3.2	3.3	3.4	3.5	3.6

Feeding cattle	0.085	4.3	4.5	4.8	5.0	5.3	5.5	5.8	6.0	6.3	6.5	6.8	7.1	7.3	7.6	7.8	8.1	8.3
Feeding animals	0.065	3.3	3.4	3.6	3.8	4.0	4.2	4.4	4.6	4.8	5.0	5.2	5.4	5.6	5.8	6.0	6.2	6.4
Forking straw bales	0.138	6.9	7.3	7.7	8.1	8.6	9.0	9.4	9.8	10.2	10.6	11.0	11.5	11.9	12.3	12.7	13.1	13.5
Milking by hand	0.054	2.7	2.9	3.0	3.2	3.3	3.5	3.7	3.8	4.0	4.2	4.3	4.5	4.6	4.8	5.0	5.1	5.3
Milking by machine	0.023	1.2	1.2	1.3	1.4	1.4	1.5	1.6	1.6	1.7	1.8	1.8	1.9	2.0	2.0	2.1	2.2	2.3
Shoveling grain	0.085	4.3	4.5	4.8	5.0	5.3	5.5	5.8	6.0	6.3	6.5	6.8	7.1	7.3	7.6	7.8	8.1	8.3
Field hockey	0.134	6.7	7.1	7.5	7.9	8.3	8.7	9.1	9.5	9.9	10.3	10.7	11.1	11.5	11.9	12.3	12.7	13.1
Fishing	0.062	3.1	3.3	3.5	3.7	3.8	4.0	4.2	4.4	4.6	4.8	5.0	5.1	5.3	5.5	5.7	5.9	6.1
Food shopping (F)	0.062	3.1	3.3	3.5	3.7	3.8	4.0	4.2	4.4	4.6	4.8	5.0	5.1	5.3	5.5	5.7	5.9	6.1
Food shopping (M)	0.058	2.9	3.1	3.2	3.4	3.6	3.8	3.9	4.1	4.3	4.5	4.6	4.8	5.0	5.2	5.3	5.5	5.7
Football	0.132	6.6	7.0	7.4	7.8	8.2	8.6	9.0	9.4	9.8	10.2	10.6	11.0	11.4	11.7	12.1	12.5	12.9
Forestry																		
Ax chopping, fast	0.297	14.9	15.7	16.6	17.5	18.4	19.3	20.2	21.1	22.0	22.9	23.8	24.7	25.5	26.4	27.3	28.2	29.1
Ax chopping, slow	0.085	4.3	4.5	4.8	5.0	5.3	5.5	5.8	6.0	6.3	6.5	6.8	7.1	7.3	7.6	7.8	8.1	8.3
Barking trees	0.123	6.2	6.5	6.9	7.3	7.6	8.0	8.4	8.7	9.1	9.5	9.8	10.2	10.6	10.9	11.3	11.7	12.1
Carrying logs	0.186	9.3	9.9	10.4	11.0	11.5	12.1	12.6	13.2	13.8	14.3	14.9	15.4	16.0	16.6	17.1	17.7	18.2
Felling trees	0.132	6.6	7.0	7.4	7.8	8.2	8.6	9.0	9.4	9.8	10.2	10.6	11.0	11.4	11.7	12.1	12.5	12.9
Hoeing	0.091	4.6	4.8	5.1	5.4	5.6	5.9	6.2	6.5	6.7	7.0	7.3	7.6	7.8	8.1	8.4	8.6	8.9
Planting by hand	0.109	5.5	5.8	6.1	6.4	6.8	7.1	7.4	7.7	8.1	8.4	8.7	9.0	9.4	9.7	10.0	10.4	10.7
Sawing by hand	0.122	6.1	6.5	6.8	7.2	7.6	7.9	8.3	8.7	9.0	9.4	9.8	10.1	10.5	10.9	11.2	11.6	12.0
Sawing, power	0.075	3.8	4.0	4.2	4.4	4.7	4.9	5.1	5.3	5.6	5.8	6.0	6.2	6.5	6.7	6.9	7.1	7.4
Stacking firewood	0.088	4.4	4.7	4.9	5.2	5.5	5.7	6.0	6.2	6.5	6.8	7.0	7.3	7.6	7.8	8.1	8.4	8.6
Trimming trees	0.129	6.5	6.8	7.2	7.6	8.0	8.4	8.8	9.2	9.5	9.9	10.3	10.7	11.1	11.5	11.9	12.3	12.6
Weeding	0.072	3.6	3.8	4.0	4.2	4.5	4.7	4.9	5.1	5.3	5.5	5.8	6.0	6.2	6.4	6.6	6.8	7.1
Furriery	0.083	4.2	4.4	4.6	4.9	5.1	5.4	5.6	5.9	6.1	6.4	6.6	6.9	7.1	7.4	7.6	7.9	8.1
Gardening																		
Digging	0.126	6.3	6.7	7.1	7.4	7.8	8.2	8.6	8.9	9.3	9.7	10.1	10.5	10.8	11.2	11.6	12.0	12.3
Hedging	0.077	3.9	4.1	4.3	4.5	4.8	5.0	5.2	5.5	5.7	5.9	6.2	6.4	6.6	6.9	7.1	7.3	7.5
Mowing	0.112	5.6	5.9	6.3	6.6	6.9	7.3	7.6	8.0	8.3	8.6	9.0	9.3	9.6	10.0	10.3	10.6	11.0
Raking	0.054	2.7	2.9	3.0	3.2	3.3	3.5	3.7	3.8	4.0	4.2	4.3	4.5	4.6	4.8	5.0	5.1	5.3
Golf	0.085	4.3	4.5	4.8	5.0	5.3	5.5	5.8	6.0	6.3	6.5	6.8	7.1	7.3	7.6	7.8	8.1	8.3
Gymnastics	0.066	3.3	3.5	3.7	3.9	4.1	4.3	4.5	4.7	4.9	5.1	5.3	5.5	5.7	5.9	6.1	6.3	6.5
Horse-grooming	0.128	6.4	6.8	7.2	7.6	7.9	8.3	8.7	9.1	9.5	9.9	10.2	10.6	11.0	11.4	11.8	12.2	12.5

(Continued.)

255

APPENDIX B (cont.)

Activity	kcal/min/kg	kg 50 / lb 110	53 117	56 123	59 130	62 137	65 143	68 150	71 157	74 163	77 170	80 176	83 183	86 190	89 196	92 203	95 209	98 216
Horse-racing																		
Galloping	0.137	6.9	7.3	7.7	8.1	8.5	8.9	9.3	9.7	10.1	10.6	11.0	11.4	11.8	12.2	12.6	13.6	13.4
Horse-racing																		
Trotting	0.110	5.5	5.8	6.2	6.5	6.8	7.2	7.5	7.8	8.1	8.5	8.8	9.1	9.5	9.8	10.1	10.5	10.8
Walking	0.041	2.1	2.2	2.3	2.4	2.5	2.7	2.8	2.9	3.0	3.2	3.3	3.4	3.5	3.6	3.8	3.9	4.0
Ironing (F)	0.033	1.7	1.7	1.8	1.9	2.0	2.1	2.2	2.3	2.4	2.5	2.6	2.7	2.8	2.9	3.0	3.1	3.2
Ironing (M)	0.064	3.2	3.4	3.6	3.8	4.0	4.2	4.4	4.5	4.7	4.9	5.1	5.3	5.5	5.7	5.9	6.1	6.3
Judo	0.195	9.8	10.3	10.9	11.5	12.1	12.7	13.3	13.8	14.4	15.0	15.6	16.2	16.8	17.4	17.9	18.5	19.1
Jumping Rope																		
70/min	0.162	8.1	8.6	9.1	9.6	10.0	10.5	11.0	11.5	12.0	12.5	13.0	13.4	13.9	14.4	14.9	15.4	15.9
80/min	0.164	8.2	8.7	9.2	9.7	10.2	10.7	11.2	11.6	12.1	12.6	13.1	13.6	14.1	14.6	14.6	15.6	16.1
125/min	0.177	8.9	9.4	9.9	10.4	11.0	11.5	12.0	12.6	13.1	13.6	14.2	14.7	15.2	15.8	16.3	16.8	17.3
145/min	0.197	9.9	10.4	11.0	11.6	12.2	12.8	13.4	14.0	14.6	15.2	15.8	16.4	16.9	17.5	18.1	18.7	19.3
Knitting, sewing (F)	0.022	1.1	1.2	1.2	1.3	1.4	1.4	1.5	1.6	1.6	1.7	1.8	1.8	1.9	2.0	2.0	2.1	2.2
Knitting, sewing (M)	0.023	1.2	1.2	1.3	1.4	1.4	1.5	1.6	1.6	1.7	1.8	1.8	1.9	2.0	2.0	2.1	2.2	2.3
Locksmith	0.057	2.9	3.0	3.2	3.4	3.5	3.7	3.9	4.0	4.2	4.4	4.6	4.7	4.9	5.1	5.2	5.4	5.6
Lying at ease	0.022	1.1	1.2	1.2	1.3	1.4	1.4	1.5	1.6	1.6	1.7	1.8	1.8	1.9	2.0	2.0	2.1	2.2
Machining-tooling																		
Machining	0.048	2.4	2.5	2.7	2.8	3.0	3.1	3.3	3.4	3.6	3.7	3.8	4.0	4.1	4.3	4.4	4.6	4.7
Operating lathe	0.052	2.6	2.8	2.9	3.1	3.2	3.4	3.5	3.7	3.8	4.0	4.2	4.3	4.5	4.6	4.8	4.9	5.1
Operating punch press	0.088	4.4	4.7	4.9	5.2	5.5	5.7	6.0	6.2	6.5	6.8	7.0	7.3	7.6	7.8	8.1	8.4	8.6
Tapping and drilling	0.065	3.3	3.4	3.6	3.8	4.0	4.2	4.4	4.6	4.8	5.0	5.2	5.4	5.6	5.8	6.0	6.2	6.4
Welding	0.052	2.6	2.8	2.9	3.1	3.2	3.4	3.5	3.7	3.8	4.0	4.2	4.3	4.5	4.6	4.8	4.9	5.1
Working sheet metal	0.048	2.4	2.5	2.7	2.8	3.0	3.1	3.3	3.4	3.6	3.7	3.8	4.0	4.1	4.3	4.4	4.6	4.7
Marching, rapid	0.142	7.1	7.5	8.0	8.4	8.8	9.2	9.7	10.1	10.5	10.9	11.4	11.8	12.2	12.6	13.1	13.5	13.9
Mopping floor (F)	0.062	3.1	3.3	3.5	3.7	3.8	4.0	4.2	4.4	4.6	4.8	5.0	5.1	5.3	5.5	5.7	5.9	6.1
Mopping floor (M)	0.058	2.9	3.1	3.2	3.4	3.6	3.8	3.9	4.1	4.3	4.5	4.6	4.8	5.0	5.2	5.0	5.5	5.7

Music playing																	
Accordion (sitting)	0.032	1.6	1.7	1.8	1.9	2.0	2.1	2.2	2.3	2.4	2.5	2.6	2.7	2.8	2.8	2.9	3.0	3.1
Cello (sitting)	0.041	2.1	2.2	2.3	2.4	2.5	2.7	2.8	2.9	3.0	3.2	3.3	3.4	3.5	3.6	3.8	3.9	4.0
Conducting	0.039	2.0	2.1	2.2	2.3	2.4	2.5	2.7	2.8	2.9	3.0	3.1	3.2	3.4	3.5	3.6	3.7	3.8
Drums (sitting)	0.066	3.3	3.5	3.7	3.9	4.1	4.3	4.5	4.7	4.9	5.1	5.3	5.5	5.7	5.9	6.1	6.3	6.6
Flute (sitting)	0.035	1.8	1.9	2.0	2.1	2.2	2.3	2.4	2.5	2.6	2.7	2.8	2.9	3.0	3.1	3.2	3.3	3.4
Horn (sitting)	0.029	1.5	1.5	1.6	1.7	1.8	1.9	2.0	2.1	2.1	2.2	2.3	2.4	2.5	2.6	2.7	2.8	2.8
Organ (sitting)	0.053	2.7	2.8	3.0	3.1	3.3	3.4	3.6	3.8	3.9	4.1	4.2	4.4	4.6	4.7	4.9	5.0	5.2
Piano (sitting)	0.040	2.0	2.1	2.2	2.4	2.5	2.6	2.7	2.8	3.0	3.1	3.2	3.3	3.4	3.6	3.7	3.8	3.9
Trumpet (standing)	0.031	1.6	1.6	1.7	1.8	1.9	2.0	2.1	2.2	2.3	2.4	2.5	2.6	2.7	2.8	2.9	2.9	3.0
Violin (sitting)	0.045	2.3	2.4	2.5	2.7	2.8	2.9	3.1	3.2	3.3	3.5	3.6	3.7	3.9	4.0	4.1	4.3	4.4
Woodwind (sitting)	0.032	1.6	1.7	1.8	1.9	2.0	2.1	2.2	2.3	2.4	2.5	2.6	2.7	2.8	2.8	2.9	3.0	3.1
Painting, inside	0.034	1.7	1.8	1.9	2.0	2.1	2.2	2.3	2.4	2.5	2.6	2.7	2.8	2.9	3.0	3.1	3.2	3.3
Painting, outside	0.077	3.9	4.1	4.3	4.5	4.8	5.0	5.2	5.5	5.7	5.9	6.2	6.4	6.6	6.9	7.1	7.3	7.5
Planting seedlings	0.070	3.5	3.7	3.9	4.1	4.3	4.6	4.8	5.0	5.2	5.4	5.6	5.8	6.0	6.2	6.4	6.7	6.9
Plastering	0.078	3.9	4.1	4.4	4.6	4.8	5.1	5.3	5.5	5.8	6.0	6.2	6.5	6.7	6.9	7.2	7.4	7.6
Printing	0.035	1.8	1.9	2.0	2.1	2.2	2.3	2.4	2.5	2.6	2.7	2.8	2.9	3.0	3.1	3.2	3.3	3.4
Racquetball	0.178	8.9	9.4	10.0	10.5	11.0	11.6	12.1	12.6	13.2	13.7	14.2	14.8	15.3	15.8	16.4	16.9	17.4
Running, cross-country	0.163	8.2	8.6	9.1	9.6	10.1	10.6	11.1	11.6	12.1	12.6	13.0	13.5	14.0	14.5	15.0	15.5	16.0
Running, horizontal																		
11 min, 30 sec/mile	0.135	6.8	7.2	7.6	8.0	8.4	8.8	9.2	9.6	10.0	10.5	10.9	11.3	11.7	12.1	12.5	12.9	13.3
9 min/mile	0.193	9.7	10.2	10.8	11.4	12.0	12.5	13.1	13.7	14.3	14.9	15.4	16.0	16.6	17.2	17.8	18.3	18.9
8 min/mile	0.208	10.8	11.3	11.9	12.5	13.1	13.6	14.2	14.8	15.4	16.0	16.5	17.1	17.7	18.3	18.9	19.4	20.0
7 min/mile	0.228	12.2	12.7	13.3	13.9	14.5	15.0	15.6	16.2	16.8	17.4	17.9	18.5	19.1	19.7	20.3	20.8	21.4
6 min/mile	0.252	13.9	14.4	15.0	15.6	16.2	16.7	17.3	17.9	18.5	19.1	19.6	20.2	20.8	21.4	22.0	22.5	23.1
5 min, 30 sec/mile	0.289	14.5	15.3	16.2	17.1	17.9	18.8	19.7	20.5	21.4	22.3	23.1	24.0	24.9	25.7	26.6	27.5	28.3
Scraping paint	0.063	3.2	3.3	3.5	3.7	3.9	4.1	4.3	4.5	4.7	4.9	5.0	5.2	5.4	5.6	5.8	6.0	6.2
Scrubbing floors (F)	0.109	5.5	5.8	6.1	6.4	6.8	7.1	7.4	7.7	8.1	8.4	8.7	9.0	9.4	9.7	10.0	10.4	10.7
Scrubbing floors (M)	0.108	5.4	5.7	6.0	6.4	6.7	7.0	7.3	7.7	8.0	8.3	8.6	9.0	9.3	9.6	9.9	10.3	10.6
Shoe repair, general	0.045	2.3	2.4	2.5	2.7	2.8	2.9	3.1	3.2	3.3	3.5	3.6	3.7	3.9	4.0	4.1	4.3	4.4
Sitting quietly	0.021	1.1	1.1	1.2	1.2	1.3	1.4	1.4	1.5	1.6	1.6	1.7	1.7	1.8	1.9	1.9	2.0	2.1

(Continued.)

APPENDIX B (cont.)

Activity	kcal/min/kg	kg 50 / lb 110	53 117	56 123	59 130	62 137	65 143	68 150	71 157	74 163	77 170	80 176	83 183	86 190	89 196	92 203	95 209	98 216
Skiing, hard snow																		
Level, moderate speed	0.119	6.0	6.3	6.7	7.0	7.4	7.7	8.1	8.4	8.8	9.2	9.5	9.9	10.2	10.6	10.9	11.3	11.7
Level, walking	0.143	7.2	7.6	8.0	8.4	8.9	9.3	9.7	10.2	10.6	11.0	11.4	11.9	12.3	12.7	13.2	13.6	14.0
Uphill, maximum speed	0.274	13.7	14.5	15.3	16.2	17.0	17.8	18.6	19.5	20.3	21.1	21.9	22.7	23.6	24.4	25.2	26.0	26.9
Skiing, soft snow																		
Leisure (F)	0.111	4.9	5.2	5.5	5.8	6.1	6.4	6.7	7.0	7.3	7.5	7.8	8.1	8.4	8.7	9.0	9.3	9.6
Leisure (M)	0.098	5.6	5.9	6.2	6.5	6.9	7.2	7.5	7.9	8.2	8.5	8.9	9.2	9.5	9.9	10.2	10.5	10.9
Skindiving, as frogman																		
Considerable motion	0.276	13.8	14.6	15.5	16.3	17.1	17.9	18.8	19.6	20.4	21.3	22.1	22.9	23.7	24.6	25.4	26.2	27.0
Moderate motion	0.206	10.3	10.9	11.5	12.2	12.8	13.4	14.0	14.6	15.2	15.9	16.5	17.1	17.7	18.3	19.0	19.6	20.2
Snowshoeing, soft snow	0.166	8.3	8.8	9.3	9.8	10.3	10.8	11.3	11.8	12.3	12.8	13.3	13.8	14.3	14.8	15.3	15.8	16.3
Squash	0.212	10.6	11.2	11.9	12.5	13.1	13.8	14.4	15.1	15.7	16.3	17.0	17.6	18.2	18.9	19.5	20.1	20.8
Standing quietly (F)	0.025	1.3	1.3	1.4	1.5	1.6	1.6	1.7	1.8	1.9	1.9	2.0	2.1	2.2	2.2	2.3	2.4	2.5
Standing quietly (M)	0.027	1.4	1.4	1.5	1.6	1.7	1.8	1.8	1.9	2.0	2.1	2.2	2.2	2.3	2.4	2.5	2.6	2.6
Steel mill, working in																		
Fettling	0.089	4.5	4.7	5.0	5.3	5.5	5.8	6.1	6.3	6.6	6.9	7.1	7.4	7.7	7.9	8.2	8.5	8.7
Forging	0.100	5.0	5.3	5.6	5.9	6.2	6.5	6.8	7.1	7.4	7.7	8.0	8.3	8.6	8.9	9.2	9.5	9.8
Hand rolling	0.137	6.9	7.3	7.7	8.1	8.5	8.9	9.3	9.7	10.1	10.6	11.0	11.4	11.8	12.2	12.6	13.0	13.4
Merchant mill rolling	0.145	7.3	7.7	8.1	8.6	9.0	9.4	9.9	10.3	10.7	11.2	11.6	12.0	12.5	12.9	13.3	13.8	14.2
Removing slag	0.178	8.9	9.4	10.0	10.5	11.0	11.6	12.1	12.6	13.2	13.7	14.2	14.8	15.3	15.8	16.4	16.9	17.4
Tending furnace	0.126	6.3	6.7	7.1	7.4	7.8	8.2	8.6	8.9	9.3	9.7	10.1	10.5	10.8	11.2	11.6	12.0	12.3
Tipping molds	0.092	4.6	4.9	5.2	5.4	5.7	6.0	6.3	6.5	6.8	7.1	7.4	7.6	7.9	8.2	8.5	8.7	9.0
Stock clerking	0.054	2.7	2.9	3.0	3.2	3.3	3.5	3.7	3.8	4.0	4.2	4.3	4.5	4.6	4.8	5.0	5.1	5.3
Swimming																		
Back stroke	0.169	8.5	9.0	9.5	10.0	10.5	11.0	11.5	12.0	12.5	13.0	13.5	14.0	14.5	15.0	15.5	16.1	16.6
Breast stroke	0.162	8.1	8.6	9.1	9.6	10.0	10.5	11.0	11.5	12.0	12.5	13.0	13.4	13.9	14.4	14.9	15.4	15.9

Activity																		
Crawl, fast	0.156	7.8	8.3	8.7	9.2	9.7	10.1	10.6	11.1	11.5	12.0	12.5	12.9	13.4	13.9	14.4	14.8	15.3
Crawl, slow	0.128	6.4	6.8	7.2	7.6	7.9	8.3	8.7	9.1	9.5	9.9	10.2	10.6	11.0	11.4	11.8	12.2	12.5
Side stroke	0.122	6.1	6.5	6.8	7.2	7.6	7.9	8.3	8.7	9.0	9.4	9.8	10.1	10.5	10.9	11.2	11.6	12.0
Treading, fast	0.170	8.5	9.0	9.5	10.0	10.5	11.1	11.6	12.1	12.6	13.1	13.6	14.1	14.6	15.1	15.6	16.2	16.7
Treading normal	0.062	3.1	3.3	3.5	3.7	3.8	4.0	4.2	4.4	4.6	4.8	5.0	5.1	5.3	5.5	5.7	5.9	6.1
Table tennis	0.068	3.4	3.6	3.8	4.0	4.2	4.4	4.6	4.8	5.0	5.2	5.4	5.6	5.8	6.1	6.3	6.5	6.7
Tailoring																		
Cutting	0.041	2.1	2.2	2.3	2.4	2.5	2.7	2.8	2.9	3.0	3.2	3.3	3.4	3.5	3.6	3.8	3.9	4.0
Hand-sewing	0.032	1.6	1.7	1.8	1.9	2.0	2.1	2.2	2.3	2.4	2.5	2.6	2.7	2.8	2.8	2.9	3.0	3.1
Machine-sewing	0.045	2.3	2.4	2.5	2.7	2.8	2.9	3.1	3.2	3.3	3.5	3.6	3.7	3.9	4.0	4.1	4.3	4.4
Pressing	0.062	3.1	3.3	3.5	3.7	3.8	4.0	4.2	4.4	4.6	4.8	5.0	5.1	5.3	5.5	5.7	5.9	6.1
Tennis	0.109	5.5	5.8	6.1	6.4	6.8	7.1	7.4	7.7	8.1	8.4	8.7	9.0	9.4	9.7	10.0	10.4	10.7
Typing																		
Electric	0.027	1.4	1.4	1.5	1.6	1.7	1.8	1.8	1.9	2.0	2.1	2.2	2.2	2.3	2.4	2.5	2.6	2.6
Manual	0.031	1.6	1.6	1.7	1.8	1.9	2.0	2.1	2.2	2.3	2.4	2.5	2.6	2.7	2.8	2.9	2.9	3.0
Volleyball	0.050	2.5	2.7	2.8	3.0	3.1	3.3	3.4	3.6	3.7	3.9	4.0	4.2	4.3	4.5	4.6	4.8	4.9
Walking, normal pace																		
Asphalt road	0.080	4.0	4.2	4.5	4.7	5.0	5.2	5.4	5.7	5.9	6.2	6.4	6.6	6.9	7.1	7.4	7.6	7.8
Fields and hillsides	0.082	4.1	4.3	4.6	4.8	5.1	5.3	5.6	5.8	6.1	6.3	6.6	6.8	7.1	7.3	7.5	7.8	8.0
Grass track	0.081	4.1	4.3	4.5	4.8	5.0	5.3	5.5	5.8	6.0	6.2	6.5	6.7	7.0	7.2	7.5	7.7	7.9
Plowed field	0.077	3.9	4.1	4.3	4.5	4.8	5.0	5.2	5.5	5.7	5.9	6.2	6.4	6.6	6.9	7.1	7.3	7.5
Wallpapering	0.048	2.4	2.5	2.7	2.8	3.0	3.1	3.3	3.4	3.6	3.7	3.8	4.0	4.1	4.3	4.4	4.6	4.7
Watch repairing	0.025	1.3	1.3	1.4	1.5	1.6	1.6	1.7	1.8	1.9	1.9	2.0	2.1	2.2	2.2	2.3	2.4	2.5
Window cleaning (F)	0.059	3.0	3.1	3.3	3.5	3.7	3.8	4.0	4.2	4.4	4.5	4.7	4.9	5.1	5.3	5.4	5.6	5.8
Window cleaning (M)	0.058	2.9	3.1	3.2	3.4	3.6	3.8	3.9	4.1	4.3	4.5	4.6	4.8	5.0	5.2	5.3	5.5	5.7
Writing (sitting)	0.029	1.5	1.5	1.6	1.7	1.8	1.9	2.0	2.1	2.1	2.2	2.3	2.4	2.5	2.6	2.7	2.8	2.8

*From McArdle WD, Katch FI: Exercise Physiology: Energy, Nutrition, and Human Performance. Philadelphia, Lea & Febiger, 1981, pp 642–649. Used by permission.

APPENDIX C: RECOMMENDED DIETARY ALLOWANCES

Food and Nutrition Board, National Academy of Sciences–National Research Council Recommended Daily Dietary Allowances,* Revised 1980: Designed for the Maintenance of Good Nutrition of Practically All Healthy People in the United States

	Age (yr)	Weight kg	Weight lb	Height cm	Height in	Protein (gm)	Fat-Soluble Vitamins Vitamin A (µg RE)†	Vitamin D (µg)‡	Vitamin E (mg α-TE)§	Water-Soluble Vitamins Vitamin C (mg)	Thiamin (mg)	Riboflavin (mg)	Niacin (mg NE)‖	Vitamin B6 (mg)	Folacin¶ (µg)	Vitamin B12 (µg)	Minerals Calcium (mg)	Phosphorus (mg)	Magnesium (mg)	Iron (mg)	Zinc (mg)	Iodine (µg)
Infants	0.0–0.5	6	13	60	24	kg × 2.2	420	10	3	35	0.3	0.4	6	0.3	30	0.5#	360	240	50	10	3	40
	0.5–1.0	9	20	71	28	kg × 2.0	400	10	4	35	0.5	0.6	8	0.6	45	1.5	540	360	70	15	5	50
Children	1–3	13	29	90	35	23	400	10	5	45	0.7	0.8	9	0.9	100	2.0	800	800	150	15	10	70
	4–6	20	44	112	44	30	500	10	6	45	0.9	1.0	11	1.3	200	2.5	800	800	200	10	10	90
	7–10	28	62	132	52	34	700	10	7	45	1.2	1.4	16	1.6	300	3.0	800	800	250	10	10	120
Males	11–14	45	99	157	62	45	1,000	10	8	50	1.4	1.6	18	1.8	400	3.0	1,200	1,200	350	18	15	150
	15–18	66	145	176	69	56	1,000	10	10	60	1.4	1.7	18	2.0	400	3.0	1,200	1,200	400	18	15	150
	19–22	70	154	177	70	56	1,000	7.5	10	60	1.5	1.7	19	2.2	400	3.0	800	800	350	10	15	150
	23–50	70	154	178	70	56	1,000	5	10	60	1.4	1.6	18	2.2	400	3.0	800	800	350	10	15	150
	51+	70	154	178	70	56	1,000	5	10	60	1.2	1.4	16	2.2	400	3.0	800	800	350	10	15	150
Females	11–14	46	101	157	62	46	800	10	8	50	1.1	1.3	15	1.8	400	3.0	1,200	1,200	300	18	15	150
	15–18	55	120	163	64	46	800	10	8	60	1.1	1.3	14	2.0	400	3.0	1,200	1,200	300	18	15	150
	19–22	55	120	163	64	44	800	7.5	8	60	1.1	1.3	14	2.0	400	3.0	800	800	300	18	15	150
	23–50	55	120	163	64	44	800	5	8	60	1.0	1.2	13	2.0	400	3.0	800	800	300	18	15	150
	51+	55	120	163	64	44	800	5	8	60	1.0	1.2	13	2.0	400	3.0	800	800	300	10	15	150
Pregnant						+30	+200	+5	+2	+20	+0.4	+0.3	+2	+0.6	+400	+1.0	+400	+400	+150	**	+5	+25
Lactating						+20	+400	+5	+3	+40	+0.5	+0.5	+5	+0.5	+100	+1.0	+400	+400	+150	**	+10	+50

*The allowances are intended to provide for individual variations among most normal persons as they live in the United States under usual environmental stresses. Diets should be based on a variety of common foods to provide other nutrients for which human requirements have been less well defined.

†Retinol equivalents. 1 retinol equivalent = 1 µg retinol or 6 µg β carotene.

‡As cholecalciferol. 10 µg cholecalciferol = 400 IU of vitamin D.

§α-Tocopherol equivalents. 1 mg d-α tocopherol = 1 α-TE. See text for variation in allowances and calculation of vitamin E activity of the diet as α-tocopherol equivalents.

‖1 NE (niacin equivalent) = 1 mg of niacin or 60 mg of dietary tryptophan.

¶The folacin allowances refer to dietary sources as determined by Lactobacillus casei assay after treatment with enzymes (conjugases) to make polyglutamyl forms of the vitamin available to the test organism.

#The recommended dietary allowance for vitamin B12 in infants is based on average concentration of the vitamin in human milk. The allowances after weaning are based on energy intake (as recommended by the American Academy of Pediatrics) and consideration of other factors, such as intestinal absorption.

**The increased requirement during pregnancy cannot be met by the iron content of habitual American diets nor by the existing iron stores of many women; therefore the use of 30 to 60 mg of supplemental iron is recommended. Iron needs during lactation are not substantially different from those of nonpregnant women, but continued supplementation of the mother for 2 to 3 months after parturition is advisable to replenish stores depleted by pregnancy.

APPENDIX D: Diet and Nutrition Guidelines for Weight Gain in Conjunction With a Qualified Weight Training Program

In General

It is important to eat 3,500 to 5,000 calories/day. To be able to consume this amount, a meal pattern of three balanced meals plus three snacks is important. Breakfast and snacks will make a considerable increase in total caloric intake.

The following are special considerations in weight gain:

1. *Caloric availability:* The primary nutritional consideration for weight gain is sufficient calories to cover metabolic, growth, and energy needs. To increase lean body mass, protein must be available for new tissue growth versus energy expenditure. There must be sufficient calories from carbohydrate and fat to "spare protein." The range of prescribed calories is usually 3,500 to 5,000 kcal/day.

2. *Protein requirements:* Protein mass is maintained at approximately 1 to 2 gm/kg/of body weight. Excessive protein intake has not been shown to increase lean body tissue beyond this amount.

3. *Vitamins:* When food selection is followed by food choices from a variety of wholesome foods, as described in the dietary exchange lists, there is theoretically no need for vitamin supplementation. However, in cases where an athlete is not eating in a nutritionally balanced way, or if he or she receives psychological benefits from supplementation, a multiple vitamin-mineral preparation may be taken.

4. *Frequency of eating:* The body works continuously and should be fueled as need arises. Nutrients can be used more efficiently if a moderate amount is ingested on a frequent basis. A variety of nutrients needs to be presented in the same manner.

5. *Selecting the diet:* The regimen is based on the dietary exchange lists (see Appendix G), a list of foods that provide selected nutrients. Choosing foods from three to four of the

groups at any one meal or snack provide more complete utilization of nutrients. The food groupings are as follows:

   a. Starch and breads
   b. Meat (includes eggs, fish, poultry, legumes, and cheese)
   c. Vegetables
   d. Fruits
   e. Milk and yogurt
   f. Fats
   g. Other (includes food supplements and sweets.)

   6. *Food supplements:* When it is difficult to eat sufficient calories to gain weight, concentrated food supplements may be eaten between meals. Many liquid supplements provide 40 calories/oz and assist in overcoming the painful feeling of being too full.

   7. *Choosing the appropriate caloric level:* To ensure that the additional weight is lean body mass and not extra fat, the rate of gain should be no more than 2 lb/week. Change of weight status should begin well before the competitive season. The first step is to determine appropriate caloric levels. A 24-hour food record will give an approximate idea of the number of calories needed daily to maintain present weight. Weight gain will occur if the number of calories is increased by 500/day until the athlete begins to gain 1 lb/week. Or, determine the appropriate new ideal body weight for the season, and multiply that weight by 15 to allow for weight gain. If weight gain does not occur (and there are times when it does not), increase calories by 500/day until weight gain occurs. Weekly visits with a dietitian will be advantageous at this point so that the diet can be monitored and adjusted as needed. If weight gain exceeds the recommended 1 to 2 lb/week, adjust calories downward. Skinfold measurements, cholesterol levels, and triglyceride levels should be noted on a monthly basis.

APPENDIX E: Guidelines for Successful Eating Behaviors

In General

1. Set up a time schedule for meals and snacks. Eat in a quiet, enjoyable atmosphere, sitting down.
2. Be aware of all foods eaten, and check portion sizes.
3. Instead of eating for recreation, substitute reading a good book, engaging in physical activity, visiting with friends, working on projects, or helping others.
4. Read labels; learn about the nutrient and caloric values of foods. Keep a food diary.
5. Find nonfood activities to reward yourself.
6. For long-term weight control, excessive coffee drinking and smoking are not effective or healthful appetite control techniques.
7. Ask family and friends to give other than food as a present or reward; ask them for their involvement and help in your goals for good health.

In the Dining Room

1. Drink at least one glass of water before eating, then eat a large portion of vegetables and salad (with low-calorie dressing).
2. Use a salad plate instead of a dinner plate.
3. Ask your friends to serve you, and you serve them.
4. After eating, clear away the dishes before having coffee or follow-up activities.
5. Dress up for dinner (you might wear a garment with fitted waistband).
6. Share dessert with several friends.

In Your Room

1. Avoid purchasing foods that are tempting and not appropriate.

2. Keep lower-calorie foods, such as fruit and vegetables, for snacks. Make them visible.

3. Prepare an emergency kit with long-lasting or low-calorie foods selected to satisfy. Dill pickles for candy cravers, air-popped popcorn for the munchers, sugar-free gum, and mints or diet pop all are satisfying alternatives.

4. Before snacking, wait up to 20 minutes or do some small tasks such as cleaning your room or brushing your teeth, or take a nap or go for a walk with a friend.

5. Ask ten friends to share one take out pizza. Send out for Mexican or Japanese food, which is lower in calories and takes more time to eat.

When Eating Out

1. Nutritious and delicious food can be found anywhere you go!

2. Plan ahead who you will eat with and what you will order. Study the menu carefully, choose wisely, and ask the waiter questions. To cut down on portion size, order a la carte or share food with a friend.

3. Look for the terms "steamed, in its own juice, garden fresh, broiled, roasted, poached, tomato juice, dry broiled."

4. Watch out for "pickled, smoked, in broth, cocktail sauce or tomato base; also buttery, sauteed, fried, au gratin, parmesan, creamed, pan fried, in cheese sauce, escalloped, in its own gravy, hollandaise."

5. For breakfast have fresh fruit or citrus juices, whole-grain bread or English muffin toasted dry, plain or hot cereals from whole grains, skim or low-fat milk, or waffles with fresh fruit and yogurt. For beverages drink sparkling water, water with lemon, seltzers, or sparkling juices. (Beer is 10 calories/oz; wine is 22 calories/oz; hard liquor is 100 to 130

calories/oz; and most sherry and brandy are 200 to 300 cal-
ories/oz! Breads are acceptable, but forget about the spreads.
For appetizers have steamed seafoods, raw vegetables, or
fresh fruit. Ask that the salted nuts, potato or tortilla chips,
crackers, and so forth be removed. Choose as entrees poultry, fish, shellfish, soups, and vegetable dishes simply prepared. Choose salads containing fresh greens, such as lettuce
and spinach, and such vegetables as cucumbers, radishes, tomatoes, carrots, and onions without cheese, eggs, meats, or
bacon unless the salad is the entree. Order dressings on the
side; request lemon wedges. For desserts have fresh fruits,
fruit ices, sherbets, gelatins, or angel food cake. A nice finish
is espresso or low-sugar dessert coffees. The best fast food
selections are salad bars, whole-grain breads, and plain ham-
burgers.

6. Avoid starving yourself all day in anticipation of the
meal. Eat a small amount of food before leaving home. If
the portion is too large, ask for a doggie bag before the
meal. Eat slowly, visit, and enjoy the meal.

APPENDIX F: Laboratory Tests and Normal Ranges for Adults and Children Affected by Exercise or Related Conditions*

Test	Normal Value	Response to Exercise	Rationale
Hemoglobin (inner core of the RBC† in a given volume)	Male 13.5–18 gm/dl (140–180 gm/l)	Decrease	Anemias, iron deficiency, excessive fluid intake
	Female 12–16 gm/dl (115–155 gm/l)	Increase	High altitude, burns, dehydration
	Athlete 16–18 gm/dl Pregnancy 11–12 gm/dl Child 11–16 gm/dl		
Hematocrit (proportion of packed cells in a given volume)	Male 40%–54% (0.40–0.54)	Decrease	Anemias
	Female 36%–46% (0.36–0.46)	Increase	Dehydration; diarrhea; drug influence: antibiotics
	Child 36%–38% (0.36–0.38)		
RBCs	Male 4.6–6.0 m/cu mm by 10–12/L	Decrease	Excessive fluid intake, intravascular hemolysis
	Female 4.0–5.0		
	Child 3.8–5.5	Increase	High altitude, dehydration
Blood volume	70–100 ml/kg of body weight	Increase	Response to regular strenuous exercise, altitudes
Plasma volume	30–50 ml/kg of body weight	Increase	Response to strenuous exercise
MCV‡	Male 80–98 cu μ Female 80–98 cu μ	Decrease	Excessive fluid intake >80, iron deficiency anemia
	Child 82–92 cu μ	Increase	Dehydration >98, pernicious anemias
Serum iron	Male 80–180 μg/dl (14–32 μmoles/L)	Increase	Excessive hemolysis (red blood cell destruction) drug influence: excessive iron supplements
	Female 60–160 μg/dl (11–29 μmoles/L)	Decrease	Blood loss, dietary deficiency
TIBC§ (measures serum iron bound with transferrin)	Adult 250–450 μg/dl (45–82 μmoles/L) or 16% saturation	Increase	Iron deficiency anemia, acute and chronic blood loss
		Decrease	Pernicious anemia; drug influence: ACTH‖, steroids

APPENDIX F   (cont.)

Test	Normal Value	Response to Exercise	Rationale
SGOT¶	Adult 5–40 µ/ml	Increase	Infections; strenuous exercise; vitamin dosage; drug influence: antibiotics, narcotics, antihypertensives, cortisone, indomethecin
		Decrease	Aspirin use, salicylates
Haptoglobin	Adult 30–160 mg/dl	Decrease	Hemolysis, pernicious anemias
Ferritin	Male 18–300 µg/dl Female 10–270 µg/dl or 60 µg/L <12 depletion >200 overload	Decrease	Bone marrow and liver storage of iron
Serum cholesterol	Adult 150–220 mg/dl (5.20–5.85 mmoles/L)	Decrease	Increased fat oxidation, also in malnutrition, anemia
VLDL#	60 mg/dl	Decrease	
LDL**	Adult 50–190 mg/dl (1.3–4.9 mmoles/L)	Decrease	
Triglycerides	Adult >150 mg/dl (<1.80 mmoles/L)	Decrease	Increased fat oxidation, protein malnutrition
	Child 10–140 mg/dl	Increase	Hypertension; uncontrolled diabetes; high-carbohydrate diet; drug influence: estrogens, alcohol
HDL††	Male 30–70 mg/dl (0.80–1.80 mmoles/L)	Decrease	Steroid use
	Female 30–90 mg/dl (0.80–2.35 mmoles/L)	Increase	Increase in hepatic enzyme activity, increased production due to exercise, or both
Bilirubin	Adult 0.1–1.2 mg/dl (2–18 µmoles/L) Child 0.2–0.8 mg/dl	Increase	RBC destruction; drug influence: steroids, increased vitamin A, C, and K, antibiotics

(Continued.)

APPENDIX F (cont.)

Test	Normal Value	Response to Exercise	Rationale
		Decrease	Iron deficiency, anemia, large amounts of caffeine, aspirin
Serum potassium	Adult 3.5–5.0 mEq/L (mmoles/L) Child 3.5–5.5 mEq/L	Decrease	Vomiting and diarrhea; dehydration; crash dieting; starvation; stress and trauma; injuries; burns; increased glucose ingestion; laxative abuse; drug influence: diuretics, thiazides, steroids, antibiotics, insulin, laxatives
		Increase	Acute renal failure, crushing injuries and burns (with kidney shutdown)
Serum sodium	Adult 135–145 mEq/L (or 135–145 mmoles/L)	Increase	Dehydration; severe vomiting and diarrhea; conjestive heart failure; drug influence: cough medicines, cortisones, antibiotics, laxatives
		Decrease	Vomiting, increased perspiration, reduced Na in diet, burns, tissue injury, large amounts of water
Serum magnesium	Adult 1.6–2.4 mEq/L	Decrease	Loss of gastrointestinal fluids, use of diuretics
Uric acid	Male 3.5–7.8 mg/dl Female 2.8–6.8 mg/dl Child 2.5–5.5 mg/dl	Decrease	Folic acid deficiency; burns; drug influence: ACTH
		Increase	Dehydration; nitrogen catabolism; stress, increased protein; weight reduction diets; gout; drug influence: megadose of vitamin C, diuretics, thiazides, aspirin, ACTH

APPENDIX F (cont.)

Test	Normal Value	Response to Exercise	Rationale
Fasting glucose	Adult 65–110 mg/dl (3.9–6.1 mmoles/L) Child 60–100 mg/dl	Decrease	Hypoglycemic response to excessive glucose/ sucrose solutions, extended strenuous exercise
		Increase	Stress, crushing injury, burns, infections, hypothermia, mild exercise, dumping syndrome, diabetes

*Adapted from Kee JL, *Laboratory and Diagnostic Tests With Nursing Implications.* New York, Appleton-Century-Crofts, 1983; Monsen ER: The journal adopts SI units for clinical laboratory values. *J Am Diet Assoc* 1987; 87:356; Tilkian SM, Conover MB, Tilkian AG: *Clinical Implications of Laboratory Tests.* St Louis, C.V. Mosby Co, 1979; Krebs PS, Scully BC, Zinkgraf SA: The acute and prolonged effects of marathon running on 20 blood parameters. *Phys Sports Med* 1983; 11:66; Martin DE, Vroom DH, May DF, et al: Physiological changes in elite male distance runners training. *Phys Sports Med* 1986; 14:152.

†RBC = red blood cell.
‡MCV = mean corpuscular volume.
§TIBC = total iron-binding capacity.
‖ACTH = adrenocorticotropic hormone.
¶SGOT = serum glutamic oxaloacetic transasminase.
#VLDL = very low-density lipoprotein.
**LDL = low-density lipoprotein.
††HDL = high-density lipoprotein.

APPENDIX G: Dietary Exchange Lists

What Are Exchange Lists?*

The exchange lists presented in Appendix G are based on material in Exchange Lists for Meal Planning, prepared by committees of the American Diabetes Association and the American Dietetic Association, in cooperation with the National Institute of Arthritis, Metabolic, and Digestive Diseases and the National Heart and Lung Institute, National Institutes of Health, Public Health Service, U.S. Department of Health, Education and Welfare.

The exchange system can be used to plan diets at many different calorie levels. Diets from 900 to 5,000 calories per day, following carbohydrate guidelines for active people, are included.

The six exchange lists help to make your meal plan work. Foods are grouped together on a list because they are alike. Every food on a list has about the same amount of carbohydrate, protein, fat, and calories. In the amounts given, all the choices on each list are equal. Any food on a list can be exchanged or traded for any other food on the same list.

The six lists are starch/bread, meat and substitutes, vegetables, fruit, milk, and fat.

Using the exchange lists and following your meal plan will provide you with a great variety of food choices and will control the distribution of calories, carbohydrate, protein, and fat throughout the day, so that your food and your insulin will be balanced.

The reason for dividing food into six different groups is that foods vary in their carbohydrate, protein, fat, and calorie content. Each exchange list contains foods that are alike; each choice contains about the same amount of carbohydrate, protein, fat, and calories.

The following chart shows the amount of these nutrients in one serving from each exchange list. As you read the exchange lists, you will notice that one choice often is a larger amount of

*From Exchange Lists for Meal Planning, prepared by the American Diabetes Association and the American Dietetic Association, 1987. Used by permission.

food than another choice from the same list. Because foods are so different, each food is measured or weighed so the amount of carbohydrate, protein, fat, and calories is the same in each choice.

If you have a favorite food that is not included in any of these groups, ask your dietitian about it. That food can probably be worked into your meal plan, at least now and then.

Exchange List	Carbohydrate (gm)	Protein (gm)	Fat (gm)	Calories
Starch/bread	15	3	Trace	80
Meat				
Lean	—	7	3	55
Medium-fat	—	7	5	75
High-fat	—	7	8	100
Vegetable	5	2	—	25
Fruit	15	—	—	60
Milk				
Skim	12	8	Trace	90
Low-fat	12	8	5	120
Whole	12	8	8	150
Fat	—	—	5	45

Starch and Bread List

Each item in this list contains approximately 15 gm of carbohydrate, 3 gm of protein, a trace of fat, and 80 calories. Whole-grain products average about 2 gm of fiber per serving. Some foods are higher in fiber.

You can choose your starch exchanges from any of the items on this list. If you wanted to eat a starch food that is not on this list, the general rule is that: (1) ½ cup of cereal, grain, or pasta is one serving; and (2) 1 oz of a bread product is one serving. Your dietitian can help you be more exact.

Exchange List		Carbohydrate (gm)	Protein (gm)	Fat (gm)	Calories
Starch/bread		15	3	Trace	80

Cereals/Grains/Pasta

Bran cereals,* concentrated	⅓ cup
Bran cereals,* flaked (e.g., Bran Buds, All Bran)	½ cup
Bulgur (cooked)	½ cup
Cooked cereals	½ cup
Cornmeal (dry)	2½ Tbsp
Grapenuts	3 Tbsp
Grits (cooked)	½ cup
Other ready-to-eat unsweetened cereals	¾ cup
Pasta (cooked)	½ cup
Puffed cereal	1½ cup
Rice, white or brown (cooked)	⅓ cup
Shredded wheat	½ cup
Wheat germ*	3 Tbsp

Dried Beans/Peas/Lentils

Beans and peas* (cooked) (e.g., kidney, white, split, black-eyed)	⅓ cup
Lentils* (cooked)	⅓ cup
Baked* beans	¼ cup

Starchy Vegetables

Corn*	½ cup
Corn on cob,* 6 in. long	1
Lima beans*	½ cup
Peas, green* (canned or frozen)	½ cup
Plantain*	½ cup
Potato, baked	1 small (3 oz)
Potato, mashed	½ cup
Squash, winter (acorn, butternut)	¾ cup
Yam, sweet potato, plain	⅓ cup

Bread

Bagel	½ (1 oz)
Bread sticks, crisp, 4 in. long by ½ in.	2 (⅔ oz)
Croutons, low fat	1 cup

Bread (cont.)

English muffin	½
Frankfurther or hamburger bun	½ (1 oz)
Pita, 6 in. across	½
Plain roll, small	1 (1 oz)
Raisin, unfrosted	1 slice (1 oz)
Rye,* pumpernickel	1 slice (1 oz)
Tortilla, 6 in. across	1
White (including French, Italian)	1 slice (1 oz)
Whole Wheat	1 slice (1 oz)

Crackers/Snacks

Animal crackers	8
Graham crackers, 2½ in. square	3
Matzoth	¾ oz
Melba toast	5 slices
Oyster crackers	24
Popcorn (popped, no fat added)	3 cups
Pretzels	¾ oz
Rye crisp, 2 in. by 3½ in.	4
Saltine-type crackers	6
Whole wheat crackers, no fat added (crisp breads, e.g., Finn, Kavli, Wasa)	2–4 slices (¾ oz)

Starch Foods Prepared With Fat†

Biscuit, 2½ in. across	1
Chow mein noodles	½ cup
Corn bread, 2-in. cube	1 (2 oz)
Cracker, round butter type	6
French fried potatoes, 2–3½ in. long	10 (1½ oz)
Muffin, plain, small	1
Pancake, 4 in. across	2
Stuffing, bread (prepared)	¼ cup
Taco shell, 6-in. across	2
Waffle, 4½-in. square	1
Whole wheat crackers, fat added (e.g., Triscuits)	4–6 (1 oz)

*3 gm or more of fiber per serving.
†Count as one starch/bread plus one fat serving.

Meat List

Each serving of meat and substitutes on this list contains about 7 gm of protein. The amount of fat and number of calories varies, depending on what kind of meat or substitute you choose. The list is divided into three parts based on the amount of fat and calories: lean meat, medium-fat meat, and high-fat meat. One ounce (one meat exchange) of each of these includes:

	Carbohydrate (gm)	Protein (gm)	Fat (gm)	Calories
Lean	0	7	3	55
Medium-fat	0	7	5	75
High-fat	0	7	8	100

Lean Meat and Substitutes*

Beef:	USDA good or choice grades of lean beef, e.g., round, sirloin, and flank steak; tenderloin; and chipped beef†	1 oz
Pork:	Lean pork, such as fresh ham; canned, cured or boiled ham,† Canadian bacon,† tenderloin	1 oz
Veal:	All cuts are lean except for veal cutlets (ground or cubed). Examples of lean veal are chops and roasts.	1 oz
Poultry:	Chicken, turkey, Cornish hen (without skin)	1 oz
Fish:	All fresh and frozen fish	1 oz
	Crab, lobster, scallops, shrimp, clams (fresh or canned in water†)	2 oz
	Oysters	6 medium
	Tuna† (canned in water)	¼ cup
	Herring (uncreamed or smoked)	1 oz
	Sardines (canned)	2 medium
Wild game:	Venison, rabbit, squirrel	1 oz
	Pheasant, duck, goose (without skin)	1 oz
Cheese:	Any cottage cheese	¼ cup
	Grated parmesan	2 Tbsp
	Diet cheese† (with less than 55 calories per ounce)	1 oz
Other:	95% fat-free luncheon meat	1 oz
	Egg whites	3 whites
	Egg substitutes with less than 55 calories per ¼ cup	¼ cup

Medium-Fat Meat and Substitutes*

Beef:	Most beef products fall into this category. Examples are all ground beef, roast (rib, chuck, rump), steak (cubed, Porterhouse, T-bone), and meatloaf.	1 oz
Pork:	Most pork products fall into this category. Examples are chops, loin roast, Boston butt, cutlets.	1 oz
Lamb:	Most lamb products fall into this category. Examples are chops, leg, and roast.	1 oz

(Continued.)

Veal:	Cutlet (ground or cubed, unbreaded)	1 oz
Poultry:	Chicken (with skin), domestic duck or goose (well-drained of fat), ground turkey	1 oz
Fish:	Tuna† (canned in oil and drained)	¼ cup
	Salmon† (canned)	¼ cup
Cheese:	Skim or part-skim milk cheeses, e.g.:	
	Ricotta	¼ cup
	Mozzarella	1 oz
	Diet cheeses† (with 56–80 calories per ounce)	1 oz
Other:	86% fat-free luncheon meat†	1 oz
	Egg (high in cholesterol, limit to three per week)	1
	Egg substitutes with 56–80 calories per ¼ cup	¼ cup
	Tofu (2½ in. by 2¾ in. by 1 in.)	4 oz
	Liver, heart, kidney, sweetbreads (high in cholesterol)	1 oz

High-Fat Meat and Substitutes*‡

Beef:	Most USDA Prime cuts of beef, such as ribs, corned beef†	1 oz
Pork:	Spareribs, ground pork, pork sausage† (patty or link)	1 oz
Lamb:	Patties (ground lamb)	1 oz
Fish:	Any fried fish product	1 oz
Cheese:	All regular cheeses,† e.g., American, Blue, Cheddar, Monterey, Swiss	1 oz
Other:	Luncheon meat,† e.g., bologna, salami, pimento loaf	1 oz
	Sausage,† e.g., Polish, Italian	1 oz
	Knockwurst, smoked	1 oz
	Bratwurst†	1 oz
	Frankfurter† (turkey or chicken)	1 frank (10/lb)
	Peanut butter (contains unsaturated fat)	1 Tbsp

One High-Fat Meat Plus One Fat Exchange

| | Frankfurter† (beef, pork, or combination) | 1 frank (10/lb) |

*One exchange is equal to any one of the following items.
†400 mg or more of sodium per exchange.
‡Remember, these items are high in saturated fat, cholesterol, and calories, and should be used only three times per week.

Vegetable List

Each vegetable serving on this list contains about 5 gm of carbohydrate, 2 gm of protein, and 25 calories. Vegetables contain 2 to 3 gm of dietary fiber.

Vegetables are a good source of vitamins and minerals. Fresh and frozen vegetables have more vitamins and less added salt. Rinsing canned vegetables will remove much of the salt.

Unless otherwise noted, the serving size for vegetables (one vegetable exchange) is ½ cup of cooked vegetables or vegetable juice or 1 cup of raw vegetables.

Exchange List	Carbohydrate (gm)	Protein (gm)	Fat (gm)	Calories
Vegetable	5	2	—	25

Artichoke (½ medium)	Mushrooms, cooked
Asparagus	Okra
Beans (green, wax, Italian)	Onions
	Pea pods
Bean sprouts	Peppers (green)
Beets	Rutabaga
Broccoli	Sauerkraut†
Brussels sprouts	Spinach, cooked
Cabbage, cooked	Summer squash
Carrots	(crookneck)
Cauliflower	Tomato (one large)
Eggplant	Tomato/vegetable
Greens (collard,	juice*
mustard, turnip)	Turnips
Kohlrabi	Water chestnuts
Leeks	Zucchini, cooked

Starchy vegetables such as corn, peas, and potatoes are found on the starch/bread list. For free vegetables, see free food table.

*400 mg or more of sodium per serving.

Fruit List

Each item on this list contains about 15 gm of carbohydrate and 60 calories. Fresh, frozen, and dry fruits have about 2 gm of fiber per serving. Fruit juices contain very little dietary fiber.

The carbohydrate and calorie content for a fruit serving are based on the usual serving of the most commonly eaten fruits. Use fresh fruits or fruits frozen or canned without sugar added. Whole fruit is more filling than fruit juice and may be a better choice for those who are trying to lose weight. Unless otherwise noted, the serving size for one fruit serving is ½ cup of fresh fruit or fruit juice or ¼ cup of dried fruit.

Exchange List	Carbohydrate (gm)	Protein (gm)	Fat (gm)	Calories
Fruit	15	—	—	60

Fresh, Frozen, and Unsweetened Canned Fruit

Apple (raw, 2 in. across)	1 apple	Pears (canned)	½ cup or 2 halves
Applesauce (unsweetened)	½ cup		
Apricots (medium, raw) or	4 apricots	Persimmon (medium, native)	2 persimmons
Apricots (canned)	½ cup, or 4 halves	Pineapple (raw)	¾ cup
Banana (9 in. long)	½ banana	Pineapple (canned)	⅓ cup
Blackberries* (raw)	¾ cup	Plum (raw, 2 in. across)	2 plums
Blueberries* (raw)	¾ cup	Pomegranate*	½ pomegranate
Cantaloupe (5 in. across)	⅓ melon	Raspberries* (raw)	1 cup
(cubes)	1 cup	Strawberries* (raw, whole)	1¼ cup
Cherries (large, raw)	12 cherries	Tangerine (2½ in. across)	2 tangerines
Cherries (canned)	½ cup	Watermelon (cubes)	1¼ cup
Figs (raw, 2 in. across)	2 figs		
Fruit cocktail (canned)	½ cup	*Dried Fruit*	
Grapefruit (medium)	½ grapefruit	Apples*	4 rings
Grapefruit (segments)	¾ cup	Apricots*	7 halves
Grapes (small)	15 grapes	Dates	2½ medium
Honeydew melon (medium)	⅛ melon	Figs*	1½
(cubes)	1 cup	Prunes*	3 medium
Kiwi (large)	1 kiwi	Raisins	2 Tbsp.
Mandarin oranges	¾ cup		
Mango (small)	½ mango	*Fruit Juice*	
Nectarine* (1½ in. across)	1 nectarine	Apple juice/cider	½ cup
Orange (2½ in. across)	1 orange	Cranberry juice cocktail	⅓ cup
Papaya	1 cup	Grapefruit juice	½ cup
Peach (2¾ in. across)	1 peach, or ¾ cup	Grape juice	⅓ cup
		Orange juice	½ cup
Peaches (canned)	½ cup, or 2 halves	Pineapple juice	½ cup
		Prune juice	⅓ cup
Pear	½ large, or 1 small		

*3 gm or more of fiber per serving.

Milk List

Each serving of milk or milk products on this list contains about 12 gm of carbohydrate and 8 gm of protein. The amount of fat in milk is measured in percent of butterfat. The calories vary, depending on what kind of milk you choose. The list is divided into three parts based on the amount of fat and calories: skim/very low-fat milk, low-fat milk, and whole milk. One serving (one milk exchange) of each of these includes:

	Carbohydrate (gm)	Protein (gm)	Fat (gm)	Calories
Skim/very low-fat	12	8	Trace	90
Low-fat	12	8	5	120
Whole	12	8	8	150

Skim and Very Low-Fat Milk		*Whole Milk*	
Skim milk	1 cup	Whole milk	1 cup
½% milk	1 cup	Evaporated whole milk	½ cup
1% milk	1 cup	Whole plain yogurt	8 oz.
Low-fat buttermilk	1 cup		
Evaporated skim milk	½ cup		
Dry nonfat milk	⅓ cup		
Plain nonfat yogurt	8 oz.		

Low-Fat Milk	
2% milk	1 cup fluid
Plain low-fat yogurt (with added nonfat milk solids)	8 oz.

Milk is the body's main source of calcium, the mineral needed for growth and repair of bones. Yogurt is also a good source of calcium. Yogurt and many dry or powdered milk products have different amounts of fat. If you have questions about a particular item, read the label to find out the fat and calorie content.

Milk is good to drink, but it can also be added to cereal, and to other foods. Many tasty dishes such as sugar-free pudding are made with milk (see the table of combination foods). Add life to plain yogurt by adding one of your fruit servings to it.

The whole milk group has much more fat per serving than the skim and low-fat groups. Whole milk has more than 3¼% butterfat. Try to limit your choices from the whole milk group as much as possible.

Fat List

Each serving on the fat list contains about 5 gm of fat and 45 calories.

The foods on the fat list contain mostly fat, although some items may also contain a small amount of protein. All fats are high in calories and should be carefully measured. Everyone should modify fat intake by eating unsaturated fats instead of saturated fats. The sodium content of these foods varies widely. Check the label for sodium information.

Exchange List	Carbohydrate (gm)	Protein (gm)	Fat (gm)	Calories
Fat	–	–	5	45

Unsaturated Fats				
Avocado	⅛ medium	Salad dressing, mayonnaise-		2 tsp
Margarine	1 tsp	type		
Margarine,* diet	1 Tbsp	Salad dressing, mayonnaise-		1 Tbsp
Mayonnaise	1 tsp	type, reduced-calorie†		
Mayonnaise,* reduced-calorie	1 Tbsp	Salad dressing* (all varieties)		1 Tbsp
Nuts and seeds		Salad dressing,‡ reduced-		2 Tbsp
Almonds, dry roasted	6 whole	calorie†		
Cashews, dry roasted	1 Tbsp.			
Pecans	2 whole	*Saturated Fats*		
Peanuts	20 small or	Butter		1 tsp
	10 large	Bacon*		1 slice
Walnuts	2 whole	Chitterlings		½ oz
Other nuts	1 Tbsp	Coconut, shredded		2 Tbsp
Seeds, pine nuts, sunflower	1 Tbsp	Coffee whitener, liquid		2 Tbsp
(without shells)		Coffee whitener, powder		4 tsp
Pumpkin seeds	2 tsp	Cream (light, coffee, table)		2 Tbsp
Oil (corn, cottonseed,	1 tsp	Cream, sour		2 Tbsp
safflower, soybean,		Cream (heavy, whipping)		1 Tbsp
sunflower, olive, peanut)		Cream cheese		1 Tbsp
Olives*	10 small or	Salt pork*		¼ oz
	5 large			

*If more than one or two servings are eaten, these foods have 400 mg or more of sodium.
†Two tablespoons of low calorie salad dressing is a free food.
‡400 mg or more of sodium per serving.

Foods for Occasional Use

Moderate amounts of some foods can be used in your meal plan in spite of their sugar or fat content as long as you can maintain blood glucose control. The following list includes average exchange values for some of these foods. Because they are concentrated sources of carbohydrate, you will notice that the portion sizes are very small. Check with your dietitian for advice on how often and when you can eat them.

Food	Amount	Exchanges
Angel food cake	1/12 cake	2 starch
Cake, no icing	1/12 cake, or a 3-in. square	2 starch, 2 fat
Cookies	2 small (1¾ in. across)	1 starch, 1 fat
Frozen fruit yogurt	⅓ cup	1 starch
Gingersnaps	3	1 starch
Granola	¼ cup	1 starch, 1 fat
Granola bars	1 small	1 starch, 1 fat
Ice cream, any flavor	½ cup	1 starch, 2 fat
Ice milk, any flavor	½ cup	1 starch, 1 fat
Sherbet, any flavor	¼ cup	1 starch
Snack chips,* all varieties	1 oz	1 starch, 2 fat
Vanilla wafers	6 small	1 starch, 1 fat

*If more than one serving is eaten, these foods have 400 mg or more of sodium.

Combination Foods

Much of the food we eat is mixed together in various combinations. These combination foods do not fit into only one exchange list. It can be quite hard to tell what is in a certain casserole dish or baked food item. This is a list of average values for some typical combination foods. This list will help you fit these foods into your meal plan. Ask your dietitian for information about any other foods you would like to eat. The *American Diabetes Association/American Dietetic Association Family Cookbooks* and the *American Diabetes Association Holiday Cookbook* have many recipes and further information about many foods, including combination foods. Check your library or local bookstore.

Food	Amount	Exchanges
Casseroles, homemade	1 cup (8 oz)	2 starch, 2 medium-fat meat, 1 fat
Cheese pizza,* thin crust	¼ of 15 oz or ¼ of 10 in.	2 starch, 1 medium-fat meat, 1 fat
Chili with beans*† (commercial)	1 cup (8 oz)	2 starch, 2 medium-fat meat, 2 fat
Chow mein*† (without noodles or rice	2 cups (16 oz)	1 starch, 2 vegetable, 2 lean meat
Macaroni and cheese*	1 cup (8 oz)	2 starch, 1 medium-fat meat, 2 fat
Soup		
Bean*†	1 cup (8 oz)	1 starch, 1 vegetable, 1 lean meat
Chunky, all varieties*	10¾-oz can	1 starch, 1 vegetable, 1 medium-fat meat
Cream* (made with water)	1 cup (8 oz)	1 starch, 1 fat
Vegetable* or broth*	1 cup (8 oz)	1 starch
Spaghetti and meatballs* (canned)	1 cup (8 oz)	2 starch, 1 medium-fat meat, 1 fat
Sugar-free pudding (made with skim milk)	½ cup	1 starch
Beans as meat substitute		
Dried beans,† peas,† lentils†	1 cup (cooked)	2 starch, 1 lean meat

*400 mg or more of sodium per serving.
†3 gm or more of fiber per serving.

Free Foods

A free food is any food (including condiments and seasonings) or drink that contains less than 20 calories per serving. You can eat as much as you want of those items that have no serving size specified. You may eat two or three servings per day of those items that have a specific serving size. Be sure to spread them out through the day.

Seasonings can be very helpful in making food taste better. Be careful of how much sodium you use. Read the label, and choose those seasonings that do not contain sodium or salt.

Drinks

- Bouillon* or broth without fat
- Bouillon, low-sodium
- Carbonated drinks, sugar-free
- Carbonated water
- Club soda
- Cocoa powder, unsweetened (1 Tbsp)
- Coffee/Tea
- Drink mixes, sugar-free
- Tonic water, sugar-free

Fruit

- Cranberries, unsweetened (½ cup)
- Rhubarb, unsweetened (½ cup)

Vegetables†
(raw, 1 cup)

- Cabbage
- Celery
- Chinese cabbage‡
- Cucumber
- Green onion
- Hot peppers
- Mushrooms
- Radishes
- Zucchini‡

Salad Greens

- Endive
- Escarole
- Lettuce
- Romaine
- Spinach

Sweet Substitutes

- Candy, hard, sugar-free
- Gelatin, sugar-free
- Gum, sugar-free
- Jam/Jelly, sugar-free (2 tsp)
- Pancake syrup, sugar-free (1–2 Tbsp)
- Sugar substitutes (saccharin, aspartame)
- Whipped topping (2 Tbsp)

Condiments

- Catsup (1 Tbsp)
- Horseradish
- Mustard
- Nonstick pan spray
- Pickles,* dill, unsweetened
- Salad dressing, low-calorie (2 Tbsp)
- Taco sauce (1 Tbsp)
- Vinegar

Seasonings

- Basil (fresh)
- Celery seeds
- Cinnamon
- Chili powder
- Chives
- Curry
- Dill
- Flavoring extracts (vanilla, almond, walnut, peppermint, butter, lemon, etc.)
- Garlic
- Garlic powder
- Herbs
- Hot pepper sauce
- Lemon
- Lemon juice
- Lemon pepper
- Lime
- Lime juice
- Mint
- Onion powder
- Oregano
- Paprika
- Pepper
- Pimento
- Spices
- Soy sauce*
- Soy sauce, low-sodium ("lite")
- Wine, used in cooking (¼ cup)
- Worcestershire sauce

*400 mg or more of sodium per serving.
†Raw, 1 cup.
‡3 gm or more of fiber per serving.

APPENDIX H: EXCHANGE PATTERNS AT SELECTED CALORIC LEVELS

The following exchange patterns meet the standard recommendations for caloric distribution for athletes: 60% carbohydrate, 15–20% protein, the remainder in fat. The athlete training for competition needs 350–500 gm/day of carbohydrates for glycogen storage. Interestingly, the caloric level must be over 2,500 kcal/day to supply this level. There is no room for weight loss regimens in competitive performance.

Meal plan prepared for 900-kcal meal pattern
Dietary requirements: 893 kcal; protein, 20% (45 gm); carbohydrate, 59% (132 gm); fat, 21% (21 gm).

Daily Meal Plan for Food Exchanges

Breakfast			Morning Snack		
1.0	Bread	exchanges			
0.5	Fat	exchanges			
0.5	Fruit	exchanges			
0.5	Milk	exchanges			
Lunch			Afternoon Snack		
0.5	Meat	exchanges			
1.0	Bread	exchanges	0.5	Bread	exchanges
0.5	Vegetable	exchanges			
1.0	Fat	exchanges	0.5	Fat	exchanges
0.5	Fruit	exchanges	1.0	Fruit	exchanges
0.5	Milk	exchanges			
Dinner			Evening Snack		
1.5	Meat	exchanges			
1.0	Bread	exchanges			
1.0	Vegetable	exchanges	0.5	Vegetable	exchanges
1.0	Fat	exchanges			
0.5	Fruit	exchanges	0.5	Fruit	exchanges
1.0	Milk	exchanges			

Meal plan prepared for 1,200-kcal meal pattern
Dietary requirements: 1,222 kcal; protein, 19% (58 gm); carbohydrate, 60% (183 gm); fat, 21% (28 gm).

Daily Meal Plan by Food Exchanges

Breakfast			Morning Snack	
2.0	Bread	exchanges		
1.5	Fat	exchanges		
0.5	Fruit	exchanges		
0.5	Milk	exchanges		
Lunch			Afternoon Snack	
1.0	Meat	exchanges	0.5 Meat	exchanges
2.0	Bread	exchanges	1.0 Bread	exchanges
0.5	Vegetable	exchanges		
1.0	Fat	exchanges	0.5 Fat	exchanges
0.5	Fruit	exchanges	1.0 Fruit	exchanges
0.5	Milk	exchanges		
Dinner			Evening Snack	
0.5	Meat	exchanges	0.5 Meat	exchanges
2.0	Bread	exchanges		
1.0	Vegetable	exchanges	0.5 Vegetable	exchanges
1.0	Fat	exchanges		
0.5	Fruit	exchanges	0.5 Fruit	exchanges
1.0	Milk	exchanges		

Meal Plan prepared for 1,800-kcal meal pattern
Dietary requirements: 1,786 kcal; protein, 19% (85 gm); carbohydrate, 60% (268 gm); fat 21% (42 gm).

Daily Meal Plan for Food Exchanges

Breakfast			Morning Snack	
3.5	Bread	exchanges		
1.5	Fat	exchanges		
0.5	Fruit	exchanges		
0.5	Milk	exchanges		
Lunch			Afternoon Snack	
1.0	Meat	exchanges	0.5 Meat	exchanges
3.0	Bread	exchanges	2.0 Bread	exchanges
0.5	Vegetable	exchanges		
1.5	Fat	exchanges	1.0 Fat	exchanges
0.5	Fruit	exchanges	1.0 Fruit	exchanges
0.5	Milk	exchanges		
Dinner			Evening Snack	
2.0	Meat	exchanges	0.5 Meat	exchanges
4.0	Bread	exchanges		
1.0	Vegetable	exchanges	0.5 Vegetable	exchanges
2.0	Fat	exchanges		
0.5	Fruit	exchanges	0.5 Fruit	exchanges
1.0	Milk	exchanges		

Meal plan prepared for 2,000-kcal meal pattern
Dietary requirements: 1,989 kcal; protein, 19% (94%); carbohydrate, 60% (298 gm); fat, 21% (46 gm).

Daily Meal Plan by Food Exchanges

Breakfast			Morning Snack		
4.5	Bread	exchanges			
1.5	Fat	exchanges			
0.5	Fruit	exchanges			
0.5	Milk	exchanges			
Lunch			**Afternoon Snack**		
1.5	Meat	exchanges	0.5	Meat	exchanges
3.5	Bread	exchanges	2.0	Bread	exchanges
0.5	Vegetable	exchanges			
2.0	Fat	exchanges	1.0	Fat	exchanges
0.5	Fruit	exchanges	1.0	Fruit	exchanges
0.5	Milk	exchanges			
Dinner			**Evening Snack**		
2.0	Meat	exchanges	0.5	Meat	exchanges
4.5	Bread	exchanges			
1.0	Vegetable	exchanges	0.5	Vegetable	exchanges
2.0	Fat	exchanges			
0.5	Fruit	exchanges	0.5	Fruit	exchanges
1.0	Milk	exchanges			

Meal plan prepared for 2,500-kcal meal pattern
Dietary requirements: 2,508 kcal; protein, 15% (94 gm); carbohydrate, 64% (401 gm); fat, 21% (58 gm).

Daily Meal Plan by Food Exchanges

Breakfast			Morning Snack		
6.5	Bread	exchanges			
2.5	Fat	exchanges			
0.5	Fruit	exchanges			
0.5	Milk	exchanges			
Lunch			**Afternoon Snack**		
0.5	Meat	exchanges			
5.5	Bread	exchanges	3.0	Bread	exchanges
0.5	Vegetable	exchanges			
3.5	Fat	exchanges	1.5	Fat	exchanges
0.5	Fruit	exchanges	1.0	Fruit	exchanges
0.5	Milk	exchanges			
Dinner			**Evening Snack**		
1.0	Meat	exchanges			
6.5	Bread	exchanges			
1.0	Vegetable	exchanges	0.5	Vegetable	exchanges
3.0	Fat	exchanges			
0.5	Fruit	exchanges	0.5	Fruit	exchanges
1.0	Milk	exchanges			

Meal plan prepared for 3,000-kcal meal pattern

Dietary requirements: 2,999 kcal; protein, 15% (112 gm), carbohydrate, 64% (480 gm); fat, 21% (70 gm).

Daily Meal Plan by Food Exchanges

Breakfast			Morning Snack		
8.0	Bread	exchanges			
3.5	Fat	exchanges			
0.5	Fruit	exchanges			
0.5	Milk	exchanges			
Lunch			Afternoon Snack		
0.5	Meat	exchanges			
6.5	Bread	exchanges	4.0	Bread	exchanges
0.5	Vegetable	exchanges			
3.5	Fat	exchanges	2.0	Fat	exchanges
0.5	Fruit	exchanges	1.0	Fruit	exchanges
0.5	Milk	exchanges			
Dinner			Evening Snack		
1.5	Meat	exchanges			
8.0	Bread	exchanges			
1.0	Vegetable	exchanges	0.5	Vegetable	exchanges
4.0	Fat	exchanges			
0.5	Fruit	exchanges	0.5	Fruit	exchanges
1.0	Milk	exchanges			

Meal plan prepared for 3,500-kcal meal pattern

Dietary requirements: 3,500 kcal; protein, 19% (166 gm); carbohydrate, 68% (595 gm); fat, 13% (51 gm).

Daily Meal Plan by Food Exchanges

Breakfast			Morning Snack		
			0.5	Meat	exchanges
6.5	Bread	exchanges	3.0	Bread	exchanges
1.5	Fat	exchanges			
1.0	Fruit	exchanges			
0.5	Milk	exchanges			
Lunch			Afternoon Snack		
2.0	Meat	exchanges	0.5	Meat	exchanges
8.0	Bread	exchanges	4.5	Bread	exchanges
1.5	Vegetable	exchanges			
1.5	Fat	exchanges	1.0	Fat	exchanges
1.0	Fruit	exchanges	1.0	Fruit	exchanges
0.5	Milk	exchanges			
Dinner			Evening Snack		
3.0	Meat	exchanges	0.5	Meat	exchanges
9.5	Bread	exchanges			
2.5	Vegetable	exchanges	1.0	Vegetable	exchanges
2.0	Fat	exchanges			
1.0	Fruit	exchanges	1.0	Fruit	exchanges
1.0	Milk	exchanges			

Meal plan prepared for 4,000-kcal meal pattern
Dietary requirements: 3,996 kcal; protein, 19% (190 gm); carbohydrate, 68% (679 gm); fat, 13% (58 gm).

Daily Meal Plan by Food Exchanges

Breakfast			Morning Snack		
			1.0	Meat	exchanges
7.5	Bread	exchanges	3.5	Bread	exchanges
2.0	Fat	exchanges			
1.0	Fruit	exchanges			
0.5	Milk	exchanges			
Lunch			Afternoon Snack		
2.5	Meat	exchanges	1.0	Meat	exchanges
9.5	Bread	exchanges	5.5	Bread	exchanges
1.5	Vegetable	exchanges			
2.0	Fat	exchanges	1.0	Fat	exchanges
1.0	Fruit	exchanges	1.0	Fruit	exchanges
0.5	Milk	exchanges			
Dinner			Evening Snack		
2.0	Meat	exchanges	1.0	Meat	exchanges
11.0	Bread	exchanges			
2.5	Vegetable	exchanges	1.0	Vegetable	exchanges
2.0	Fat	exchanges			
1.0	Fruit	exchanges	1.0	Fruit	exchanges
1.0	Milk	exchanges			

Meal plan prepared for 4,500-kcal meal pattern
Dietary requirements: 4,503 kcal; protein, 20% (225 gm); carbohydrate, 67% (754 gm); fat, 13% (65 gm).

Daily Meal Plan by Food Exchanges

Breakfast			Morning Snack		
			1.0	Meat	exchanges
8.5	Bread	exchanges	4.0	Bread	exchanges
1.5	Fat	exchanges			
1.0	Fruit	exchanges			
0.5	Milk	exchanges			
Lunch			Afternoon Snack		
3.0	Meat	exchanges	1.0	Meat	exchanges
10.5	Bread	exchanges	6.5	Bread	exchanges
1.5	Vegetable	exchanges			
2.0	Fat	exchanges	1.0	Fat	exchanges
1.0	Fruit	exchanges	1.0	Fruit	exchanges
0.5	Milk	exchanges			
Dinner			Evening Snack		
4.5	Meat	exchanges	1.0	Meat	exchanges
12.5	Bread	exchanges			
2.5	Vegetable	exchanges	1.0	Vegetable	exchanges
2.0	Fat	exchanges			
1.0	Fruit	exchanges	1.0	Fruit	exchanges
1.0	Milk	exchanges			

Meal plan prepared for 5,000-kcal meal pattern
Dietary requirements: 4,999 kcal; protein, 20% (250 gm); carbohydrate, 67% (837 gm); fat, 13% (72 gm).

Daily Meal Plan by Food Exchanges

Breakfast			Morning Snack		
			1.0	Meat	exchanges
9.5	Bread	exchanges	5.0	Bread	exchanges
2.0	Fat	exchanges			
1.0	Fruit	exchanges			
0.5	Milk	exchanges			
Lunch			Afternoon Snack		
3.5	Meat	exchanges	1.0	Meat	exchanges
12.0	Bread	exchanges	7.0	Bread	exchanges
1.5	Vegetable	exchanges			
2.0	Fat	exchanges	1.0	Fat	exchanges
1.0	Fruit	exchanges	1.0	Fruit	exchanges
0.5	Milk	exchanges			
Dinner			Evening Snack		
5.0	Meat	exchanges	1.0	Meat	exchanges
14.0	Bread	exchanges			
2.5	Vegetable	exchanges	1.0	Vegetable	exchanges
2.5	Fat	exchanges			
1.0	Fruit	exchanges	1.0	Fruit	exchanges
1.0	Milk	exchanges			

Meal plan prepared for female/male diabetic 15 to 18 years old, 2,000 kcal
Dietary requirements: 2,066 kcal; protein, 15% (77 gm); carbohydrate, 55% (284 gm); fat, 30% (69 gm).

Daily Meal Plan by Food Exchanges

Breakfast			Morning Snack	
4.5	Bread	exchanges		
2.5	Fat	exchanges		
1.0	Fruit	exchanges		
1.0	Milk	exchanges		
Lunch			Afternoon Snack	
2.0	Meat	exchanges		
4.0	Bread	exchanges		
1.5	Vegetable	exchanges		
4.5	Fat	exchanges		
			2.0	Fruit exchanges
Dinner			Evening Snack	
4.0	Meat	exchanges		
4.0	Bread	exchanges		
2.0	Vegetable	exchanges		
2.0	Fat	exchanges		
			1.0	Fruit exchanges
			1.0	Milk exchanges

Diet prepared for female/male diabetic 15 to 18 years old, 2,000 kcal

Day 1

Breakfast

1 slice	Bread, pumpernickel, toasted with raspberry jelly
1½ cups	Cereal, cream of wheat, enriched
2 pats	Butter, unsalted
¾ cup	Grapefruit sections, raw
1 cup	Milk, 2% fat/low-fat

Lunch

1½ slices	Pizza, pepperoni, baked
2	Carrots, raw, whole, scraped
1 Tbsp	Salad dressing, Italian, low fat
¼ head	Lettuce, iceberg, raw, leaves

Dinner

4 oz	Pork chop, lean/fat, broiled
1 cup	Squash
2 cups	Rice
2 tsp	Salad dressing, vinegar and oil, homemade
1 cup	Lettuce, avocado, tomato and artichoke salad

Morning Snack

Afternoon Snack

⅓ cup	Prunes, dried, uncooked

Evening Snack

1	Peach, raw, whole
⅔ cup	Yogurt, plain, nonfat

Diet prepared for female/male diabetic 15 to 18 years old, 2,000 kcal

Day 2

Breakfast

3 cups	Total, Wheaties
1	Bran Muffin
2 tsp	Margarine, corn/soy
1 cup	Strawberries, raw
1 cup	Milk, 2% fat/low-fat

Lunch

2 oz	Chicken breast, no skin, roasted
1½ cups	Green beans with water chestnuts
1 cup	Corn, frozen, boiled, kernels
2 cups	Salad of cucumbers, peppers, cabbage
2 tbsp	Low fat dressing

Dinner

1¼ oz	Fish, striped bass, broiled
1	Small baked potato
1 tbsp	Margarine
1 cup	Broccoli
1 cup	Layered vegetable salad (onions, celery, carrots, peas), cucumber dressing
8 oz	Seltzer water
2	Ginger snaps

Morning Snack

Afternoon Snack

⅔ cup	Cranapple juice, canned

Evening Snack

6 oz	Cranberry juice, bottled
⅔ cup	Yogurt, plain, nonfat

288

Meal plan prepared for female vegetarian more than 23 years old, 2,200 kcal
Dietary requirements: 2,199 kcal; protein, 15% (82 gm); carbohydrate, 65% (385 gm); fat,
20% (37 gm).

Daily Meal Plan by Food Exchanges

Breakfast		Morning Snack
4	French toast slices, powdered sugar	6 oz V8 juice
3 tsp	Margarine	
	Hot spicy apple sauce	
	Yogurt	
Lunch		**Afternoon Snack**
2½ cups	Seashell macaroni stuffed with Feta cheese and spinach with parmesan cheese	4 oz orange juice raw vegetables
1 cup	Tomato slices, marinated in French dressing	
1 cup	Frozen raspberry yogurt	
Dinner		**Evening Snack**
2 cups	Split pea soup with legumes, carrots, onions, sprinkled with parsley	"Milkshake" made with ¾ cup plain yogurt, ½ cup strawberries
	Cornbread, margarine	
	Apple/swiss cheese Waldorf salad	

Diet Prepared for Pregame Meal, 600 kcal*

6 oz	Zucchini lasagna with cheese	2 meat + 1 milk + 1.5 bread
1 cup	Carrots and parsley	1 vegetable
2 cups	Tossed salad with oil-free dressing	Free exchange
10 oz	Skim milk	1 milk
1 slice	Angel food cake with strawberries	1 bread + 1 fruit

*Contains 578 kcal; 31% protein, 60% carbohydrate, and 9% fat.

APPENDIX I: Cholesterol in Some Common Foods*

The amount of fat in a food is also a consideration in planning the cholesterol-lowering diets.

Food	Cholesterol (mg)
Beef†	94
Pork†	89
Lamb†	98
Chicken†	79
Turkey†	89
Veal†	99
Liver†	438
Halibut†	60
Trout†	55
Clams†	50
Crab†	100
Lobster†	85
Scallops†	53
Shrimp†	150
Egg, 1 large	252
Milk, whole, 1 cup	34
Milk, 2%, 1 cup	22
Milk, skim, 1 cup	5
Cheese, blue, 1 oz	24
Cheese, cheddar, 1 oz	28
Cheese, cottage, low-fat, ½ cup	12
Cheese, mozzarella, 1 oz	27
Cheese, swiss, 1 oz	35
Butter, 1 Tbsp	35
Fruits	None
Vegetables	None
Peanut butter	None

*From American Heart Association of Washington. Used by permission.
†3.5 oz cooked (100 gm).

REFERENCES

1. Bowes, Church: Food Values of Portions Commonly Used, ed 14. Philadelphia, JB Lippincott Co, 1985.
2. Feeley RM, Criner PE, Watt BK: Cholesterol content of foods. *J Am Diet Assoc* 1972; 61:134–149.

APPENDIX J: Foods High in Iron*

Food	Average Serving Weight (gm)	Approximate Measure		Iron (mg) Per Serving	Iron (mg) Per 100 gm
Almonds	15	12–15		0.7	4.4
Apricots, dried	30	5	halves	1.5	4.9
Bacon, cooked	25	4–5	slices	0.8	3.3
Beans, dried	30 (dry)	½	cup (cooked)	2.1	6.9
Lima, dried	30 (dry)	½	cup (cooked)	2.3	7.5
Beef, rib roast, cooked	60	2	oz	1.8	3.0
Corned, medium fat	60	2	oz	2.6	4.3
Dried	30	1	oz	1.5	5.1
Beet greens, cooked	75	½	cup	2.4	3.2
Bologna	30	1	slice	0.7	2.2
Bran flakes, 40%	15	½	cup	0.8	5.1
Brazil nuts	15	2	medium	0.5	3.4
Bread, whole wheat	25	1	slice	0.6	2.2
Cashews	15	6–8		0.8	5.0
Chard	75	½	cup	1.9	2.5
Chocolate, bitter	30	1	square	1.3	4.4
Sweetened, plain	30	1	square	0.8	2.8
Clams	60	2	oz	4.2	7.0
Cocoa	7	1	Tbsp	0.8	11.6
Coconut, fresh	15	½	oz	0.3	2.0
Dried	15	2	Tbsp	0.5	3.6
Cornmeal, degermed, enriched	15 (dry)	½	cup (cooked)	0.4	2.9
Cress, garden	10	5–8	sprigs	0.3	2.9
Currants, dried	30	2	Tbsp	0.8	2.7
Dandelion greens	75	½	cup	2.3	3.1
Dates	30	3–4		0.6	2.1
Egg, whole	50	1		1.4	2.7
Yolk	20	1		1.4	7.2
Figs, dried	30	2	small	0.9	3.0
Flour, all-purpose, enriched	15	2	Tbsp	0.4	2.9
Flour, whole wheat	15	2	Tbsp	0.5	3.3
Ham, smoked	60	2	oz	1.7	2.9
Hazelnuts	15	10–12		0.6	4.1
Heart, beef	60	2	oz	2.8	4.6
Kale	75	¾	cup	1.7	2.2
Kidney, beef	60	2	oz	4.7	7.9
Lamb, leg	60	2	oz	1.9	3.1
Lentils, dry	30 (dry)	½	cup (cooked)	2.2	7.4
Liver, beef	60	2	oz	4.7	7.8
Liver sausage	30	1	slice	1.6	5.4
Molasses, light	20	1	Tbsp	0.9	4.3
Oatmeal	15 (dry)	½	cup (cooked)	0.7	4.5

(Continued.)

APPENDIX J: Foods High in Iron* (cont.)

Food	Weight (gm)	Approximate Measure		Per Serving	Per 100 gm
		Average Serving		Iron (mg)	
Oysters, raw	60	2	oz	3.4	5.6
Parsley	10	10	small sprigs	0.4	4.3
Peaches, dried	30	3	halves	1.9	6.9
Peas, dry	30 (dry)	½	cup (cooked)	1.4	4.7
Pecans	15	12	halves	0.4	2.4
Popcorn	15	1	cup, popped	0.4	2.7
Pork loin, cooked	60	2	oz	1.8	3.0
Pork sausage	60	2	oz	1.4	2.3
Prunes, dried	30	4	prunes	1.2	3.9
Raisins, dried	50	5	Tbsp	1.7	3.3
Rice, brown	15 (dry)	½	cup (cooked)	0.3	2.0
Rye, whole meal	15	1	Tbsp	0.6	3.7
Sardines	60	2	oz	1.6	2.7
Shrimp, canned	60	2	oz	1.9	3.1
Syrup, table blends	20	1	Tbsp	0.8	4.1
Soybeans, dried	25	2	Tbsp	2.0	8.0
Flour, medium fat	15	3	Tbsp	2.0	13.0
Spinach, cooked	75	½	cup	1.5	2.0
Sugar, brown	15	1	Tbsp	0.4	2.6
Tongue, beef	60	2	oz	1.7	2.8
Turkey	60	2	oz	2.3	3.8
Turnip greens	75	½	cup	1.8	2.4
Veal roast, cooked	60	2	oz	2.2	3.6
Walnuts	15	8–15	halves	0.3	2.1
Wheat flakes	15	½	cup	0.5	3.0
Shredded, plain	30	1	biscuit	1.1	3.5
Whole meal	15	½	cup (cooked)	0.5	3.4
Yeast, compressed	30	1	oz	1.5	4.9
Dried brewer's	15	2	Tbsp	2.7	18.2

*From Krause MV, Mahan KL: *Food, Nutrition, and Diet Therapy,* ed 7. Philadelphia, WB Saunders Co, 1984. Used by permission.

APPENDIX K: Dietary Fiber and Carbohydrate Content of Foods Per 100 gm of Edible Portion*

Food	Total (gm)	Carbohydrate Sugar† (gm)	Starch (gm)	Dietary Fiber‡ (gm)
Cereals and breads				
Arrowroot	94.0	Trace	94.0	—
Barley (pearl), raw	83.6	Trace	83.6	6.5
Barley, boiled	27.6	Trace	27.6	2.2
Bemax	44.7	16.0	28.7	—
Bran (wheat)	26.8	3.8	23.0	44.0
Corn flour	92.0	Trace	92.0	—
Custard powder	92.0	Trace	92.0	—
Flour (whole meal 100%)	65.8	2.3	63.5	9.6
Flour, brown (85%)	68.8	1.9	66.9	7.5
Flour, white (72%)	74.8	1.5	73.3	3.0
Flour, household, plain	80.1	1.7	78.4	3.4
Flour, self-rising	77.5	1.4	76.1	3.7
Patent (40%)	78.0	1.4	76.6	—
Macaroni, raw	79.2	Trace	79.2	—
Macaroni, boiled	25.2	Trace	25.2	—
Oatmeal, raw	72.8	Trace	7.28	7.0
Porridge	8.2	Trace	8.2	0.8
Rice, polished, raw	86.8	Trace	86.8	2.4
Rice, boiled	29.6	Trace	26.9	0.8
Rye flour (100%)	75.9	Trace	15.9	—
Sago, raw	94.0	Trace	94.0	—
Semolina, raw	77.5	Trace	77.5	—
Soya flour, full fat	23.5	11.2	12.3	11.9
Soya flour, low fat	28.2	13.4	14.8	14.3
Spaghetti, raw	84.0	2.7	81.3	—
Spaghetti, boiled	26.0	0.8	25.2	—
Spaghetti, canned, in tomato sauce	12.2	3.4	8.8	—
Tapioca, raw	95.0	Trace	95.0	—
Bread				
Whole meal	41.8	2.1	39.7	8.5
Brown	44.7	1.8	42.9	5.1
Hovis	45.1	2.4	42.7	4.6
White	49.7	1.8	47.9	2.7
White, fried	51.3	1.7	49.6	(2.2)
Toasted	64.9	2.1	62.8	(2.8)
Dried crumbs	77.5	2.6	74.9	(3.4)
Currant	51.8	13.0	38.8	(1.7)
Malt	49.4	18.6	30.8	—
Soda	56.3	3.0	53.3	2.3
Rolls, brown, crusty	57.2	2.1	55.1	(5.9)
Rolls, brown, soft	47.9	1.9	46.0	(5.4)

(Continued.)

APPENDIX K: Dietary Fiber and Carbohydrate Content of Foods (cont.)

Food	Carbohydrate			Dietary Fiber‡ (gm)
	Total (gm)	Sugar† (gm)	Starch (gm)	
Bread *(continued)*				
Rolls, white, crusty	57.2	2.1	55.1	(3.1)
Rolls, white, soft	53.6	1.9	51.7	(2.9)
Rolls, starch reduced	45.7	1.6	44.1	(2.0)
Chapatis with fat	50.2	1.8	46.5	3.7
Chapatis without fat	43.7	1.6	42.1	(3.4)
Breakfast cereals				
All-Bran	43.0	15.4	27.6	26.7
Corn Flakes	85.1	7.4	77.7	11.0
Grape Nuts	75.9	9.5	66.4	7.0
Muesli	66.2	26.2	40.0	7.4
Puffed Wheat	68.5	1.5	67.0	15.4
Ready Brek	69.9	2.2	67.7	7.6
Rice Krispies	88.1	9.0	79.1	4.5
Shredded wheat	67.9	0.4	67.5	12.3
Special K	78.2	9.6	68.6	5.5
Sugar Puffs	84.5	56.5	28.0	6.1
Weeta Bix	70.3	6.1	66.5	12.7
Biscuits				
Chocolate, full coated	67.4	43.4	24.0	3.1
Cream crackers	68.3	Trace	68.3	(3.0)
Crisp bread, rye	70.6	3.2	67.4	11.7
Crisp wheat, starch reduced	36.9	7.4	29.5	4.9
Digestive, plain	66.0	16.4	49.6	(5.5)
Digestive, chocolate	66.5	28.5	38.0	3.5
Ginger nuts	79.1	35.8	43.3	2.0
Homemade	65.5	26.8	38.7	1.7
Matzo	86.6	4.2	82.4	3.9
Oatcakes	63.0	3.1	59.9	4.0
Sandwich	69.2	30.2	39.0	1.2
Semisweet	74.8	22.3	52.5	2.3
Short-sweet	62.2	24.1	38.1	1.7
Shortbread	65.5	17.2	48.3	2.1
Wafers, filled	66.0	44.7	21.3	1.6
Wafer biscuits	75.8	2.3	73.5	(3.2)
Fruits				
Apples, just flesh	11.9	11.8	0.1	2.0
Apples, flesh, skin, core	9.2	9.1	0.1	1.5
Apples, cooking, raw	9.6	9.2	0.4	2.4
Apples, stewed, no sugar	8.2	7.9	0.3	2.1
Apples, stewed, with sugar	17.3	17.0	0.3	1.9
Apricots, fresh raw	6.7	6.7	0	2.1
Apricots, stewed, no sugar	5.7	5.6	0	1.7
Apricots, stewed, with sugar	15.6	15.6	0	1.6

Food	Carbohydrate Total (gm)	Carbohydrate Sugar† (gm)	Carbohydrate Starch (gm)	Dietary Fiber‡ (gm)
Fruits *(continued)*				
Apricots, dried, raw	43.4	43.4	0	24.0
Apricots, dried, stewed, without sugar	16.1	16.1	0	8.9
Apricots, dried, stewed, with sugar	19.9	19.9	0	8.5
Apricots, canned	27.7	27.7	0	1.3
Avocados	1.8	1.8	Trace	2.0
Bananas, raw	19.2	16.2	3.0	3.4
Blackberries, raw	6.4	6.4	0	7.3
Blackberries, stewed, no sugar	5.5	5.5	0	6.3
Blackberries, stewed, with sugar	14.8	14.8	0	5.7
Cherries, eating, raw	11.9	11.9	0	1.7
Cherries, cooking, raw	11.6	11.6	0	1.7
Cherries, stewed, no sugar	9.8	9.7	0	1.4
Cherries, stewed, with sugar	20.1	19.7	0	1.2
Cranberries, raw	3.5	3.5	0	4.2
Currants, black, raw	6.6	6.6	0	8.7
Currants, black, stewed, no sugar	5.6	5.6	0	7.4
Currants, black, stewed, with sugar	15.0	15.0	0	6.8
Currants, red, raw	4.4	4.4	0	8.2
Currants, red, stewed, no sugar	3.8	3.8	0	7.0
Currants, red, stewed, with sugar	13.3	13.3	0	6.4
Currants, white, raw	5.6	5.6	0	6.8
Currants, stewed, no sugar	4.8	4.8	0	5.8
Currants, stewed, with sugar	14.2	14.2	0	5.3
Currants, dried	63.1	63.1	0	6.5
Dates, dried	63.9	63.9	0	8.7
Dates, dried, with pits	54.9	54.9	0	7.5
Figs, green, raw	9.5	9.5	0	2.5
Figs, dried, raw	52.9	52.9	0	18.5
Figs, stewed, no sugar	29.4	29.4	0	10.3
Figs, stewed, with sugar	34.3	34.3	0	9.7
Fruit pie filling, canned	25.1	23.2	1.9	(1.8)
Fruit salad, canned	25.0	25.0	0	1.1
Gooseberries, green, raw	3.4	3.4	0	3.2
Gooseberries, stewed, no sugar	2.9	2.9	0	2.7
Gooseberries, stewed, with sugar	12.5	12.5	0	2.5
Gooseberries, ripe, raw	9.2	9.2	0	3.5
Grapes, black, raw	15.5	15.5	0	0.4
Grapes, white, raw	16.1	16.1	0	0.9
Grapefruit, raw	5.3	5.3	0	0.6
Grapefruit, canned	15.5	15.5	0	0.4
Green gages	11.8	11.8	0	2.6
Green gages, stewed, no sugar	10.0	10.0	0	2.2
Green gages, stewed, with sugar	19.4	19.2	0	2.1
Guavas, canned	15.7	15.7	Trace	3.6
Lemons, whole	3.2	3.2	0	5.2

(Continued.)

APPENDIX K: Dietary Fiber and Carbohydrate Content of Foods   (cont.)

Food	Carbohydrate			Dietary Fiber‡ (gm)
	Total (gm)	Sugar† (gm)	Starch (gm)	
Fruits *(continued)*				
Lemon juice, fresh	1.6	1.6	0	0
Loganberries, raw	3.4	3.4	0	6.2
Loganberries, stewed, no sugar	3.1	3.1	0	5.7
Loganberries, stewed, with sugar	13.4	13.4	0	5.2
Loganberries, canned	26.2	26.2	0	3.3
Lychees, raw	16.0	16.0	0	(0.5)
Lychees, canned	17.7	17.7	0	0.4
Mandarin oranges, canned	14.2	14.2	0	0.3
Mangoes, raw	15.3	15.3	Trace	(1.5)
Mangoes, canned	20.3	20.2	0.1	1.0
Melons				
Cantaloupe, raw	5.3	5.3	0	1.0
Yellow honeydew, raw	5.0	5.0	0	0.9
Watermelon, raw	5.3	5.3	0	—
Mulberries, raw	8.1	8.1	0	1.7
Nectarines, raw	12.4	12.4	0	2.4
Olives, in brine	Trace	Trace	0	4.4
Oranges, raw	8.5	8.5	0	2.0
Orange juice, fresh	9.4	9.4	0	0
Passion fruit, raw	6.2	6.2	0	15.9
Pawpaw, canned	17.0	17.0	0	0.5
Peaches, fresh, raw	9.1	9.1	0	1.4
Peaches, dried, raw	53.0	53.0	0	14.3
Peaches, stewed, no sugar	19.6	19.6	0	5.3
Peaches, stewed, with sugar	23.3	23.3	0	5.1
Peaches, canned	22.9	22.9		1.0
Pears, eating	10.6	10.6	0	2.3
Pears, cooking, raw	9.3	9.3	Trace	2.9
Pears, stewed, no sugar	7.9	7.9	Trace	2.5
Pears, stewed, with sugar	17.1	17.1	Trace	2.3
Pears, canned	20.0	20.0	0	1.7
Pineapple, fresh	11.6	11.6	0	1.2
Pineapple, canned	20.2	20.2	0	0.9
Plums, Victoria dessert, raw	9.6	9.6	0	2.1
Plums, cooking, raw	6.2	6.2	0	2.5
Plums, stewed, no sugar	5.2	5.2	0	2.2
Plums, stewed, with sugar	15.3	15.1	0	1.9
Pomegranate juice	11.6	11.6	0	0
Prunes, dried, raw	40.3	40.3	0	16.1
Prunes, stewed, no sugar	20.4	20.4	0	8.1
Prunes, stewed, with sugar	26.5	26.5	0	7.7
Raisins, dried	64.4	64.4	0	6.8
Raspberries, raw	5.6	5.6	0	7.4

Food	Carbohydrate Total (gm)	Sugar† (gm)	Starch (gm)	Dietary Fiber‡ (gm)
Fruits *(continued)*				
Raspberries, stewed, no sugar	5.9	5.9	0	7.8
Raspberries, stewed, with sugar	17.3	17.3	0	7.0
Raspberries, canned	22.5	22.5	0	(5.0)
Rhubarb, raw	1.0	1.0	0	2.6
Rhubarb, stewed, no sugar	0.9	0.9	0	2.4
Rhubarb, stewed, with sugar	11.4	11.4	0	2.2
Strawberries, raw	6.2	6.2	0	2.3
Strawberries, canned	21.1	21.1	0	1.0
Sultanas, dried	64.7	64.7	0	7.0
Tangerines, raw	8.0	8.0	0	1.9
Nuts				
Almonds	4.3	4.3	0	14.3
Barcelona nuts	5.2	3.4	1.8	10.3
Brazil nuts	4.1	1.7	2.4	9.0
Chestnuts	36.6	7.0	29.6	6.8
Cob or hazelnuts	6.8	4.7	2.1	6.1
Coconut, fresh	3.7	3.7	0	13.6
Coconut, milk	4.9	4.9	0	(Trace)
Coconut, desiccated	6.4	6.4	0	23.5
Peanuts, fresh	8.6	3.1	5.5	8.1
Peanuts, roasted, salted	8.6	3.1	5.5	8.1
Peanut butter, smooth	13.1	6.7	6.4	7.6
Walnuts	5.0	3.2	1.8	5.2
Vegetables				
Artichokes, globe, boiled	2.7	—	0	—
Asparagus, boiled	1.1	1.1	0	1.5
Aubergine, raw	3.1	2.9	0.2	2.5
Beans, French, boiled	1.1	0.8	0.3	3.2
Beans, runner, raw	3.9	2.8	1.1	2.9
Beans, broad, boiled	7.1	0.6	6.5	4.2
Beans, red kidney, raw	45.0	(3.0)	(42.0)	(25.0)
Bean sprouts, canned	0.8	0.4	0.4	3.0
Broccoli, tops, raw	2.5	2.5	Trace	3.6
Broccoli, boiled	1.6	1.5	0.1	4.1
Brussel sprouts, raw	2.7	2.6	0.1	4.2
Brussel sprouts, boiled	1.7	1.6	0.1	2.9
Cabbage, red, raw	3.5	3.5	Trace	3.4
Cabbage, white, raw	3.5	3.7	0.1	2.7
Carrots, old, raw	5.4	5.4	0	2.9
Carrots, boiled	4.3	4.2	0.1	3.1
Carrots, young, boiled	4.5	4.4	0.1	3.0
Carrots, canned	4.4	4.4	Trace	3.7
Cauliflower, raw	1.5	1.5	Trace	2.1
Cauliflower, boiled	0.8	0.8	Trace	1.8
Celery, raw	1.3	1.2	0.1	1.8
Celery, boiled	0.7	0.7	0	2.2

(Continued.)

APPENDIX K: Dietary Fiber and Carbohydrate Content of Foods   (cont.)

Food	Total (gm)	Sugar† (gm)	Starch (gm)	Dietary Fiber‡ (gm)
		Carbohydrate		
Vegetables *(continued)*				
Chicory, raw	1.5	—	0	—
Corn, sweet, on-the-cob, raw	23.7	1.7	22.0	3.7
Corn, sweet, on-the-cob, boiled	22.8	1.7	21.1	4.7
Corn, sweet, canned, kernels	16.1	8.9	7.2	5.7
Cucumber, raw	1.8	1.8	0	0.4
Endive, raw	1.0	1.0	0	2.2
Horseradish, raw	11.0	7.3	3.7	8.3
Leeks, raw	6.0	6.0	0	3.1
Leeks, boiled	4.6	4.6	0	3.9
Lentils, raw	53.2	2.4	50.8	11.7
Lentils, split, boiled	17.0	0.8	16.2	3.7
Lettuce, raw	1.2	1.2	Trace	1.5
Mushrooms, raw	0	0	0	2.5
Mustard and cress, raw	0.9	0.9	0	3.7
Okra, raw	2.3	2.3	Trace	(3.2)
Onions, raw	5.2	5.2	0	1.3
Onions, boiled	2.7	2.7	0	1.3
Parsley, raw	Trace	Trace	0	9.1
Parsnips, raw	11.3	8.8	2.5	4.0
Parsnips, boiled	13.5	2.7	10.8	2.5
Peas, fresh, raw	10.6	4.0	6.6	5.2
Peas, fresh, boiled	7.7	1.8	5.9	5.2
Peas, frozen, raw	7.2	4.1	3.4	7.8
Peas, frozen, boiled	4.3	1.0	3.3	12.0
Peas, canned, garden	7.0	3.6	3.4	6.3
Peas, processed	13.7	1.3	12.4	7.9
Peas, dried, raw	50.0	2.4	47.6	16.7
Peas, dried, boiled	19.1	0.9	18.2	4.8
Peas, split, dried, raw	56.6	1.9	54.7	11.9
Peas, split, dried, boiled	21.9	0.9	21.0	5.1
Peas, chick Bengal gram, raw	50.0	(10.0)	(40.0)	(15.0)
Peas, red pidgeon, raw	54.0	(9.0)	(45.0)	(15.0)
Peppers, green, raw	2.2	2.2	Trace	0.9
Peppers, green, boiled	1.8	1.7	0.1	0.9
Plantain, green, raw	28.3	0.8	27.5	(5.8)
Plantain, green, boiled	31.1	0.9	30.2	6.4
Potatoes, old, raw	20.8	0.5	20.3	2.1
Potatoes, boiled	19.7	0.4	19.3	1.0
Potatoes, mashed, with margarine and milk	18.0	0.6	17.4	0.9
Potatoes, baked	25.0	0.6	24.4	2.5
Potatoes, new, boiled	18.3	0.7	17.6	2.0

Food	Carbohydrate			Dietary Fiber‡ (gm)
	Total (gm)	Sugar† (gm)	Starch (gm)	
Vegetables *(continued)*				
Potatoes, new, canned	12.6	0.4	12.2	2.5
Potatoes, instant powder	73.2	2.2	71.0	16.5
Potatoes, instant powder, made up	16.1	0.5	15.6	3.6
Potato chips	49.3	0.7	48.6	11.9
Pumpkin, raw	3.4	2.7	0.7	0.5
Radishes, raw	2.8	2.8	0	1.0
Spinach, boiled	1.4	1.2	0.2	6.3
Spring greens, boiled	0.9	0.9	0	3.8
Sweet potatoes, raw	21.5	(9.7)	(11.8)	(2.5)
Sweet potatoes, boiled	20.1	9.1	11.0	2.3
Tomatoes, raw	2.8	2.8	Trace	1.5
Tomatoes, canned	2.0	2.0	Trace	0.9
Turnips, raw	3.8	3.8	0	2.8
Turnips, boiled	2.8	2.3	0	2.2
Turnip tops, boiled	0.1	0	0.1	3.9
Watercress, raw	0.7	0.6	0.1	3.3
Yams, raw	32.4	1.0	31.4	(4.1)
Yams, boiled	29.8	0.2	29.6	3.9

*From Krause MV, Mahan KL: *Food, Nutrition, and Diet Therapy,* ed 7. Philadelphia, WB Saunders Co, 1984. Used by permission.
†Sugar includes all free monosaccharides and disaccharides.
‡Values in parentheses are taken from the literature.

APPENDIX L: Calcium and Phosphorus Content of Foods

Food	Amount	Calcium (mg)	Phosphorus (mg)
Cereal and grain products			
Macaroni, spaghetti, noodles	½ cup cooked	8	47
Rice	½ cup cooked	7	21
Vegetables	100 gm (about) ½ cup cooked		
Artichokes		51	69
Asparagus		21	50
Bean sprouts		17	48
Broccoli		88	62
Brussel sprouts		32	72
Cabbage		44	20
Corn		4	48
Cress		61	48
Greens			
Beet greens		99	25
Collards		152	39
Dandelion greens		140	42
Kale		134	46
Mustard greens		183	50
Spinach		98	30
Swiss chard		73	24
Turnip greens		184	37
Leeks		52	50
Lima beans		47	121
Mushrooms		6	116
Okra		92	41
Parsnips		45	62
Peas		20	66
Potatoes, white		9	65
Rutabagas		59	31
Winter squash		28	48
Other vegetables, average		25	26
Fruit			
Blackberries	⅝ cup	32	19
Orange	1 small	41	20
Raspberries	⅔ cup	30	22
Rhubarb	⅜ cup	78	15
Tangerine	1 large	40	18
Fresh fruit, average	½ cup or 1 medium	16	20
Canned fruit, average	½ cup	10	12
Fruit juice	½ cup	10	13

Food	Amount	Calcium (mg)	Phosphorus (mg)
Fats and oils			
Butter or margarine	1 tsp	1	1
Nondairy cream substitute, nondairy powder	1 tsp	Trace	8
French dressing	1 Tbsp	2	2
Gravy	1 Tbsp	—	2
Mayonnaise	1 tsp	1	1
Sweets			
Candy, sugar	½ oz	—	—
Candy, milk chocolate	½ oz	26	28
Honey	1 Tbsp	4	3
Jelly	1 Tbsp	2	2
Sugar, white	1 Tbsp	—	—
Sugar, brown	1 Tbsp	9	6
Syrup, maple	1 Tbsp	33	3
Desserts			
Assorted cookies	1 2-in.	7	32
Cake, white	2 in. by 3 in. by 2 in.	34	46
Pie, cream	⅛ of 9-in. pie	62	88
Pie, fruit	⅛ of 9-in. pie	23	30
Snack foods			
Popcorn	1 cup	2	39
Potato chips	5	3	15
Beverages			
Beer	8 oz	10	62
Carbonated beverages			
Colas, average	8 oz	7	42
Ginger ale, average	8 oz	3	—
Coffee	6 oz	5	5
Tea	6 oz	5	4

*From Krause MV, Mahan KL: *Food, Nutrition, and Diet Therapy,* ed 7. Philadelphia, WB Saunders Co, 1984. Used by permission.

APPENDIX M: Foods Grouped According to Purine Content*

GROUP 1: HIGH PURINE CONTENT
(100–1000 mg of purine nitrogen/100 gm of food)

Anchovies	Mackerel
Bouillon	Meat extracts
Brains	Mincemeat
Broth	Mussels
Consommé	Partridge
Goose	Roe
Gravy	Sardines
Heart	Scallops
Herring	Sweetbreads
Kidney	Yeast, baker's and
Liver	brewer's

Foods in this list should be omitted from the diet of patients who have gout (acute and remission stages).

GROUP 2: MODERATE PURINE CONTENT
(9–100 mg of purine nitrogen/100 gm of food)

Meat and Fish
(except those in group 1):	*Vegetables*
Fish	Asparagus
Poultry	Beans, dried
Meat	Lentils
Shellfish	Mushrooms
	Peas, dried
	Spinach

One serving (2–3 oz) of meat, fish or fowl or 1 serving (½ cup) vegetable from this group is allowed each day or 5 days/week (depending on condition) during remissions.

GROUP 3: NEGLIGIBLE PURINE CONTENT

Bread, enriched white and
crackers
Butter or fortified margarine
(in moderation)
Cake and cookies
Carbonated beverages
Cereal beverage
Cereals and cereal products
(refined and enriched)
Cheese
Chocolate
Coffee
Condiments
Cornbread
Cream (in moderation)
Custard
Eggs
Fats (in moderation)

Fruit
Gelatin desserts
Herbs
Ice cream
Milk
Macaroni products
Noodles
Nuts
Oil
Olives
Pickles
Popcorn
Puddings
Relishes
Rennet desserts
Rice
Salt
Sugar and sweets
Tea
Vegetables (except those
in group 2)
Vinegar
White sauce

Foods included in this group may be used daily.

*From Krause MV, Mahan KL: *Food, Nutrition, and Diet Therapy,* ed 7. Philadelphia, WB Saunders Co, 1984. Used by permission.

APPENDIX N: Increased Protein Content of the Daily Meal Plan*†

Daily Meal Plan To increase the protein content of the day's meals from 100 gm to 125 or 150, use the allowances of dried milk solids indicated in columns 2 and 3.	Protein Content (gm)		
	100 (approx.)‡	125 (approx.)§	150 (approx.) ‖
Breakfast			
Fruit juice, citrus, ½ cup	0.5	0.5	0.5
Cereal, enriched, ½ cup, cooked or prepared, with	2.5	2.5	2.5
½ cup whole milk	4.2	4.2	4.2
Plus 2 Tbsp dried nonfat milk solids	—	6.0	6.0
Egg, 1	6.5	6.5	6.5
Bread (white, enriched, or whole-wheat), 1 slice	2.5	2.5	2.5
Butter or enriched margarine (as desired)			
Whole milk, 1 cup	8.5	8.5	8.5
Lunch			
Meat, poultry, fish, 2 oz cooked; or cheese	15.2	15.2	15.2
Salad, ½ cup (with dressing)	0.5	0.5	0.5
Cooked vegetable, green or yellow, ½ cup	2.0	2.0	2.0
Bread (white, enriched or whole-wheat), 1 slice	2.5	2.5	2.5
Butter or enriched margarine (as desired)			
Simple dessert,¶ fruit	0.5	0.5	0.5
Whole milk, 1 cup	8.5	8.5	8.5
Plus 2 Tbsp dried nonfat milk solids	—	6.0	6.0
Midafternoon snack			
Whole milk, 1 cup	—	8.5	8.5
Plus 2 Tbsp dried nonfat milk solids	—	—	6.0
Graham crackers, 2	—	—	2.5
Dinner			
Meat, poultry, fish (liver once/week); or cheese:			
4 oz raw weight; 3 oz cooked	22.8	22.8	22.8
Cooked vegetable, ½ cup	2.0	2.0	2.0
Potato	2.0	2.0	2.0
Plus 2 Tbsp dried nonfat milk solids	—	6.0	6.0
Bread (white, enriched or whole-wheat), 1 slice	2.5	2.5	2.5
Butter or enriched margarine (as desired)			
Simple dessert,¶ pudding	4.5	4.5	4.5
Plus 2 Tbsp dried nonfat milk solids	—	—	6.0
Whole milk, 1 cup	8.5	8.5	8.5
Evening snack			
Whole milk, 1 cup	8.5	8.5	8.5
Plus 2 Tbsp dried nonfat milk solids	—	—	6.0
Total Protein, gm	104.7	131.2	151.7

*From Krause MV, Mahan KL: *Food, Nutrition, and Diet Therapy*, ed 7. Philadelphia, WB Saunders Co, 1984. Used by permission.

†If additional calories are needed to maintain body weight, concentrated foods such as sugar, jelly, sauces and salad dressings may be added. To make these meal plans low in sodium, omit all salt in cooking and at the table, omit the cheese, substitute unsalted butter or fortified margarine, and replace all or part of the whole milk and dried nonfat milk solids with low-sodium milk, available in fresh fluid and canned forms and in powdered whole milk (Lonalac, Mead Johnson) and powdered skim milk (Cellu, Chicago Dietetic Supply House).

‡2,400 kcal.

§2,700 kcal.

‖ 3,000 kcal.

¶Desserts: custards, puddings, plain ice cream, fruit.

APPENDIX O: Suggestions for Increasing Energy Intake in Steps of 500 kcal*

Additional Foods	Weight (gm)	kcal	Protein
Plus 500 kcal (served between meals)			
1. 1 cup dry cereal	28	110	2
1 banana	100	80	
1 cup whole milk	244	159	8
1 slice toast	23	60	2
1 Tbsp peanut butter	15	86	4
		495	16
2. 8 saltine crackers	23	99	3
1 oz cheese	28	113	7
1 cup ice cream	133	290	6
		502	16
3. 6 graham cracker squares	42	165	3
2 Tbsp peanut butter	30	172	8
1 cup orange juice	249	122	
2 Tbsp raisins	18	52	
		511	11
Plus 1,000 kcal (served between meals)			
1. 8 oz fruit-flavored yogurt	227	240	9
1 slice bread	23	60	2
2 oz cheese	56	226	14
1 apple	150	87	
¼ of 14-in. cheese pizza	130	306	16
1 small banana	140	81	1
		1,000	42
2. Instant Breakfast with whole milk	276	280	15
1 cup cottage cheese	225	239	31
½ cup pineapple	128	95	
1 cup apple juice	248	117	
6 graham cracker squares	42	165	3
1 pear	180	100	1
		996	50

(Continued.)

APPENDIX O: Suggestions for Increasing Energy Intake in Steps of 500 kcal* (cont.)

Additional Foods	Weight (gm)	kcal	Protein
Plus 1,500 kcal (served between meals)			
1. 2 slices bread	46	120	4
2 Tbsp peanut butter	30	172	8
1 Tbsp jam	20	110	
4 graham cracker squares	28	110	2
8 oz fruit-flavored yogurt	227	240	9
¾ cup roasted peanuts	108	628	28
1 cup apricot nectar	251	143	1
		1,523	52
2. 1 baked custard	248	285	13
Instant Breakfast with whole milk	276	280	15
1 cup dry cereal	28	110	2
1 banana	100	80	
1 cup whole milk	244	159	8
1 cup orange juice	249	122	
4 Tbsp raisins	36	104	
1 bagel	55	165	6
2 Tbsp cream cheese	28	99	2
2 Tbsp jam	40	110	—
		1,514	46

*From Krause MV, Mahan KL: *Food, Nutrition, and Diet Therapy*, ed 7. Philadelphia, WB Saunders Co, 1984. Used by permission.

APPENDIX P: Nutrients Significantly Affected by Selected Drugs

Nutrient	Drug Action	Drugs
Vitamin B_6	Function as vitamin B_6 antagonists or increase the turnover of B_6 in the body	Isoniazid, cycloserine and other antituberculous drugs Hydralazine Penicillamine L-Dopa Oral contraceptives Alcohol
Folic acid	Function as folic acid antagonists; affect the absorption of folic acid or increase the turnover or loss of folate from the body	p-Aminosalicylic acid Methotrexate Pyrimethamine Isoniazid Anticonvulsants Triamterene Trimethoprim Oral contraceptives Cycloserine Salicylazosulfapyridine Acetylsalicylic acid Pentamidine Alcohol
Vitamin B_{12}	Affect the absorption of vitamin B_{12}	Neomycin Biguanides p-Aminosalicylic acid Cholestyramine Potassium chloride Alcohol

(Continued.)

APPENDIX P: Nutrients Significantly Affected by Selected Drugs   (cont.)

Nutrient	Drug Action	Drugs
Niacin	By antagonizing Vitamin B_6, cause depletion, because vitamin B_6 is a necessary coenzyme in the synthesis of niacin from tryptophan	Isoniazid
Riboflavin	Decreases riboflavin absorption by increasing gastrointestinal motility	Thyroxine
	Displaces riboflavin from plasma binding site and causes hyperexcretion of riboflavin	Boric acid
Thiamin	Impairs absorption of thiamin or impairs the formation of the coenzyme form of the vitamin	Alcohol
Ascorbic acid	Increase requirements	Digitalis alkaloids
	Decrease the absorption or stimulate the metabolism of the vitamin	Oral contraceptives
	Deplete the tissues of the vitamin	Acetylsalicylic acid Alcohol Anorectic agents Anticonvulsants Tetracycline Adrenal corticosteroids
	Depletes adrenal ascorbic acid	
Vitamin A	Acts as a solvent for carotene and vitamin A and thus prevents absorption	Mineral oil
	Decrease absorption by damage to mucosa; inhibition of pancreatic lipase and inactivation of bile salts	Cholestyramine Neomycin Alcohol Colchicine (affects carotene)

Vitamin D	Affect absorption or metabolism of vitamin D	Cholestyramine Laxatives Antacids Mineral oil Phenolphthalein Anticonvulsants Glutethimide
	Accelerate the degradation of 25-OHD$_3$	Diphosphonates Corticosteroids
	Block the production of 1,25-OH$_2$D$_3$ in the kidney	Clofibrate Mineral oil Isoniazid
Vitamin E	Diminishes the carrier lipoprotein for vitamin E Decreases absorption	
Vitamin K	Decrease synthesis of vitamin K$_2$ by intestinal bacteria, but no effect on vitamin status unless vitamin K intake is inadequate	Tetracyclines and other broad-spectrum antibiotics
	Decrease absorption of vitamin K	Mineral oil Neomycin Cholestyramine
	Cause vitamin K deficiency	Coumarin anticoagulants Aspirin and other salicylates
Iron	Depresses iron absorption	Bicarbonate
	Increases iron absorption	Isoniazide
	Impairs the uptake of iron into protoporphyrin; capable of causing sideroblastic anemia	Cholestyramine

(Continued.)

APPENDIX P: Nutrients Significantly Affected by Selected Drugs (cont.)

Nutrient	Drug Action	Drugs
Zinc	Cause excessive urinary excretion of zinc	Alcohol D-Penicillamine Corticosteroids Estrogen component of oral contraceptives Chlorthalidone Thiazides Furosemide
Magnesium	Increase urinary excretion of magnesium	Chlorothiazide Hydrochlorothiazide Ethacrynic acid Ammonium chloride Mercurial diuretics Alcohol
	Drug-induced steatorrhea causes formation of magnesium soaps and excessive fecal excretion of magnesium	
Calcium	Cause malabsorption of calcium	Prednisone and other glucocorticoids Phenobarbital Phenytoin Primidone Glutethimide Diphosphonates Phenolphthalein Neomycin

Nutrient	Action	Drug
	Cause excessive urinary excretion of calcium	Furosemide Ethacrynic acid Triamterene Alcohol
	Increase intestinal absorption of calcium	Combination oral contraceptives
Protein	Cause malabsorption of protein	Neomycin Actinomycin D
	Inhibit protein synthesis	Corticosteroids
Fat	Cause malabsorption of fat	Neomycin Colchicine Cholestyramine p-Aminosalicylic acid
Carbohydrate	Cause malabsorption of lactose	Neomycin Colchicine
	Causes malabsorption of sucrose	Neomycin
Sodium and potassium	Increase fecal excretion	Neomycin Colchicine
Phosphate	Increase fecal excretion	Aluminum hydroxide antacids

*From Krause MV, Mahan KL: *Food, Nutrition, and Diet Therapy*, ed 7. Philadelphia, WB Saunders Co, 1984. Used by permission.

APPENDIX Q: Effects of Some Drugs on Nutritional Status

Drug	Possible Mechanism	Nutritional Implication
Amphetamines		
Dextroamphetamine	Central nervous system effect on appetite	Weight loss
Methylphenidate	Central nervous system effect on appetite	Decreased rate of growth in children due to decreased intake
Analgesics		
Alcohol	Toxic effect on intestinal mucosa Impairs pancreatic enzyme secretion	Decreased absorption of thiamin, folic acid, vitamin B_{12} Increased urinary excretion of magnesium and zinc Decreased serum vitamin B_{12}
Aspirin (salicylates)	Decreases leukocyte uptake of ascorbic acid and alters ascorbic acid distribution May uncouple energy source necessary for renal tubular resorption of amino acids	Decreased plasma and platelet ascorbic acid levels Increased urinary loss of ascorbic acid, potassium and amino acids Decreased absorption of tryptophan, possibly other amino acids and glucose
Colchicine	Decreases activity of intestinal disaccharidases Damages gastrointestinal mucosa by blocking mucosal cell replication	Decreased absorption of vitamin B_{12}, fat, carotene, sodium, potassium, lactose, xylose, protein Decreased serum cholesterol, carotene and vitamin B_{12}
Indomethacin	Increases rate of gastric emptying May uncouple energy source for mucosal active transport of amino acids	Decreased plasma and platelet ascorbic acid levels Dyspepsia Decreased absorption of amino acids and xylose May cause anemia
Antacids		
Aluminum hydroxide	Decreases absorption of phosphate	Phosphate depletion Decreased vitamin A absorption

Drug	Possible Mechanism	Nutritional Implication
Others	Basic environment inactivates thiamin and prevents formation of ferrous from ferric iron	Inadequate amount of thiamin Decreased absorption of iron
Anticoagulants		
Coumarins	Antagonize vitamin K and vice versa Drug effect antagonized by high doses of vitamin E	Increased prothrombin time
Anticonvulsants		
Phenobarbital Phenytoin Primidone	Increase turnover of vitamin D, may block hydroxylation of vitamin D May increase biliary excretion of vitamin D	Decreased serum levels of 25-hydroxy-vitamin D_3 and calcium and magnesium Possible osteomalacia or rickets Decreased serum levels of folate, vitamin B_{12}, pyridoxine Can cause megaloblastic anemia
Barbiturates	Accelerate inactivation of vitamin D	Increased need for vitamin D and folic acid with long-term use Decreased absorption of thiamin Increased urinary excretion of vitamin C Decreased serum vitamin B_{12} Can cause megaloblastic anemia
Antidepressants		
Amitriptyline Imipramine		Interfere with riboflavin metabolism
Lithium carbonate	May increase appetite May inhibit magnesium-dependent enzymes or alter magnesium distribution	Possible weight gain Altered blood glucose Increased plasma magnesium Increased calcium excretion Decreased calcium uptake by bone

(Continued.)

APPENDIX Q: Effects of Some Drugs on Nutritional Status   (cont.)

Drug	Possible Mechanism	Nutritional Implication
Antifungals Amphotericin B	Nephrotoxicity	Increased urinary excretion of potassium and nitrogen Decreased serum magnesium and potassium Increased blood urea nitrogen (BUN)
Antimicrobials Chloramphenicol	Decreases protein synthesis by blocking mRNA-ribosome bond	Possibly increased need for riboflavin, pyridoxine and vitamin B_{12} Possible peripheral neuritis, optic neuropathy Can antagonize response to folate, iron, and vitamin B_{12} therapy
Penicillins	Carry potassium with them into urine Possibly induce hyperaldosteronism	Hypokalemia
Tetracyclines	Chelate divalent ions May decrease synthesis of mucosal iron-carrier protein	Decreased absorption of calcium, iron, magnesium, zinc, xylose, amino acids and fat; net effect with minerals not clinically significant Increased urinary excretion of vitamin C, riboflavin, nitrogen, folic acid, and niacin Decreased synthesis of vitamin K by intestinal bacteria
Neomycin (Some of these changes also seen with kanamycin and paromomycin)	Decreases activity of disaccharidases Causes mucosal injury Precipitates bile acids and disrupts micelle formation	Decreased absorption of fat, medium-chain triglycerides (MCT), carbohydrate, protein, fat-soluble vitamins A, D, and K, vitamin B_{12}, calcium, and iron

Drug	Possible Mechanism	Nutritional Implication
Gentamicin	Nephrotoxicity	Increased urinary excretion of magnesium and potassium
Viomycin	Induces hyperaldosteronism	May cause hypomagnesemia, hypokalemia, hypocalcemia, alkalosis
Cephalosporins	Nephrotoxicity	May cause hypokalemia
	Damages gastrointestinal mucosa	May cause vitamin K deficiency with prolongation of prothrombin time
Antineoplastics	Cytotoxic	
Antitubercular agents		
p-Aminosalicyclic acid	Affects mucosal transport mechanism	Decreased absorption of vitamin B_{12}, iron, folate, fat and xylose
	Decreases intestinal mucosal disaccharidases	Possible peripheral neuritis
Isoniazid	Structurally related to pyridoxine and niacin	Increased urinary excretion of pyridoxine
		Causes pyridoxine depletion
		Can cause polyneuropathy, megaloblastic anemia
		Causes niacin depletion, pigmented rash, cheilosis, and diarrhea
		Decreased serum folate
Cycloserine	Acts as a pyridoxine antagonist	Decreased protein synthesis
		May decrease absorption of calcium and magnesium
		May decrease serum folate, vitamin B_{12}, and pyridoxine
Antivitamins		
Methotrexate	Inhibits dihydrofolate reductase; decreased formation of active folate	Malabsorption of vitamin B_{12}, folate, fat, and xylose

(Continued.)

APPENDIX Q: Effects of Some Drugs on Nutritional Status   (cont.)

Drug	Possible Mechanism	Nutritional Implication
Methotrexate *(continued)*	Causes gastrointestinal mucosal injury	Weight loss, diarrhea, nausea, anorexia, vomiting, gingivitis, and stomatitis
Biguanides		
Metformin	Decreases activity of maltase, isomaltase, and sucrase in jejunum	Decreased absorption of glucose, xylose, vitamin B_{12} Decreased serum folate, vitamin B_{12}
Phenformin	May affect active transport mechanisms	Decreased rate of glucose absorption in human ileum Decreased absorption of vitamin B_{12}, fat, calcium and amino acids
Cardiac drugs		
Propranolol		Decreased carbohydrate tolerance Increased BUN
Digitalis glycosides	Inhibit glucose absorption	Diarrhea; cachexia Increased urinary excretion of magnesium, calcium, and potassium
Cathartics	Can cause intestinal hyperperistalsis May irritate intestine	Can cause steatorrhea Can increase intestinal calcium and potassium loss Decreased glucose absorption
Phenolphthalein		Decreased absorption of vitamin D
Chelating agents		
Penicillamine	Chelates with pyridoxine Chelates with zinc and copper	Increased urinary excretion of pyridoxine, zinc, and copper Can cause pyridoxine depletion Decreased taste acuity; unpleasant taste

Drug	Possible Mechanism	Nutritional Implication
Corticosteroids	Stimulate protein catabolism Depress protein synthesis	Decreased absorption of calcium and phosphorus Increased urinary excretion of ascorbic acid, calcium, potassium, zinc, and nitrogen Decreased serum zinc Increased blood glucose, serum triglycerides, and serum cholesterol Increased need for vitamin B_6, ascorbic acid, folate, and vitamin D Decreased bone formation Decreased wound healing
Diuretics		
Ethacrynic acid	May interfere with glucose-carrier complex	Decreased carbohydrate tolerance Increased urinary excretion of calcium, magnesium, potassium; possible hypokalemia and hypomagnesemia
Furosemide		Increased urinary excretion of calcium, magnesium, potassium, and zinc Decreased serum and muscle magnesium and potassium Decreased carbohydrate tolerance
Mercurials	Renal tubule damage	Increased urinary excretion of thiamin, magnesium, calcium, and potassium Possibly induced magnesium depletion and bone resorption

(Continued.)

APPENDIX Q: Effects of Some Drugs on Nutritional Status   (cont.)

Drug	Possible Mechanism	Nutritional Implication
Spironolactone		Increased urinary excretion of calcium and magnesium
Thiazides	May increase intestinal calcium absorption or increase bone resorption	Increased urinary excretion of potassium, magnesium, zinc, and riboflavin Decreased carbohydrate tolerance Possible potassium and magnesium depletion Decreased serum folate
Triamterene	Competitive inhibition of dihydrofolate reductase; reduces activation of folic acid	Possibly increased calcium excretion
Hypocholesterolemics Cholestyramine	Binds bile salts and disrupts micelles Binds intrinsic factor at ileal pH Binds iron	Decreased absorption of cholesterol, vitamins A, D, K, and B_{12}, folate, fat, MCT, glucose, xylose, carotene and iron Decreased calcium absorption Decreased serum calcium and vitamin B_{12} Increased urinary excretion of calcium
Clofibrate	May decrease activity of intestinal disaccharidases	Decreased taste acuity, unpleasant aftertaste Decreased absorption of carotene, glucose, iron, MCT, vitamin B_{12}, and electrolytes
Colestipol	Bile acid sequestrant	Reduced serum cholesterol Lowered plasma and serum levels of vitamins A and E

Drug	Possible Mechanism	Nutritional Implication
Hypotensive Agents		
Hydralazine	Inactivates pyridoxine May chelate trace metals	Increased excretion of pyridoxine; pyridoxine depletion Possible peripheral neuritis
Diazoxide	May cause pancreatic damage	Hyperglycemia Decreased tubular excretion of uric acid
Reserpine		Increased gastrointestinal motility and secretion May cause weight gain
Sodium nitroprusside	Binds vitamin B_{12}	Increased urinary B_{12} excretion Decreased plasma B_{12}
Laxatives		
Mineral oil (petrolatum, liquid)	Dissolves fat-soluble vitamins Increases intestinal motility	Decreased absorption of carotene, vitamins A, D, E, and K, calcium, and phosphate
L-*Dopa* (levodopa)	Pyridoxine involved in metabolism of L-dopa Antagonizes pyridoxine	Possible polyneuropathy related to pyridoxine depletion Increased need for ascorbic acid and pyridoxine Decreased absorption of tryptophan and other amino acids Increased urinary excretion of sodium and potassium
Oral contraceptives	May increase catabolism, decrease absorption or alter tissue uptake of vitamin C May inhibit folate conjugase May increase transport proteins for vitamin A	Altered tryptophan metabolism Decreased serum vitamin C levels Possibly decreased serum vitamin B_{12}, folate, pyridoxine, riboflavin, magnesium, and zinc

(Continued.)

APPENDIX Q: Effects of Some Drugs on Nutritional Status   (cont.)

Drug	Possible Mechanism	Nutritional Implication
Oral Contraceptives (continued)		
	Estrogens increase the rate of conversion of tryptophan to niacin	Increased hemoglobin, hematocrit, serum levels of vitamins A and E, total lipids, triglycerides, iron, total iron-binding capacity (TIBC), and plasma copper Possible polyneuropathy, peripheral neuritis, and megaloblastic anemia
Parasympatholytic agents		
Atropine	Decreases gastric acidity	May decrease iron absorption
Potassium supplements	Slow release of potassium chloride causes decrease of ileal pH (acidification)	Decreased absorption of vitamin B_{12}
Sedative-hypnotics		
Glutethimide	Possibly increases inactivation of 25-hydroxy vitamin D_3	Increased vitamin D turnover Increased bone resorption Polyneuropathy
Sulfonamides		
Salicylazosulfapyridine (Sulfasalazine)	Inhibits intestinal transport of folate Inhibits action of polyglutamyl folate conjugase	Decreased absorption of folate Decreased serum folate and serum iron Decreased response to folate supplement
Other sulfonamides		Peripheral neuritis Increased urinary excretion of ascorbic acid
Tranquilizers		
Chlorpromazine	Hepatotoxic May interfere with riboflavin metabolism	Can reduce physical activity Possible weight gain Increased serum cholesterol

Drug	Possible Mechanism	Nutritional Implication
Uricosuric agents		
Probenecid	Action on renal tubule	Increased urinary excretion of riboflavin, calcium, magnesium, sodium, potassium, phosphate, and chloride
		Decreased urinary excretion of pantothenic acid
		Decreased absorption of riboflavin and amino acids
Urinary germicides		
Nitrofurantoin	May inhibit intestinal folate conjugase	Decreased serum folate
		Possible megaloblastic anemia and peripheral neuritis

*From Krause MV, Mahan KL: *Food, Nutrition, and Diet Therapy,* ed 7. Philadelphia, WB Saunders Co, 1984. Used by permission.

APPENDIX R: The Metric System and Equivalents*

A meter is a yard—plus a little extra.
A kilogram is two pounds—plus a little extra.
A liter is a quart—plus a little extra.

The metric system is a standarized system of measurement that is used internationally. However, the United States also employs another system of measurement based on the old English system. In the field of dietetics, both systems are used. The following charts give equivalents for common household measures. With this information it is possible to calculate measure and weigh in either system.

Equivalent Level Measures and Weights

60 drops	= 1 tsp
	5 cc
	5 gm
1 tsp	= 5 gm
3 tsp	= 1 Tbsp
	15 cc
	15 gm
1 dessert spoon	= 10 cc
2 Tbsp	= 30 cc
	30 gm
	1 oz (fluid)
4 Tbsp	= ¼ cup
	60 cc
	60 gm
8 Tbsp	= ½ cup
	120 cc
	120 gm
16 Tbsp	= 1 cup
	240 gm
	250 ml
	8 oz (fluid)
	½ lb

*Modified from Krause MV, Mahan KL: *Food, Nutrition, and Diet Therapy*, ed 7. Philadelphia, WB Saunders Co, 1984. Used by permission.

2 cups	= 1 pint
	480 gm
	500 ml
	16 oz (fluid)
	1 lb
4 cups	= 2 pints
	1 quart
	1,000 or 960 cc
	1,000 ml
	1 kg
	2.2 lb
4 quarts	= 1 gallon
8 quarts	= 1 peck
2 gallons	= 1 peck
4 pecks	= 1 bushel
8 gallons	= 1 bushel

Equivalents in Grams

For easy computing purposes, the cubic centimeter (cc) is considered equivalent to 1 gm (1 cc = 1 gm).

Also for easy computing purposes, 1 oz equals 30 gm or 30 cc.

1 quart	= 960 gm
1 pint	= 480 gm
1 cup	= 240 gm
½ cup	= 120 gm
1 soup cup	= 120 gm
1 glass (8 oz)	= 240 gm
½ glass (4 oz)	= 120 gm
1 orange juice glass	= 100–120 gm
1 Tbsp	= 15 gm
1 tsp	= 5 gm

Units of Length

Metric Unit	Equivalent Metric Unit	Equivalent English Unit
meter (m)	100 cm	39.37 in.
	1,000 mm	(3.28 ft; 1.09 yd)
centimeter (cm)	0.01 m	0.3937 in.
	10 mm	
millimeter (mm)	0.001 m	0.03937 in.
	0.1 cm	

Units of Weight

Metric Unit	Equivalent Metric Unit	Equivalent English Unit
kilogram (kg)	1,000 gm	35.3 oz
	1,000,000 mg	(2.2046 lb)
gram (gm)	0.001 kg	
	1,000 mg	0.0353 oz
milligram (mg)	0.000001 kg	
	0.001 gm	0.0000353 oz

Units of Volume

Metric Unit	Equivalent Metric Unit	Equivalent English Unit
liter (L)	1,000 ml	1.057 quart
milliliter (ml)	0.001 L	0.001057 quart
or		
cubic centimeter (cc)		

Temperature

To convert a Fahrenheit temperature to centigrade:
$$°C = (°F - 32)/1.8$$

To convert a centigrade temperature to Fahrenheit:
$$°F = (1.8 × °C) + 32$$

With the Fahrenheit scale, the freezing point of water is 32°F and the boiling point 212°F. On the centigrade scale, the freezing point of water is 0°C and the boiling point is 100°C.

Units of Speed

Miles/hr	km/hr	M/Sec	Miles/hr	km/hr	M/Sec
1	1.6	0.47	11	17.7	5.17
2	3.2	0.94	12	19.3	5.64
3	4.8	1.41	13	20.9	6.11
4	6.4	1.88	14	22.5	6.58
5	8.0	2.35	15	24.1	7.05
6	9.6	2.82	16	25.8	7.52
7	11.2	3.29	17	27.4	7.99
8	12.8	3.76	18	29.0	8.46
9	14.4	4.23	19	30.6	8.93
10	16.0	4.70	20	32.2	9.40

Common Expressions of Work, Energy, and Power

Watts	Kilocalories (kcal)	Foot-Pounds (ft-lb)
1 watt = 0.73756 ft-lb/sec	1 kcal = 3086 ft-lb	1 ft-lb = 3.2389×10^{-3} kcal
1 watt = 0.01433 kcal/min	1 kcal = 426.8 kg-m	1 ft-lb = 0.13825 kg-m
1 watt = 1.341×10^{-3} hp or 0.0013 hp	1 kcal = 3087.4 ft-lb	1 ft-lb = 5.050×10^{-3} hp/hr
1 watt = 6.12 kg-m/min	1 kcal = 1.5593×10^{-3} hp/hr	

Conversion Factors for Use in the Exercise Sciences

To convert	Into	Multiply by
centimeters	feet	3.281×10^{-2}
centimeters	inches	0.3937
centimeters	kilometers	1×10^{-5}
centimeters	yards	1.094×10^{-2}
centimeters of mercury	pounds/sq ft	27.85
centimeters of mercury	pounds/sq in	0.1934
cubic centimeters	cu feet	3.531×10^{-5}
cubic centimeters	cu inches	0.06102
cubic centimeters	cu meters	1×10^{-6}
cubic centimeters	cu yards	1.308×10^{-6}
cubic centimeters	liters	0.001
cubic feet	liters	28.32
cubic feet	pints (U.S. liq.)	59.84
cubic feet	quarts (U.S. liq.)	29.92
days	seconds	86,400.0
deciliters	liters	0.1
drams	ounces	0.0625
feet	centimeters	30.48

(Continued.)

Conversion Factors for Use in the Exercise Sciences   (cont.)

To convert	Into	Multiply by
feet	kilometers	3.048×10^{-4}
feet	meters	0.3048
feet	millimeters	304.8
feet/min	meters/min	0.3048
gallons	cu feet	0.1337
gallons	liters	3.785
grams	kilograms	0.001
grams	milligrams	1,000.0
inches	centimeters	2.540
joules	kilogram-calories	2.389×10^{-4}
kilograms	pounds	2.205
liters	gallons (U.S. liquid)	0.2642
liters	pints (U.S. liquid)	2.113
liters	quarts (U.S. liquid)	1.057
meters	centimeters	100.0
meters	feet	3.281
meters	inches	39.37
meters	miles (nautical)	5.396×10^{-4}
miles/hr	feet/min	88.0
miles/hr	kms/min	0.02682
miles/hr	knots	0.8684
miles/hr	meters/min	26.82
miles/min	feet/sec	88.0
milligrams	grains	0.01543236
milligrams	grams	0.001
milligrams/liter	parts/million	1.0
milliliters	liters	0.001
millimeters	centimeters	0.1
millimeters	feet	3.281×10^{-3}
millimeters	inches	0.03937
millimeters	kilometers	1×10^{-6}
millimeters	meters	0.001
millimeters	yards	1.094×10^{-3}
newton	dynes	1×10^{5}
ohm (international)	ohm (absolute	1.005
ohms	megohms	1×10^{-6}
ounces	grams	28.349527
ounces	pounds	0.0625
pints (liquid)	gallons	0.125
pints (liquid)	liters	0.4732
pints (liquid)	quarts (liquid)	0.5
pounds	kilograms	0.4536

To convert	Into	Multiply by
pounds	ounces	16.0
pounds of water	gallons	0.1198
quarts (liquid)	gallons	0.25
quarts (liquid)	liters	0.9463
revolutions	degrees	360.0
revolutions/min	degrees/sec	6.0
revolutions/sec	revs/min	60.0
tons (metric)	kilograms	1,000.0
tons (metric)	pounds	2,205.0
yards	centimeters	91.44
yards	kilometers	9.144×10^{-4}
yards	meters	0.9144
yards	miles (nautical)	4.934×10^{-4}
yards	miles (statute)	5.682×10^{-4}
yards	millimeters	914.4

Terminology and Units of Measurement

The American College of Sports Medicine suggests that the following terminology and units of measurement be used in scientific endeavors to promote consistency and clarity of communications, and to avoid ambiguity. The terms defined below utilize the units of measurement of the Système International d'Unités (SI).

Exercise: Any and all activity involving generation of force by the activated muscle(s) which results in a disruption of a homeostatic state. In dynamic exercise, the muscle may perform shortening (concentric) contractions or be overcome by external resistance and perform lengthening (eccentric) contractions. When muscle force results in no movement, the contraction should be termed static or isometric.

Exercise Intensity: A specific level of maintenance of muscular activity that can be quantified in terms of power (energy expenditure or work performed per unit of time), isometric force sustained, or velocity of progression.

Endurance: The time limit of a person's ability to maintain either a specific isometric force or a specific power level involving combinations of concentric or eccentric muscular contractions.

Mass: A quantity of matter of an object, a direct measure of the object's inertia (note: mass equals weight/acceleration due to gravity; units: gram or kilogram).

Weight: The force with which a quantity of matter is attracted toward Earth by normal acceleration of gravity (traditional unit: kilogram of weight).

Energy: The capability of producing force, performing work, or generating heat (unit: joule or kilojoule).

Force: That which changes or tends to change the state of rest or motion in matter (unit: newton).

Speed: Total distance travelled per unit of time (units: meter per second).

Velocity: Displacement per unit of time. A vector quantity requiring that direction be stated or strongly implied (units: meter per second or kilometer per hour).

Work: Force expressed through a distance but with no limitation on time (unit: joule or kilojoule). Quantities of energy and heat expressed independently of time should also be presented in joules. The term "work" should not be employed synonymously with muscular exercise.

Power: The rate of performing work; the derivative of work with respect to time; the product of force and velocity (unit: watt). Other related processes such as energy release and heat transfer should, when expressed per unit of time, be quantified and presented in watts.

Torque: The effectiveness of a force to produce rotation about an axis (unit: newton · meter).

Volume: A space occupied, for example, by a quantity of fluid or a gas (unit: liter or milliliter). Gas volumes should be indicated as ATPS, BTPS, or STPD.

Amount of a substance: That amount of the particular substance containing the same number of particles as there are in 12 gm (1 mole) of the nuclide ^{12}C (unit: mole of millimole). For respiratory gases, 1 mole of the gas at STPD is equal to 22.4 L.

APPENDIX S: Nutrition Knowledge Assessment Quiz

Answer true or false to the following statements:

_____ 1. In children and adults, there is no single food that contains all the nutrients required for proper growth and health.

_____ 2. Protein is the principle source of energy for the body.

_____ 3. All nutrients required by the body can be provided by food.

_____ 4. Vitamins and minerals are good sources of energy for the body.

_____ 5. Fat provides more calories per gram than does either protein or carbohydrate.

_____ 6. Bread and potatoes should be avoided during a weight loss program.

_____ 7. Sherbet provides calories and a good variety of nutrients.

_____ 8. As caloric requirements decrease, nutrient needs lessen as well.

_____ 9. All chemicals must be listed on food labels.

_____10. "Dietetic" foods are always low in their caloric content.

_____11. Additives are dangerous to health because they are chemicals.

_____12. Natural and synthetic vitamin supplements are of equal nutritional value.

_____13. "Organic" foods are higher in nutrient content than are foods grown in chemically fertilized soil.

_____14. Honey is nutritionally superior to table sugar.

_____15. Intake of nutrients above recommended allowances guarantees good health.

_____16. Alcohol and beer contain a large amount of B vitamins.

_____17. As much protein as desired may be consumed without contributing to weight gain.

_____18. Margarine has less calories than does butter.

_____19. White table sugar is a toxin for all people.

_____20. During exercise, thirst is an accurate indicator of how much water you need to drink.

21. Nutrient   Major Food Source
_____ A. Vitamin A   1. Citrus fruits
_____ B. Vitamin C   2. Milk
_____ C. Calcium   3. Meat and legumes
_____ D. Iron   4. Deep yellow fruits and vegetables

Answers:
1. True
2. False
3. True
4. False
5. True
6. False
7. False
8. False
9. False
10. False
11. False
12. True
13. False
14. False
15. False
16. False
17. False
18. False
19. False
20. False
21. A—4
    B—1
    C—2
    D—3

APPENDIX T: Nutrition in the Physical Education Setting

Class Objectives

1. Identify sport:
   a. School—team related
   b. Lifetime—individual
2. Understanding ideal body weight.
3. Identify problems associated with the sport:
   a. Energy demands
   b. Fluid needs
   c. Special problems
4. Plan a 1-week menu:
   a. 60% carbohydrate, 15% protein, 15%–25% fat
5. Plan a preevent meal and a postevent meal.
6. Compare individual diet history with no. 4. Add improvements or make suggestions.
7. Knock down a myth.

Daily Objectives

1. Developing skills in understanding nutrition's role in performance, discussing psychological and health benefits of sports, and discussing health problems related to sports.
2. Understanding ideal body weight, understanding a laboratory session, examining height and weight charts, skinfold, and hydrostatis assessment.
3. Understanding energy calculations.
4. Understanding the dietary exchange system and four food groups.
5. Taking a diet history.
6. Understanding myths and why are they so common in athletics.

APPENDIX U: Glossary (Chalk Talk: A Nutrition Vocabulary for Athletes)

The game jargon is a tool for communication in sports. The words do not mean much by themselves, but in the context of athletic events, they take on special meanings. They are shortcuts in conversation, and outsiders sometimes feel left out without knowledge of their meaning. Like sports, nutrition has its own language. Many of the words are familiar, but they have a special meaning when applied to athletic performance.

Acid-base balance:
: Equilibrium between acid and base concentration in the body fluids; regulation becomes difficult in vigorous exercise

Acne:
: A skin condition usually associated with the maturation of young adults; can be caused by unsanitary athletic equipment (e.g., wrestler's headgear or excessive sweating)

Aerobic exercise:
: Exercise during which the heart rate is increased to a target zone and remains in this zone for longer than 20 minutes; determination of the target zone is dependent on age and resting heart rate; when energy is delivered to the exercise muscle in the presence of oxygen, as in long distance running.

Alcohol:
: An ingredient in a variety of beverages, including beer, wine, liqueurs, cordials, and mixed and straight drinks; pure alcohol yields about 7 calories/gm, of which 75% is available to the body; athletic concerns are its diuretic effects and action on glycogen storage

Amenorrhea:

Failure to menstruate, reflecting a halted ovulatory cycle

Amino acids

The chemicals that make up protein; about 20 amino acids are found in the protein of living tissues

Anaerobic exercise:

Exercise performed at an intensity that overrides oxygen intake and transport, as in sprinting

Anemia (sports)

Dilutional anemia, characterized by low-normal hemoglobin levels; found in all levels of training; an increase of red blood cell mass and plasma volume

Anabolic steroids:

Hormones produced in males during puberty; sometimes the synthetic forms are used by athletes to try to promote extra muscular development; also known as androgens

Anorexia:

Lack of appetite

Anorexia nervosa:

Intentional lack of appetite, occurring mostly in young women; life threatening; requires skilled professional treatment

Anthropometrics:

Measurements of the body including height, weight, arm circumferences, or skinfold thickness; used in evaluation of nutrition

Antioxidant:

A compound that reacts with oxygen, thus protecting other compounds from oxidizing

Appetite:

The desire to eat normally

Athlete:

Anyone participating in exercises, sports, or games requiring physical strength, agility, or stamina

Balanced diet:

A diet in which each nutrient and each food group is supplied in appropriate quantities relative to the others

Basal metabolic rate:

The amount of energy used by the body at rest over a specific period of time and after a 12-hour fast

Behavior modification:

Systematic substitution of one set of behaviors for another with reward of desired behavior

Bioelectrical impedence:

A method of determining the percentage of total body fat

Blood:

The fluid circulating through the body, carrying oxygen and nutrients to the body cells; consists of the liquid portion (plasma) and the more solid elements (red blood cells, white blood cells, and platelets)

Blood doping:

Infusion of the recipient's own blood to achieve higher endurance performance

Brown fat:

Fat found in hibernating mammals (and to some extent in humans) in which energy is oxidized without being stored

Bulimia:

Continuous, never-satisfied hunger, associated with a binge and purge syndrome

Calorie:

A unit used to express the heat or energy value of food; a kilocalorie is the amount of heat or energy necessary to raise the temperature of 1,000 gm of water 1° C.

Carbohydrate:
: One of three major sources of energy in food; most common are sugars and starches, containing about 4 calories/gm

Carbohydrate loading:
: A method of increasing carbohydrate consumption; also called glycogen loading (carbohydrate is stored in muscles and liver as glycogen); it has been documented that an increased glycogen store in muscles is an advantage in endurance activities

Carcinogen:
: A cancer-causing substance

Cholesterol:
: An essential fatlike substance found in all living cells, especially the brain, liver, kidneys, adrenals, and myelin sheaths that surround nerves; produced in the liver

Complementary proteins:
: Two or more proteins whose amino acid assortments complement each other in such a way that the essential amino acids missing from each are supplied by the other

Complete proteins:
: A protein that contains all the essential amino acids in sufficient amounts and ratio to permit growth, nitrogen equilibrium, or both

Complex carbohydrate:
: The polysaccharides—starches, glycogen, and celluloses

Dehydration:
: The loss of water from the body

Diabetes:
: A metabolic disorder characterized by an inadequate supply of effective insulin; one symptom is unregulated blood glucose

Diet history: An interview that is used to determine the adequacy of a person's diet

Diuretic: A medication or food substance that causes increased water excretion

Drug: Food, supplement, or preparation containing elements greater than 150% normal to the human body

Edema: The swelling of body tissues caused by leakage of fluid from the blood vessels

Electrolyte balance: Distribution of electrolytes (salts) among the body fluids

Elite athlete: An athlete who is able to perform at the very highest possible level

Energy: The capacity to do work; every food contains protein, carbohydrate, fat, or a combination of these nutrients available for energy production; the energy needs of the body are the first priority of life

Enrichment: The addition of nutrients to foods that contain a particular nutrient; commonly done in foods where the nutrient value is lost or decreased due to processing or storage

Ergogenic aid: A food or drug that offers the hope of greatly improved performance

Exchange: A food serving equivalent in energy nutrient composition and calorie content to another on the exchange lists (e.g., one small apple is a fruit exchange equivalent to 12 grapes in carbohydrate content and calories)

Fat:

A lipid usually is solid at room temperature, insoluble in water

Fatty acid:

An organic acid composed of a carbon chain with hydrogens and an acid group attached

Fiber:

The indigestible part of plant food, important in the diet as roughage or bulk

Fortification:

The addition of nutrient or nutrients to food, whether or not they are naturally present or at levels higher than those naturally present; milk is fortified with vitamin D

Fructose:

A monosaccharide sometimes known as fruit sugar

Galactose:

Part of the disaccharide lactose

Glucose:

A monosaccharide sometimes known as blood sugar or grape sugar, also "dextrose"

Glycogen:

The storage form of carbohydrate in the body; the body makes glycogen from glucose and stores it in the liver and muscles; normal storage provides approximately 1.5 hours of energy to work at 65% maximum effort

Gram:

A unit of mass; 1 oz is 28.25 gm

High-density lipoprotein:

Lipoproteins that return cholesterol from the storage places to the liver for dismantling and disposal

Hemoglobin:

The oxygen-carrying protein of the blood; found in rcd blood cells

Hormone:

A chemical messenger, secreted by one organ in response to a condition

Hormone   *(cont.)*:   in the body, that acts on another organ or organs and elicits a specific response

Hydrostatic weighing: A method of determining body density

Hypertension: High blood pressure

Hypoglycemia: An abnormally low blood glucose concentration (<60 mg/100 ml); "reactive" is a temporary hypoglycemia that may be exhibited by any normal person; "spontaneous" is rare, seen in cases of abnormal carbohydrate metabolism

Hyponatremia: Low blood sodium

Ideal body weight: Estimated weight considered best for optimal health, based on age, height, and body weight

Insulin   A hormone secreted by the pancreas in response to increased blood glucose concentration

Ketones: Molecules produced by condensing together the incompletely oxidized fragments of fat, formed when carbohydrate is not available

Joule: SI-derived unit of work, energy, and quantity of heat; symbol is J; to convert kcal to kJ, multiply kcal by 4.2

Lactic acid: An acid produced when oxygen is not available to completely oxidize pyruvic acid to carbon dioxide and water; lactic acid then accumulates in muscles

Lipids: A grouping of compounds soluble in organic solvents, including triglycer-

Lipids *(cont.)*:   ides, phospholipids, and sterols; commonly called fats

Lipoprotein: A compound made of protein and lipid; in this form, insoluble cholesterol is transported in blood

Metabolism: The sum total of all chemical reactions in living cells

Mineral: A naturally occurring inorganic, homogeneous substance; an element; required for building and repairing body tissue or controlling functions of the body; calcium, iron, magnesium, phosphorus, potassium, sodium, and zinc are major minerals

Monosaccharide: A single sugar—glucose, fructose, galactose

Myoglobin: The oxygen-holding protein of the muscles

Nitrogen balance: The amount of nitrogen consumed compared with the amount excreted in a given time

Nutrient: A substance obtained from food and used in the body for growth, maintenance, or repair; approximately 50 known nutrients are needed to survive, and that must be supplied by the foods eaten; all foods contain a variety of nutrients, but no food contains all the nutrients we need, the best approach for adequate nutrition is to eat a variety of foods

Nutrient density: A characteristic of food that provides a high quantity of one or more essential nutrients, with a small quantity of calories

Nutrition:	A combination of processes by which the body uses food for energy, growth, tissue replacement, and maintenance of body functions
Obesity:	Body weight more than 15% to 25% above desirable body weight
Osteoporosis:	Porous bone; or bone loss
Overweight:	Body weight more than 10% above desirable body weight
Peristalsis:	The wave like motions of the gut that pushes the contents along the digestive tract
Physical examination:	Medical examination that includes careful study of the body
Pica:	Eating of nonnutritious substances; often the symptom of iron deficiency
Polysaccharide:	Many monosaccharides linked together
Polyunsaturated fats:	Fats from vegetables such as corn, cottonseed, sunflower, safflower, and soybean oil; these oils have more double bonds and may be beneficial in lowering blood cholesterol
Protein:	A compound—composed of carbon, hydrogen, oxygen, and nitrogen—arranged as amino acids linked in a chain, usually about 300 units long
RDA (recommended dietary allowances):	Nutrient intakes suggested by the Food and Nutrition Board of the National Academy of Sciences, National Research Council, for the maintenance of health in people in the United States
RE (retinol equivalents):	Newer units that measure vitamin A and E

Saturated fat:	A fat carrying the maximum possible number of double bonds; solid at room temperature
Set point:	Considered to be the body's preferred weight, to which it tends to return naturally after any disturbance
Skinfold test:	A clinical test of body fatness that measures, by caliper, the thickness of a fold of skin on the back of the arm, below the shoulder blade, or in other places
Supplement:	A preparation in pill, powder, or liquid form containing nutrients used to supplement the diet
Toxicity:	Levels of substance where it causes harmful effects
Triglycerides:	The major class of dietary lipids; a compound where three fatty acids are attached to a molecule of glycerol
U.S. RDA:	The RDA figures used on labels, usually the highest RDAs suggested for any age-sex group for each unit
Underweight:	Body weight more than 10% below desirable weight
Unsaturated fat:	A fat in which one or more points of unsaturation occur; usually liquid at room temperature
Vitamin:	A noncaloric organic compound needed in very small amounts in the diet, which perform specific and individual functions to promote growth or reproduction, or to maintain health and life

APPENDIX V: Eating Your Way
to Good Health*

The ideal diet is low in fat, sugar, sodium, and cholesterol. The following numbers indicate the presence of these substances in the following foods: 1—moderate saturated fat; 2—moderate unsaturated fat; 3—high unsaturated fat; 4—high saturated fat; 5—high sugar; 6—high salt/sodium; 7—may be high in salt/sodium; 8—high cholesterol; 9—refined grains.

	Anytime	In Moderation	Now and Then
Group 1: Milk products Children: three–four servings/day Adult: two—three servings/day	Buttermilk made from skim milk Low-fat cottage cheese Low-fat milk, 1% milkfat Low-fat yogurt Nonfat dry milk Low-sodium skim milk/cheeses Skim milk Skim milk and banana shake	Cocoa made with skim milk[5] Cottage cheese, regular 4% milkfat[1] Frozen low-fat yogurt[5] Ice milk[5] Low-fat milk, 2% milkfat[1] Low-fat yogurt, sweetened[5] Mozzarella cheese, part-skim type only[1, 7]	Cheesecake[4, 5] Cheese fondue[4, 7] Cheese soufflé[4, 7, 8] Eggnog[1, 5, 8] Hard cheeses: blue, brick, camembert, cheddar muenster, swiss[4, 7] Ice cream[4, 5] Processed cheeses[4, 6] Whole milk[4]
Group 2: Poultry, fish, meat, and eggs Two servings/day	Fish 　Cod, flounder, haddock, halibut, perch, rockfish, shellfish (except shrimp), sole, low-sodium water-packed tuna Egg products 　egg whites only Poultry 　Chicken or turkey, baked, roasted, or poached in skin	Fish (drained well, if canned) 　Fresh fish[1, 2] 　Herring[3, 6] 　Mackerel, canned[2, 7] 　Pink salmon, canned[2, 7] 　Sardines[2, 7] 　Shrimp[8] 　Tuna, oil-packed[2, 7] Poultry 　Chicken liver; baked or broiled[8] 　Fried chicken, homemade in vegetable oil[3] 　Chicken or turkey, baked 　Roasted or poached (with skin)[2]	Poultry-fried chicken, commercially prepared[4] Eggs 　Cheese omelet[4, 8] 　Egg yolk or whole egg (about 3/week)[3, 8] Red meats 　Bacon[4, 7] 　Beef liver, fried[1, 8] 　Bologna[4, 6] 　Corned beef[4, 6] 　Ground beef[4] 　Ham, trimmed well[1, 6] 　Hot dogs[4, 6] 　Liverwurst[4, 6] 　Pig's feet[4]

(Continued.)

343

	Anytime	In Moderation	Now and Then
Group 2: Poultry, fish, meat, and eggs *(continued)*		Red meats (trimmed of all outside fat)[1] Flank steak[1] Leg or loin of lamb[1] Ground steak or ground round[1] Rump roast[1] Sirloin steak, lean[1] Veal[1]	Red meats, untrimmed[4] Salami[4,6] Sausage[4,6] Spareribs[4]
Group 3: Fruits and vegetables Four or more servings/day	All fruits and vegetables except those listed at right Applesauce (unsweetened) Unsweetened fruit juices Unsalted vegetable juices White or sweet potatoes	Avocado[3] Coleslaw[3] Cranberry sauce (canned)[5] French fries, homemade in vegetable oil[2], commercial[1] fried eggplant (vegetable oil)[2] Fruit canned in syrup[5] Gazpacho[2,7] Glazed carrots[5,7] Guacamole[3] Potatoes au gratin[1,7] Salted vegetable juices[6] Sweetened fruit juices[5] Vegetables canned with salt[7]	Palm[4] Coconut[4] Pickles[6]

344

Group 4: Grains and legumes
Four or more servings/day

Whole grain bread and milk	Cornbread[9]	Croissant[4, 9]
Dried beans and peas (legumes)	Flour tortilla[9]	Doughnut (yeast-leavened)[3]
Lentils	Granola cereals[1] or hominy grits[9]	Presweetened breakfast cereals[5, 9]
Oatmeal	Macaroni and cheese[1, 7, 9]	Sticky buns[1]
Whole-wheat pasta	Matzo[9]	Stuffing (made with butter)[4, 7, 9]
Brown rice	Nuts[3]	
Rye bread	Pasta, except whole wheat[9]	
Sprouts	Peanut butter[3]	
Whole-grain hot and cold cereal	Pizza[6, 9]	
Whole-wheat matzo	Refined, unsweetened cereals[9]	
	Refined beans, commercial[1]	
	homemade in oil[2]	
	Seeds[3]	
	Soybeans[2]	
	Tofu[2]	
	Waffles or pancakes with syrup[5, 7, 9]	
	White bread and rolls[9]	
	White rice[9]	

*Reprinted with permission from the *New American Eating Guide*, which is available from the Center for Science in the Public Interest, 1755 S Street, NW, Washington, DC, 20009, for $3.00 ($6.00 laminated), copyright 1979.

APPENDIX W: Nutrition Questionnaire

Name _____ Date of birth _____

Team or address _____

Brief competitive history _____

_____

Brief family history _____

_____

Brief health history _____

_____

Are you:

Pleased with your present eating habits? _____

Willing to change your present eating habits? _____

Following a special diet at this time? _____

Describe your present diet: _____

_____

_____

Describe supplements, dosage if known: _____

_____

_____

Height _____, Weight _____

Heaviest weight (lightest) _____, when _____

How much would you like to weigh? _____

Describe your normal training diet _____

Describe your preevent meal _____

Have your eating habits changed recently? _____

Do you ever go on fasts or rigid diets? _____

Do you always eat at regular times during the day? _____

Do you chew tobacco, starch, gum, ice, or any other nonfood?

_____

Do you lose your appetite if you are stressed, or upset? _____

What are your ten favorite foods? _____

_____

What are your three least favorite foods? _____

_____

What meal or snack do you like the best? _____

Where and with whom do you normally eat your meals? _____

_____

Write down any questions you may have regarding nutritional practices? _____

_____

Dietary recommendations for _____

For any other additional information, please contact me.

APPENDIX X: Nutrition Quiz

1. An appropriate way to decide if your weight is "ideal" is to compare it to: a, your friends' weight; b, the amount of food that you eat; c, reputable charts of growth velocity at your age; d, your dream goal.
2. You are considering eating candy bars for quick energy food before work-out because: a, candy bars have a lot of sugar; b, you like them; c, they are convenient; d, you decide against candy as there are other snacks which provide energy and greater amounts of other nutrients at the same time.
3. What do you need to know about the "Bikini Diet" before you could decide if it is safe? a, that it provides all the essential nutrients you need; b, that you could still eat all your favorite foods; c, that it was fun to talk about; d, how much it will cost.
4. How does your level of activity relate to the number of calories you need to maintain a constant weight? a, if you rarely exercise you need more calories; b, if you don't eat much you need more calories; c, if you exercise a lot you need more calories; d, if you are very active you need fewer calories.
5. Total caloric needs are determined mostly by: a, basal metabolism, growth and physical activity; b, last year's bathing suit; c, your current weight and how much you eat; d, the way you play sports.
6. How could you find out if you are eating correctly? a, determine the amount of fat you have on your body; b, determine your height and weight; c, count your calories each day; d, analyze the nutritive value of the food you eat over a period of time.
7. What would be most important when planning a diet for your sport? a, add large doses of vitamins to the diet; b, increase protein intake; c, avoid snacks; d, plan adequate energy intake, carbohydrates and fluids.
8. Which of the following foods is a complete source of protein? a, bread; b, corn flakes; c, eggs; d, green beans.

9. Which of the following foods is not a good source of carbohydrate? a, fish; b, orange; c, pasta; d, angel food cake.
10. The basic four food groups help in planning and evaluating diets because they: a, recommend foods good for certain organs; b, tell what foods are not good for us; c, list what to eat, how much, and when to eat it; d, recommend the types and amounts of foods which are appropriate for us at certain ages.
11. You and your dad both want to lose weight. Your weight plan is different than his because: a, your dad has different nutritional requirements; b, your dad should not exercise; c, you like different foods; d, you are sick of fresh fruit and vegetables.
12. During which two stages in the life cycle are nutrient and calorie needs highest in relation to body weight? a, infant and teenage; b, adolescent and adult; c, teenage and elderly; d, infant and elderly.
13. The advertisement suggests that taking a mega vitamin and mineral supplement will lead to superior athletic ability. Which statement is true? a, supplements are needed to increase endurance; b, vitamins and minerals have little to do with athletic performance; c, supplements are not needed if body needs for vitamins and minerals are met through diet; d, supplements are the best way for athletes to get nutrients.
14. The temperature is over 85°F and the humidity is 80%. You need to; a, withdraw from the race; b, sip fluids every 5 miles or at least each 30 minutes; c, run faster and get the race over with; d, take a salt tablet so you won't sweat.
15. One reason why drugs and alcohol affect nutritional status of the athlete is that: a, they increase the body's absorption of nutrients; b, they cause hunger; c, they reduce absorption of nutrients and impair carbohydrate metabolism; d, they deaden feelings so you don't know you need nutrients.

Answers.
1. c
2. d
3. a
4. c
5. a
6. d
7. d
8. c
9. a
10. d
11. a
12. a
13. c
14. a
15. c

APPENDIX Y: Sodium and Potassium Content of Foods

Food	Approximate Amount	Weight (gm)	Sodium (mEq)	Potassium (mEq)
Meat				
Meat (cooked)				
Beef	1 ounce	30	0.8	2.8
Ham	1 ounce	30	14.3	2.6
Lamb	1 ounce	30	0.9	2.2
Pork	1 ounce	30	0.9	3.0
Veal	1 ounce	30	1.0	3.8
Liver	1 ounce	30	2.4	3.2
Sausage, pork	2 links	40	16.5	2.8
Beef, dried	2 slices	20	37.0	1.0
Cold cuts	1 slice	45	25.0	2.7
Frankfurters	1	50	24.0	3.0
Fowl				
Chicken	1 ounce	30	1.0	3.0
Goose	1 ounce	30	1.6	4.6
Duck	1 ounce	30	1.0	2.2
Turkey	1 ounce	30	1.2	2.8
Egg	1	50	2.7	1.8
Fish	1 ounce	30	1.0	2.5
Salmon				
Fresh	¼ cup	30	0.6	2.3
Canned	¼ cup	30	4.6	2.6
Tuna				
Fresh	¼ cup	30	0.5	2.2
Canned	¼ cup	30	10.4	2.3
Sardines	3 medium	35	12.5	4.5
Shellfish				
Clams	5 small	50	2.6	2.3
Lobster	1 small tail	40	3.7	1.8
Oysters	5 small	70	2.1	1.5
Scallops	1 large	50	5.7	6.0
Shrimp	5 small	30	1.8	1.7
Cheese				
Cheese, American or Cheddar type	1 slice	30	9.1	0.6
Cheese foods	1 slice	30	15.0	0.8
Cheese spreads	2 tablespoons	30	15.0	0.8
Cottage cheese	¼ cup	50	5.0	1.1
Peanut butter	2 tablespoons	30	7.8	5.0
Peanuts, unsalted	25	25	. . .	4.5
Fat				
Avocado	⅛	30	. . .	4.6
Bacon	1 slice	5	2.2	0.6
Butter or margarine	1 teaspoon	5	2.2	. . .

(Continued.)

APPENDIX Y: Sodium and Potassium Content of Foods   (cont.)

Food	Approximate Amount	Weight (gm)	Sodium (mEq)	Potassium (mEq)
Fat *(continued)*				
Cooking fat	1 teaspoon	5	. . .	. . .
Cream				
Half and half	2 tablespoons	30	0.6	1.0
Sour	2 tablespoons	30	0.4	. . .
Whipped	1 tablespoon	15	0.3	1.0
Cream cheese	1 tablespoon	15	1.7	. . .
Mayonnaise	1 teaspoon	5	1.3	. . .
Nuts	5 (2 teaspoons)	6	. . .	0.8
Almonds, slivered				
Pecans	4 halves	5	. . .	0.8
Walnuts	5 halves	10	. . .	1.0
Oil, salad	1 teaspoon	5	. . .	. . .
Olives, green	3 medium	30	31.3	0.4
Bread				
Bread	1 slice	25	5.5	0.7
Biscuit	1 (2″ diameter)	35	9.6	0.7
Muffin	1 (2″ diameter)	35	7.3	1.2
Cornbread	1 (1½″ cube)	35	11.3	1.7
Roll	1 (2″ diameter)	25	5.5	0.6
Bun	1	30	6.6	0.7
Pancake	1 (4″ diameter)	45	8.8	1.1
Waffle	½ square	35	8.5	1.0
Cereals				
Cooked	⅔ cup	140	8.7	2.0
Dry, flake	⅔ cup	20	8.7	0.6
Dry, puffed	1½ cups	20	. . .	1.5
Shredded wheat	1 biscuit	20	. . .	2.2
Crackers				
Graham	3	20	5.8	2.0
Melba toast	4	20	5.5	0.7
Oyster	20	20	9.6	0.6
Ritz	6	20	9.5	0.5
Rye-Krisp	3	30	11.5	3.0
Saltines	6	20	9.6	0.6
Soda	3	20	9.6	0.6
Dessert				
Commercial gelatin	½ cup	100	2.2	. . .
Ice cream	½ cup	75	2.0	3.0
Sherbet	⅓ cup	50	. . .	. . .
Angel food cake	1½″ × 1½″	25	3.0	0.6
Sponge cake	1½″ × 1½″	25	1.8	0.6
Vanilla wafers	5	15	1.7	. . .

Food	Approximate Amount	Weight (gm)	Sodium (mEq)	Potassium (mEq)
Flour products†				
Cornstarch	2 tablespoons	15	. . .	. . .
Macaroni	¼ cup	50	. . .	0.8
Noodles	¼ cup	50	. . .	0.6
Rice	¼ cup	50	. . .	0.9
Spaghetti	¼ cup	50	. . .	0.8
Tapioca	2 tablespoons	15	. . .	. . .
Vegetable†				
Beans, dried (cooked)	½ cup	90	. . .	10.0
Beans, lima	½ cup	90	. . .	9.5
Corn				
Canned‡	⅓ cup	80	8.0	2.0
Fresh	½ ear	100	. . .	2.0
Frozen	⅓ cup	80	. . .	3.7
Hominy (dry)	¼ cup	36	4.1	. . .
Parsnips	⅔ cup	100	0.3	9.7
Peas				
Canned†	½ cup	100	10.0	1.2
Dried	½ cup	90	1.5	6.8
Fresh	½ cup	100	. . .	2.5
Frozen	½ cup	100	2.5	1.7
Popcorn	1 cup	15	. . .	. . .
Potato				
Potato chips	1 oz	30	13.0	3.7
White, baked	½ cup	100	. . .	13.0
White, boiled	½ cup	100	. . .	7.3
Sweet, baked	¼ cup	50	0.4	4.0
Milk				
Whole milk	1 cup	240	5.2	8.8
Evaporated whole milk	½ cup	120	6.0	9.2
Powdered whole milk	¼ cup	30	5.2	10.0
Buttermilk	1 cup	240	13.6	8.5
Skim milk	1 cup	240	5.2	8.8
Powdered skim milk	¼ cup	30	6.9	13.5
Vegetable A†				
Asparagus				
Cooked	½ cup	100	. . .	4.7
Canned‡	½ cup	100	10.0	3.6
Frozen	½ cup	100	. . .	5.5
Bean sprouts	½ cup	100	. . .	4.0
Beans, green or wax				
Fresh or frozen	½ cup	100	. . .	4.0
Canned‡	½ cup	100	10.0	2.5
Beet greens	½ cup	100	3.0	8.5
Broccoli	½ cup	100	. . .	7.0
Cabbage, cooked	½ cup	100	0.6	4.2
Raw	1 cup	100	0.9	6.0

(Continued.)

APPENDIX Y: Sodium and Potassium Content of Foods (cont.)

Food	Approximate Amount	Weight (gm)	Sodium (mEq)	Potassium (mEq)
Vegetable A *(continued)*				
Cauliflower, cooked	1 cup	100	0.4	5.2
Celery, raw	1 cup	100	5.4	9.0
Chard, Swiss	⅗ cup	100	3.7	8.0
Collards	½ cup	100	0.8	6.0
Cress, garden (cooked)	½ cup	100	0.5	7.2
Cucumber	1 medium	100	0.3	4.0
Eggplant	½ cup	100	. . .	3.8
Lettuce	Varies	100	0.4	4.5
Mushrooms, raw	4 large	100	0.7	10.6
Mustard greens	½ cup	100	0.8	5.5
Pepper, green or red				
Cooked	½ cup	100	. . .	5.5
Raw	1	100	0.5	4.0
Radishes	10	100	0.8	8.0
Sauerkraut	⅔ cup	100	32.0	3.5
Spinach	½ cup	100	2.2	8.5
Squash	½ cup	100	. . .	3.5
Tomatoes	½ cup	100	. . .	6.5
Tomato juice‡	½ cup	100	9.0	5.8
Turnip greens	½ cup	100	0.7	3.8
Turnips	½ cup	100	1.5	4.8
Vegetable B†				
Artichokes	1 large bud	100	1.3	7.7
Beets	½ cup	100	1.8	5.0
Brussel sprouts	⅔ cup	100	. . .	7.6
Carrots, cooked	½ cup	100	1.4	5.7
Raw	1 large	100	2.0	8.8
Dandelion greens	½ cup	100	2.0	6.0
Kale, cooked	¾ cup	100	2.0	5.6
Frozen	½ cup	100	1.0	5.0
Kohlrabi	⅔ cup	100	. . .	6.6
Leeks, raw	3–4	100	. . .	9.0
Okra	½ cup	100	. . .	4.4
Onions, cooked	½ cup	100	. . .	2.8
Pumpkin	½ cup	100	. . .	6.3
Rutabagas	½ cup	100	. . .	4.4
Squash, winter				
Baked	½ cup	100	. . .	12.0
Boiled	½ cup	100	. . .	6.5
Fruit				
Apple				
Fresh	1 small	80	. . .	2.3
Sauce	½ cup	120	. . .	2.5
Juice	½ cup	120	. . .	3.1

Food	Approximate Amount	Weight (gm)	Sodium (mEq)	Potassium (mEq)
Fruit *(continued)*				
Apricots				
Canned	½ cup	120	. . .	6.0
Dried	4 halves	20	. . .	5.0
Fresh	3 small	120	. . .	8.0
Nectar	⅓ cup	80	. . .	3.0
Banana	½ small	60	. . .	4.8
Berries, fresh				
Blackberries	¾ cup	100	. . .	3.0
Blueberries	½ cup	80	. . .	1.5
Boysenberries	1 cup	120	. . .	3.2
Gooseberries	¾ cup	120	. . .	4.0
Loganberries	¾ cup	100	. . .	4.4
Raspberries	¾ cup	100	. . .	4.5
Strawberries	1 cup	150	. . .	6.3
Cherries				
Canned	½ cup	120	. . .	4.0
Fresh	15 small	80	. . .	2.7
Dates				
Pitted	2	15	. . .	2.5
Figs				
Canned	½ cup	120	. . .	4.6
Dried	1 small	15	. . .	2.5
Fresh	1 large	60	. . .	3.0
Fruit cocktail	½ cup	120	. . .	5.0
Grapes				
Canned	⅓ cup	80	. . .	2.2
Fresh	15	80	. . .	3.2
Juice				
Bottled	¼ cup	60	. . .	2.8
Frozen	⅓ cup	80	. . .	2.4
Grapefruit				
Fresh	½ medium	120	. . .	3.6
Juice	½ cup	120	. . .	4.1
Sections	¾ cup	150	. . .	5.1
Mandarin orange	¾ cup	200	. . .	6.5
Mango	½ small	70	. . .	3.4
Melon				
Cantaloupe	½ small	200	. . .	13.0
Honeydew	¼ medium	200	. . .	13.0
Watermelon	½ slice	200	. . .	5.0
Nectarine	1 medium	80	. . .	6.0
Orange				
Fresh	1 medium	100	. . .	5.1
Juice	½ cup	120	. . .	5.7
Sections	½ cup	100	. . .	5.1
Papaya	½ cup	120	. . .	7.0

(Continued.)

APPENDIX Y: Sodium and Potassium Content of Foods (cont.)

Food	Approximate Amount	Weight (gm)	Sodium (mEq)	Potassium (mEq)
Fruit *(continued)*				
Peach				
Canned	½ cup	120	. . .	4.0
Dried	2 halves	20	. . .	5.0
Fresh	1 medium	120	. . .	6.2
Nectar	½ cup	120	. . .	2.4
Pear				
Canned	½ cup	120	. . .	2.5
Dried	2 halves	20	. . .	3.0
Fresh	1 small	80	. . .	2.6
Nectar	⅓ cup	80	. . .	0.9
Pineapple				
Canned	½ cup	120	. . .	3.0
Fresh	½ cup	80	. . .	3.0
Juice	⅓ cup	80	. . .	3.0
Plums				
Canned	½ cup	120	. . .	4.5
Fresh	2 medium	80	. . .	4.1
Prunes	2 medium	15	. . .	2.6
Juice	¼ cup	60	. . .	3.6
Raisins	1 tablespoon	15	. . .	2.9
Rhubarb	½ cup	100	. . .	6.5
Tangerines				
Fresh	2 small	100	. . .	3.2
Juice	½ cup	120	. . .	5.5
Sections	½ cup	100	. . .	3.2

*From Krause MV, Mahan KL: *Food, Nutrition, and Diet Therapy,* ed 7. Philadelphia, WB Saunders Co, 1984. Used by permission.
†Value for products without added salt.
‡Estimated average based on addition of salt, approximately 0.6% of the finished product.

Index

A

Acid-base balance, definition of, 332
Acidophilus milk, analysis of, 93
Acne, definition of, 332
Addictive behavior, nutritional
    intervention for, 230–236
Adenosine triphosphate (ATP),
    metabolic pathways for,
    19–20
Adolescent growth spurt, nutritional
    intervention for, 228–229
Adult, young, performance of,
    conditions affecting, 64–65
Aerobic exercise
  definition of, 332
  in weight maintenance, 161–162,
    163
Age, basal metabolism and, 36–37
Aids, ergogenic, 80–82, 110–112 (see
    also Ergogenic aids)
Alcohol
  abuse of, physician
    recommendations for,
    186–187
  in childhood, 42

definition of, 332
diabetes and, 42
driving and, 43
fuel utilization and, 38–43
hypertension and, 42
in lactation, 42
nutritional implications of, 312
in pregnancy, 41–42
premenstrual syndrome and, 42
weight loss and, 42
Alfalfa, analysis of, 83
Allergies, food, physician
    recommendations for,
    187–188
Aloe vera, analysis of, 83
Altitude
  change in, in caloric needs
    estimation, 164
  high, response to, 74–76
Aluminum hydroxide, nutritional
    implications of, 312
Amenorrhea
  in athlete, 65–66
  definition of, 333
  physician recommendations for,
    188–189

eating, successful, guidelines for, 263–265

Behavior modification, definition of, 334

Behavioral objectives, establishing, in nutrition education, 6

Benefits and risks of ergogenic aids, 81–82

Biguanides, nutritional implications of, 316

Bile in digestive process, 13, 15

Biochemical index in nutritional status assessment, 121

Bioelectrical impedence, definition of, 334

Biotin, 107

Blackstrap molasses, analysis of, 85

Blood, definition of, 334

Blood doping
  definition of, 334
  fuel utilization and, 43

Blood pressure, elevated, physician recommendations for, 215–216

Body composition
  in adaptation to cold environments, 77
  in nutritional and physical assessment, 140–145

Body fat, determination of percentage of, 140–145

Body frame type in appropriate weight determination, 135–138

Body mass index in appropriate weight determination, 138–139

Body weight, ideal, definition of, 338

Bran, analysis of, 85

Bread, exchange list for, 271

Brewer's yeast, analysis of, 86

Bronchitis, physician recommendations for, 196–197

Brown fat, definition of, 334

Bulimia
  definition of, 334
  physician recommendations for, 195–196

Burns, physician recommendations for, 197–199

C

Caffeine, fuel utilization and, 43–44

Calcium, 102
  absorption of, 16
  for child athlete, 62–63
  daily needs of athletes for, 179
  drug effects on, 310–311
  in foods, 300–301

Caloric support for child athlete, 55, 61–62

Calorie(s)
  definition of, 334
  levels of, exchange patterns of selected, 282–289 (*see also* Meal plan)
  needs for
    daily of athletes, 179
    estimation of, 159–167
      altitude changes in, 164
      for competition, 165–166
      dorm food and, 167
      endurance in, 164
      for injury, illness, or hospitalization, 167
      for off-season, 164–165
      for postseason, 166
      practice schedules and, 167
      for preseason, 165
      for short-term taper, 166
      strength in, 162, 164

Carbohydrate(s) (*see also* Glycogen stores)
  for child athlete, 63
  complex, definition of, 335
  daily needs of athletes for, 179
  definition of, 335
  drug effects on, 311
  as energy nutrients, 16–17
  in foods, 293–299
  metabolism of, 24–31
  performance and, 25–27
  studies on, 17–18

Carbohydrate loading
  alcohol and, 44
  definition of, 335

Premenstrual syndrome (PMS)
alcohol and, 42
physician recommendations for,
189–190
Preseason, caloric needs estimation
for, 165
Primidone, nutritional implications
of, 313
Probenecid, nutritional implications
of, 321
Propranolol, nutritional implications
of, 316
Protein(s)
in athlete's diet, 32
for vegetarian, 32–34
complementary, definition of, 335
complete, definition of, 335
daily needs of athletes for, 179
definition of, 340
drug effects on, 311
as energy nutrients, 16, 17
increased, in daily meal plan, 304
metabolism of, 32–34
needs of athletes for, 2
recommended dietary allowances
for, 33
requirements for, in individual
nutrition care, 155
Protein supplements, analysis of, 98
Purine content, foods grouped by
302–303
Pyridoxine, 106
daily needs of athletes for, 181

R

Recommended dietary allowances
(RDAs)
definition of, 340
in nutritional assessment, 131–132
Recommended Dietary Allowances,
260
Recreational activities, energy
expenditure in, 253–259
Reserpine, nutritional implications of,
319
Resource list, nutrition, 246–252
Restaurants, meal planning and,
173–175

Retinol, 108
Retinol equivalents (RE), definition
of, 340
Riboflavin, 106
daily needs of athletes for, 181
drug effects on, 308
Risks and benefits of ergogenic aids,
81–82
Road, meal planning on, 172–173
Royal jelly, analysis of 98–99

S

Salicylates, nutritional implications of,
312
Salicylazosulfapyridine, nutritional
implications of, 320
Saturated fat, definition of, 341
School lunch, meal planning and,
176–177
Seaweed, analysis of, 99–100
Sedative-hypnotics, nutritional
implications of, 320
Selenium, 104
Self-awareness in food behavior
pattern change, 150–151
Self-encouragement in food behavior
pattern change, 151
Set point, definition of, 341
Sex, basal metabolism and, 36–37
Short-term taper, caloric needs
estimation for, 166
Sickle cell anemia, physician
recommendations for,
192–193
Silicon, 104
Skinfold measurement in body fat
percentage determination,
142, 143, 144
Skinfold test, definition of, 341
Slow-twitch muscle fibers, 24, 25
Snacking in event planning, 171–172
Sodium, 103
drug effects on, 311
in foods, 351–356
Sodium nitroprusside, nutritional
implications of, 319
Sound nutrition of ergogenic aids,
110–112